AAOS

Symposium on

Total joint replacement
of the upper extremity

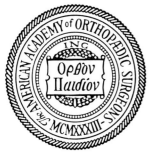

American Academy
of
Orthopaedic Surgeons

Symposium on
Total joint replacement
of the upper extremity

New York, New York
September 1979

Edited by

Allan E. Inglis, M.D.

Professor of Clinical Surgery and Clinical Professor of Anatomy,
Departments of Surgery and Anatomy, Cornell University Medical College,
New York, New York

with 319 *illustrations*

The C. V. Mosby Company

ST. LOUIS · TORONTO · LONDON   1982

MOSBY

A TRADITION OF PUBLISHING EXCELLENCE

Editor: Eugenia A. Klein
Assistant editor: Kathryn H. Falk
Manuscript editor: Carl Masthay
Design: Staff
Production. Kathleen Teal

Printed in the United States of America

The C.V. Mosby Company
11830 Westline Industrial Drive, St. Louis, Missouri 63141

Library of Congress Cataloging in Publication Data

Symposium on Total Joint Replacement of the Upper
    Extremity (1979: New York, N.Y.)
    Symposium on Total Joint Replacement of the
Upper Extremity, New York, New York, September
1979.

    Includes index.
    1. Artificial joints—Congresses. 2. Extremities,
Upper—Surgery—Congresses. 3. Orthoplasty—
Congresses. I. Inglis, Allan E. II. American
Academy of Orthopaedic Surgeons. [DNLM: 1. Joint
prosthesis—Congresses. 2. Arm—Surgery—Congress-
es. WE 805 S9896s 1979]
RD686.S89 1979   617'.570592   81-18677
ISBN 0-8016-0017-0   AACR2

C/CB/B 9 8 7 6 5 4 3 2 1   01/D/038

Contributors

Robert D. Beckenbaugh, M.D.
Assistant Professor of Orthopedic Surgery, Department of Orthopedics, Mayo Medical School, Rochester, Minnesota

William P. Cooney III, M.D.
Assistant Professor of Orthopedic Surgery, Department of Orthopedic Surgery, Mayo Medical School, Rochester, Minnesota

Ralph W. Coonrad, M.D.
Associate Clinical Professor of Orthopaedic Surgery, Duke University School of Medicine; Medical Director and Chief Surgeon, Lenox Baker Children's Hospital, Durham, North Carolina

Roger Dee, M.D., F.R.C.S., F.A.A.O.S.
Professor and Chairman, Department of Orthopaedics, School of Medicine, Health Sciences Center, State University of New York at Stony Brook, Stony Brook, New York

James H. Dobyns, M.D.
Associate Professor of Orthopedic Surgery, Department of Orthopedic Surgery, Mayo Medical School, Rochester, Minnesota

Frederick C. Ewald, M.D.
Assistant Clinical Professor, Harvard Medical School; Surgeon, Brigham and Women's Hospital, Boston, Massachusetts

Neil A. Green, M.D.
Fellow, Hand-Upper Extremity Service, The Hospital for Special Surgery, New York, New York

Anthony G. Gristina, M.D.
Professor and Chairman, Section on Orthopaedic Surgery, Department of Surgery, Bowman-Gray School of Medicine of Wake Forest University, Winston-Salem, North Carolina

Michael Harty, M.Ch., M.A., F.R.C.S.(Eng.)
Professor of Anatomy and Orthopaedic Surgery, Department of Anatomy and Orthopaedic Surgery, University of Pennsylvania School of Medicine, Philadelphia, Pennsylvania

Allan E. Inglis, M.D.
Professor of Clinical Surgery and Clinical Professor of Anatomy, Departments of Surgery and Anatomy, Cornell University Medical College, New York, New York

Judy Leonard, O.T.R.
Jennison, Michigan

Ronald L. Linscheid, M.D.
Professor of Orthopedic Surgery, Department of Orthopedic Surgery, Mayo Medical School, Rochester, Minnesota

Stephen A. Paget, M.D., F.A.C.P.
Assistant Professor of Medicine, Department of Rheumatic Disease, New York Hospital–Cornell University Medical Center; Attending Physician, The Hospital for Special Surgery, New York, New York

Chitranjan S. Ranawat, M.D.
Professor of Orthopaedic Surgery, Department of Orthopaedics, Cornell University Medical Center; Director of Hand Services and Attending Physician, The Hospital for Special Surgery, New York, New York

Robert J. Schultz, M.D.
Professor and Chairman, Department of Orthopaedic Surgery, and Director, Sylvester Carter Hand Service, New York Medical College, Valhalla, New York

Arthur Steffee, M.D.
Chief of Orthopedics, St. Vincent Charity Hospital Cleveland; Geauga Community Hospital, Chardon, Ohio.

Lee Ramsay Straub, M.D.
Professor of Clinical Surgery (Orthopaedics), Cornell University Medical College; Attending Orthopaedic Surgeon, The Hospital for Special Surgery, New York, New York

Alfred B. Swanson, M.D., F.A.C.S.
Clinical Professor of Surgery, Michigan State University, Lansing; Director, Orthopaedic and Hand Surgery Training Program, Blodgett-Butterworth Hospitals; Director, Orthopaedic Research Department, Blodgett Memorial Medical Center, Grand Rapids, Michigan

Genevieve de Groot Swanson, M.D.
Assistant Clinical Professor of Surgery, Michigan State University, Lansing; Coordinator, Orthopaedic Research Department, Blodgett Memorial Hospital, Grand Rapids, Michigan

Peter A. Torzilli, Ph.D.
Associate Scientist, Department of Biomechanics, The Hospital for Special Surgery, New York; Assistant Professor, Department of Surgery (Orthopaedics), Cornell University Medical College, New York, New York

Robert G. Volz, M.D., F.A.C.S.
Professor of Surgery, Department of Surgery, Section of Orthopaedic Surgery, University of Arizona, Tucson, Arizona

Peter S. Walker, Ph.D.
Director of Orthopedic Biomechanics, Department of Orthopaedic Surgery, Brigham and Women's Hospital affiliated with Harvard Medical School, Boston, Massachusetts

Russell F. Warren, M.D.
Assistant Professor of Orthopaedic Surgery, Cornell University Medical College; Director, Sports Medicine Service and Attending Physician, Shoulder Service, The Hospital for Special Surgery, Department of Orthopaedics, New York, New York

Lawrence Webb, M.D.
Resident in Orthopaedic Surgery, Bowman-Gray School of Medicine of Wake Forest University, Winston-Salem, North Carolina

Preface

Papers selected for inclusion in this book represent the work of authors who participated in a two-day course, Total Joint Replacement of the Upper Extremity, sponsored by the American Academy of Orthopaedic Surgeons and held at The Waldorf-Astoria Hotel, New York, on September 27 and 28, 1979.

Educational programs sponsored by the Academy and others during the last decade have provided up-to-date information related to the technology of total joint replacement in which implants are used. Although conditions affecting the hip and knee have drawn most attention during that period of time, many biomedical research findings in lower extremity technology are also applicable to major non-weightbearing joints in the upper extremity.

This course program represented a forum for authors to present biomedical information along with relevant basic science in connection with diagnosis, indications for and against treatment, and surgical techniques and rehabilitative measures for use in implant arthroplasty of joints of the upper extremity. The shoulder, elbow, wrist, and the smaller joints of the hand and digits were the subjects of the program represented in this text.

On behalf of the Academy, gratitude is expressed to the faculty members who have so generously taken time to prepare papers for both presentation and publication. Deep appreciation is also expressed for the contributions of the several secretaries who devoted many hours in preparation of the manuscripts.

Allan E. Inglis, *Editor*

Contents

Introduction

The Committee on Continuing Education of the American Academy of Orthopaedic Surgeons had the sagacity to note that upper extremity implant arthroplasty was being performed in certain major centers in the past three to five years. Further, they had noted that reports concerning the successes and problems in upper extremity implant surgery were beginning to emanate from these centers. They suggested to the Upper Extremity Committee, presided over by Dr. Herbert Stark, that an Academy-sponsored course be designed to cover total joint replacement of the upper extremity with the usual preparation. Such a course was given in September 1970. An attempt was made to place upper extremity total joint arthroplasties in place and time with particular respect to the bioengineering anatomic resources, surgical technology, complications, and predicted results, even though the follow-up study was necessarily short. The speakers at this meeting followed their assignments and stayed on course, providing the other speakers and audience with a superb picture of their work. Complications and successes were emphasized. All those who attended came away with a much clearer view of what was available to the public in the form of upper extremity implant arthroplasties.

The Academy has given permission for certain portions of this meeting to be published. We are most grateful that The C.V. Mosby Company has agreed to go forward with this project. They have been most patient with these speakers and essayists.

PART ONE

Rheumatic therapy and upper arm anatomy

1. Therapy of rheumatic diseases

Stephen A. Paget, M.D.

Rheumatoid arthritis (RA) is the most common cause of destructive joint disease of sufficient severity to necessitate upper extremity joint replacement. However, other disorders such as degenerative joint disease, the seronegative spondyloarthropathies (ankylosing spondylitis, psoriatic arthritis, Reiter's syndrome, inflammatory bowel disease–associated arthritis), crystal-induced arthritis (gout, pseudogout), and systemic lupus erythematosus (SLE) can, because of basic pathogenetic mechanisms or therapeutic side effects, lead to a similar outcome.

To understand the therapeutic modalities employed in these arthropathies and their potential sites of action, one should be cognizant of the basic immunopathologic events hypothesized to lead to joint destruction. Table 1-1 and Fig. 1-1 summarize these basic principles (such principles have been best defined in rheumatoid arthritis and systemic lupus erythematosus but probably also apply to other inflammatory arthropathies). Employing these concepts, Table 1-2 lists the therapeutic modalities of rheumatoid arthritis and describes the site or sites of action. It further notes whether the agents have the potential to bring about a disease remission (that is, change the course of the disease; alter the basic pathogenetic mechanisms). Although such drugs can help significantly in the management of rheumatoid and other forms of arthritis (see the first box), all have potentially mild to severe side effects or specific problems relating to surgery (Table 1-2). Finally, the second box lists some of the newer modalities of therapy. Most of these remain experimental but give hope to the future. Certainly, elucidation of the basic pathogenetic mechanisms leading to diseases such as rheumatoid arthritis is necessary before specific therapy will be found.

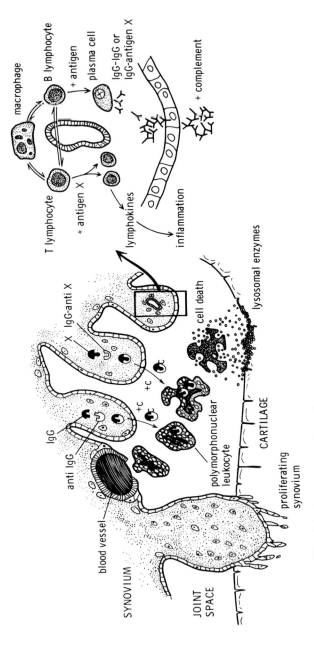

Fig. 1-1. An attractive hypothesis concerning the pathogenesis of inflammation in rheumatoid arthritis is shown schematically. It postulates that the main event is an antigen-antibody reaction in the joints (such as IgG–anti-IgG or an unknown antigen X–anti-X). Such immune complexes activate the cascade of complement-generating factors that promote chemotactic migration of polymorphs. The latter phagocytose the complexes and release lysosomal enzymes causing articular damage. More recent evidence has put into question the destructive potential of the enzymes liberated into the synovial fluid and has demonstrated that as the proliferative lesion of rheumatoid arthritis progresses, tissue is destroyed in areas contiguous with the surface of cells of the advancing proliferating synovium. (From Paget, S.A., and Gibofsky, A.: Am. J. Med. **67**: 961-970, Dec. 1979.)

Table 1-1. Basic immunopathologic factors involved in joint destruction in rheumatoid arthritis

Immunopathologic factor	Source of factor	Participation in tissue damage
1. Arachidonic acid derivatives (prostaglandins)	Synovial tissue	Promotion of inflammation
2. Pannus	Proliferating synovium	Production of destructive enzymes
3. Immune complexes (antigen-antibody complexes)	Synovial membrane, plasma cells	Bind complement and lead to polymorph chemotaxis; polymorph lysosomal enzymes lead to tissue damage
4. Immunoreactive mononuclear cells		
a. T-lymphocytes	Synovial membrane	Liberate lymphokines that lead to inflammation; enhance or suppress B-lymphocyte and plasma cell antibody production
b. B-lymphocytes	Synovial membrane	Transform into plasma cells that secrete antibodies that form into immune complexes
c. Macrophages	Synovial membrane	Modulate T- and B-lymphocyte response to antigen

Table 1-2. Therapeutic modalities employed in rheumatoid arthritis

Modality	Sites of action	Remittive agent	Surgical considerations
Nonsteroid anti-inflammatory agents	Prostaglandin synthesis	No	Bleeding (platelet effect)
Antimalarial drugs	Unknown	No	None
Gold salts (including Auranofin)	Macrophage	Yes	None
Penicillamine	T-lymphocyte	Yes	Delayed wound healing*
Corticosteroids	Lymphocyte Monocyte Polymorphonuclear leukocyte	No	Wound healing, infection, osteoporosis, aseptic necrosis, thromboembolism*
Immunosuppressive agents	T- and B-lymphocytes	Yes	Infection, delayed wound healing*

*Some might debate whether this is true.

THERAPEUTIC MODALITIES IN VARIOUS FORMS OF ARTHRITIS

1. Systemic lupus erythematosus
   a. Polyarthritis—NSAID (nonsteroidal anti-inflammatory drugs), steroids
   b. Aseptic necrosis—prevention, decompression
2. Seronegative spondylarthropathies
   a. Peripheral joint—NSAID, gold salts, immunosuppressives
   b. Spine disease—NSAID
3. Crystal-induced arthritis
   a. Gout—NSAID, colchicine, probenecid, allopurinol
   b. Pseudogout—NSAID, treat underlying disease
4. Osteoarthritis—NSAID

NEWER MODALITIES OF ARTHRITIS THERAPY

1. Immunomodulators
   a. Immunostimulators
      (1) Levamisole
      (2) Tilorone
      (3) BCG vaccine
   b. Immunosuppressors
      (1) Frentizole
2. Techniques for the removal of immunoreactive elements
   a. Thoracic duct drainage—T-lymphocytes
   b. Lymphopheresis—lymphocytes
   c. Plasmapheresis—humoral factors
3. Miscellaneous
   a. Dapsone—action unknown
   b. Chemical synovectomy—isotope, steroids
   c. Enzyme inhibitors—action unknown

2. Basic anatomy of the shoulder and elbow

Michael Harty

"There is but little room for inexactness in the field of surgery, a deviation of even a centimeter or two from the correct approach may change early success into diaster." LORD BROCK

Knowledge of anatomy still forms an essential prerequisite for correct clinical diagnosis, the sine qua non of successful treatment. Appreciation of the changes in anatomic relationships that occur during the normal range of joint motion forms an indispensible adjunct to an accurate evaluation of symptoms and a precise diagnosis.

BASIC AXIOMS FOR SURGICAL EXPOSURE

Complete orientation is necessary at all times. If the surgeon becomes confused, he must determine his precise anatomic position before proceeding further. The position and draping of the patient must allow easy access to the operative site and free mobility of the limb at all stages. Suitable movement of the limb will permit relaxation of muscles, ligaments, capsule, and tendons, thus reducing the amount of forced retraction. By following close to the skin creases, by avoiding bone prominences, and by making the incision adequate, excessive pressure with subsequent maceration of the wound edge is avoided. A neat, mobile, pain-free scar will reward such efforts. Use of the natural cleavage planes provided by the intermuscular septa, and preferably those cleavages between nerve territories, helps reduce hemorrhage and the resultant postoperative adherent muscle scars. Hemorrhage should be controlled by a tourniquet when ever possible, selection of a dry route, isolation and ligation of the larger vessels in the field, and the use of electrocautery for the control of smaller vessels. One should protect the vital structures at the operative site either by placing the exposure at a safe distance from them or by identifying them and gently retracting them out of the field. Excessive amounts of suture material and closure of the wound under tension should be avoided because they invite infection and disruption. The edges of a carefully selected and well-placed incision will readily approximate each other at closure. The functional integrity of

7

the surrounding muscle groups and their innervation facilitate the early postoperative activity so essential for a tranquil and rapid recovery.

Adequate equipment must be available for the operation. Improvised devices or hastily contrived gadgets are usually time-wasting and ineffectual. The patient must not be forced to fit the equipment. Preoperative inspection by the surgeon of the available materials will avoid delay and difficulty. Trained personnel are essential to the smooth functioning of any operating team. The scrub nurse should always be one step ahead of the surgeon. Only in this way can needless and frustrating delays be avoided. The surgical assistants should be sufficiently advanced in their training to take an intelligent interest and to participate in the procedure. The precision demanded in orthopaedic surgery requires that new residents be initiated under supervision and be well versed in germane gross anatomy.[6]

For many years the diagrams of Langer's lines have been suggested as the most appropriate direction for a skin incision.[1] Webster[8] and other surgeons have advocated incisions that parallel the wrinkle or natural crease lines. The crease lines are attached by fibrous septa placed at right angles to the pull of the underlying muscles or tendons, as seen typically at the palmar and digital creases. Holmstrand[5] and his colleagues demonstrated that the majority of collagenous fibers in the dermis are parallel to the wrinkle lines, and, furthermore, the collagen fibers that form in scar tissue are invariably parallel to the scar. Therefore incisions made perpendicular to the direction of the muscle pull heal with their collagenous fibers parallel to those in the normal dermis. The wrinkle lines may be emphasized by active or passive contraction of the underlying muscle.[5]

Man's hand is his major grasping and tactile organ, and for that purpose it is placed at the end of a very mobile upper limb. Full arm movements demand free mobility at the scapulohumeral, the acromioclavicular, and the sternoclavicular joints, coupled with an adequate active scapulothoracic muscle slide and rotation.

SHOULDER
Anatomic features

The free shoulder mobility is achieved only at the expense of stability. The shallow glenoid socket can accomodate only one third of the humeral head, and so shoulder stability is maintained mainly by the cuff muscles, which reinforce the inelastic lax capsule and the fibrous labrum glenoidale. More distally the overhanging acromion and coracoid process with their connecting ligament give additional protection on the superior aspect. The vulnerable brachial plexus and axillary vessels skirt closely to the anteroinferior aspect of the shoulder capsule. The general anatomic principle that the neurovascular bundle passes on the flexor and more protected side of the limb is matched by the surgical corollary that joints are commonly exposed from their extensor or collateral aspects.

The palpable osseous prominences about the shoulder are essential in the precise anatomic orientation required for surgical approaches. Posteriorly the inferior scapular angle, the acromion, and the spine, terminating at the level of the third thoracic spine, are easily identified (Fig. 2-1). The acromion, the clavicle, and the

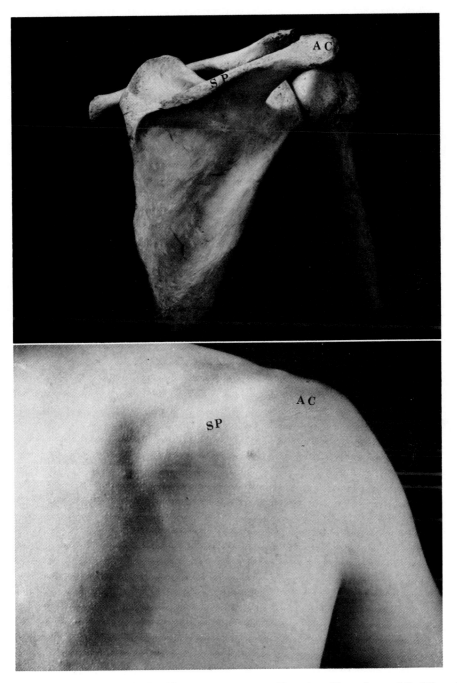

Fig. 2-1. Posterior aspect of shoulder, *AC*, Acromion; *SP*, spine. (From Joyce, J.J., III, and Harty, M.: J. Bone Joint Surg. **49A:** 547-552, 1967.)

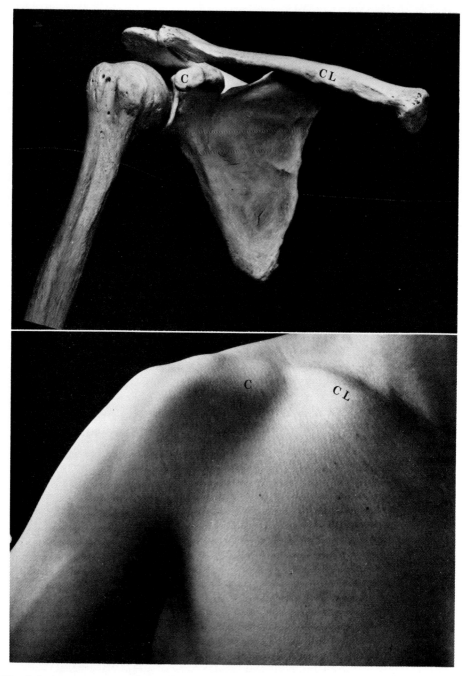

Fig. 2-2. Anterior aspect of shoulder. *C*, Coracoid process; *CL*, clavicle. (From Joyce, J.J., III, and Harty, M.: J. Bone Joint Surg. **49A:**547-552, 1967.)

proximal humerus covered by the deltoid muscle form the basic points of reference anteriorly (Fig. 2-2). The double-curved clavicle, which maintains the separation of the acromion from the sternum, gives a bony covering to the neurovascular bundle in the cervicoaxillary canal. The surgeon can readily locate the coracoid tip, hidden by the anterior deltoid margin, by placing the contralateral hand and fingers on the shoulder prominence when the thumb falls comfortably on the coracoid (Fig. 2-3). Alterations in the classical anatomic relationship are associated with all joint motion, and the shoulder is no exception. The glenoid surface does not face directly laterally; it is tilted anterolaterally at 45 degrees to the sagittal plane, and for this reason posterior approaches to the shoulder provide a poor view of the glenoid cavity. The subdeltoid or subacromial bursa intervenes between the deltoid, acromion, and coracoacromial ligament superficially and the humeral tuberosities with their attached cuff muscles deeply. A loose areolar space, which may communicate with the bursa, extends distally over the lateral aspect of the proximal humerus over the infraspinatus and subscapularis tendons and may overlie the coracoid tip (Fig. 2-4). Medial retraction of the short bicipital and coracobrachialis muscles exposes the subscapularis tendon, which always has the anterior humeral circumflex vessels parallel to its inferior border (Fig. 2-5). The coracobrachialis must be retracted gently because it conceals the musculocutaneous nerve, and still more important it covers the neurovascular bundle to the upper limb.[4]

The rotator-cuff muscles provide the major stabilizers of the shoulder joint by passing anterolaterally from the scapula to the articular margins of the humeral head, where they commonly blend with the capsule. The anteriorly situated sub-

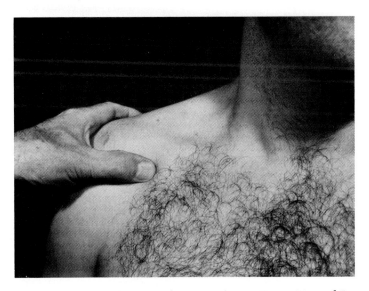

Fig. 2-3. Method of locating right coracoid process. (From Harty, M., and Joyce, J.J.: Orthop. Clin. North Am. **6**(2):553-564, 1975.)

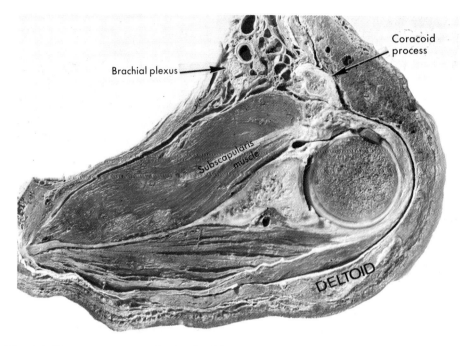

Fig. 2-4. Transverse section of right shoulder (view from above). Note extensive subdeltoid bursa.

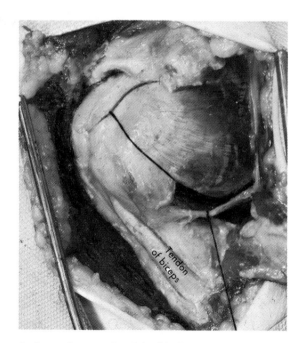

Fig. 2-5. Tendon of subscapularis enclosed by black suture. Note anterior humeral circumflex artery (retracted). (From Harty, M., and Joyce, J.J.: Orthop. Clin. North Am. **6**(2):553-564, 1975.)

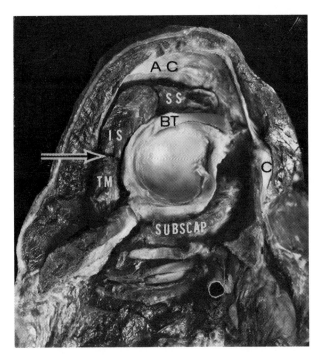

Fig. 2-6. Rotator cuff on joint capsule. *AC*, Acromion; *BT*, biceps tendon; *C*, coracoid; *IS*, infraspinatus; *SS*, supraspinatus; *TM*, teres minor. Note that axillary nerve and posterior circumflex artery pass inferior to subscapularis. *Arrow*, Area of posterior approach. (From Harty, M., and Joyce, J.J.: Orthop. Clin. North Am. 6(2):553-564, 1975.)

scapularis attaches to the lesser tuberosity of the humerus, whereas the supraspinatus, the infraspinatus, and the teres minor insert into the greater tuberosity (Fig. 2-6). They provide a graduated synergic activity that maintains the humeral head in the shallow glenoid cavity. Although the long head of the triceps and the tendon of the teres major are closely related to the inferior aspect of the shoulder, they provide little support to joint stability because their insertion is too far removed from the axis of motion. The anterior aspect of the joint capsule lies immediately beneath the subcapularis tendon, but a subscapular bursa may communicate with the joint cavity (Fig. 2-4). The suprascapular nerve enters the superior margin of the infraspinatus muscle and the axillary nerve enters the inferior aspect of the teres minor muscle; hence retraction of the infraspinatus proximally and the teres minor distally exposes the posterior joint capsule without jeopardizing any muscular innervations[3] (Fig. 2-7).

Surgical approaches

Careful dissection, clean muscle reflection, and atraumatic handling of the neurovascular structures are essential steps in obtaining adequate visualization and good functional recovery. The anterosuperior and posterior aspects of the gleno-

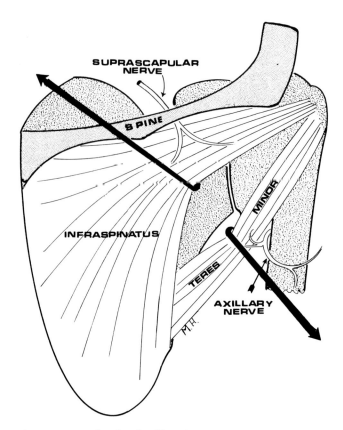

Fig. 2-7. Posterior exposure of right shoulder. (From Harty, M., and Joyce, J.J.: Orthop. Clin. North Am. **6**(2):553-564, 1975.)

humeral joint are those that most frequently require surgical procedures. More rarely the clavicle with its acromioclavicular and sternoclavicular joints may require exposure. The basic anatomic landmarks are indicated in Figs. 2-1 and 2-2. Most of the shoulder area is enveloped by the usually prominent and variably developed deltoid muscle, which is also an important guideline and obstruction in the shoulder area. Resisted muscular contraction emphasizes the outline of the deltoid, the pectoralis major, and the muscles of the posterior axillary field.

Anterior approaches to glenohumeral joint. The versatile anterior route provides excellent access to the anterior capsule and to the anterior and inferior aspects of the glenohumeral joint. In addition, extension of the incision will permit viewing of the insertion of the musculotendinous cuff. Recurrent anterior dislocations or fracture-dislocations of the glenohumeral joint, repair of the proximal tendon of the biceps, excision of bone tumors, treatment of bone infections, and certain shoulder reconstructions, constitute the main indications for the anterior glenohumeral exposure.

Limitations. A true anterior route to the shoulder affords visualization of only the anterior and, to a limited degree, the superior aspects of the glenohumeral joint. The increased wound depth in obese or very muscular subjects often restricts full visualization of the area.

Landmarks. The most valuable surface landmarks in planning the skin incision for exposure of the front of the shoulder joint are the acromion process, the outer third of the clavicle, the coracoid tip, the deltoid tuberosity, and the deltopectoral groove.

Danger points. Beneath the skin, the cephalic vein and branches of the thoracoacromial axis may be encountered. Forcible retraction of the coracobrachialis can injure the neurovascular bundle to the arm that lies immediately under the muscle. Zealous manipulation of the arm may stretch the axillary nerve, which skirts the inferior capsule. The thick multipennate deltoid covering and concealing the shoulder has tough fibrous condensations at its proximal and distal bony attachments, which provide firm anchorage for sutures. Because the axillary nerve enters the deep posterior surface of the deltoid, the anterior two thirds of that muscle can be reflected without fear of denervation. The deeper sheet of the pectoralis major, which attaches to the lateral lip of the bicipital groove, sends a fascial layer up to the greater tuberosity. When the arm is abducted, deliberate incision is often needed to penetrate this semitranslucent but tough fibrous barrier. Development of the deltopectoral interval exposes the coracobrachialis and short head of the biceps. By osteotomy of the tip of the coracoid process or by division of the conjoined tendon, the coracobrachialis and short head of the biceps can be retracted medially to expose the subscapularis tendon, which is often adherent to the underlying anterior capsule. External rotation of the shoulder facilitates visualization of the anterior part of the shoulder with the overlying structures. The capsule-tendon complex is divided approximately 1 to 2 cm medial to its humeral attachment. An excellent view of the anterior aspect of the glenohumeral joint is obtained. Osteotomy of the outer inch of the acromion process affords a more extensive view of the superior aspect of the humerus (Fig. 2-8).

Superolateral approach. The restricted visualization afforded through the deltoid-splitting exposure and the potential danger of injury to the circumflex nerve limit the value of this approach. Although some fractures of the greater tuberosity of the humerus and small rotator-cuff tears are said to be accessible through the superolateral approach, it is usually reserved for the evacuation of calcium deposits in the rotator cuff.

Limitations. Although the deltoid-splitting incision may be extended anteriorly and posteriorly in the form of an inverted L or T and detachment of the deltoid from the acromion and clavicle, poor healing and an unsightly scar frequently follow such a maneuver.[7] Distal separation of the deltoid fibers is limited by the axillary nerve, which lies 3.8 to 5 cm below the acromial tip.

Posterior approach. Tumors in the posterior aspect of the shoulder, reconstructions, certain arthrodeses, or repair of posterior shoulder dislocations constitute the

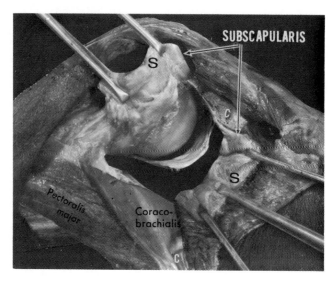

Fig. 2-8. Anterior exposure of right shoulder. Subscapularis tendon, *S*, cut and reflected. Coracobrachialis cut and reflected over pectoralis major. *C*, Coracoid process. (From Harty, M., and Joyce, J.J.: Orthop. Clin. North Am. **6**(2):553-564, 1975.)

common indications for use of the posterior approach to the scapulohumeral joint.

Limitations. Only the posterior aspect of the shoulder is accessible through the posterior route.

Position of patient. Generally the patient is prone, or nearly so. A sandbag under the anterior aspect of the chest on the side of operation and an arm support make the operative site more accessible. The limb must be draped to permit full maneuverability of the shoulder and arm.

Landmarks. The most important guides are the acromion, the spine of the scapula, the inferior scapular angle, and the posterior axillary fold. Damage to the axillary and suprascapular nerves and vessels constitute the main danger points in the posterior approach.

Technique. Although many skin incisions are recommended, often a V-shaped cut is used with its limbs paralleling the scapular spine and the posterior deltoid border. After the deep fascia is opened, the posterior deltoid margin is recognized. The muscle is detached from the scapular spine and retracted laterally. The interval between the infraspinatus and teres minor muscles is identified carefully and opened. Retraction of the infraspinatus superiorly is aided by division of its capsular attachment. Protection of the suprascapular nerve as it curves around the scapular notch is essential. Distal displacement of the teres minor further exposes the posterior shoulder capsule, which is opened to expose the posterior glenohumeral joint (Fig. 2-7).

THE ELBOW

Many surgical approaches to the elbow region have been described, but only a few are presently used by the orthopaedic surgeon. Adequate hand and forearm function depend on the anatomic integrity of the neurovascular structures passing close to the elbow joint. Disturbance of muscle function with limitation of movements or pain and weakness may follow a poorly planned or executed surgical exposure.[2]

Anatomic features

Any surgical exposure is influenced and commonly governed by the overlying gross anatomy. At the elbow, the joint is superficial on the extensor, lateral, and medial aspects, where it is covered only by skin and tendon or aponeurosis, but remember the site of the ulnar nerve. This is in sharp contrast to the flexor surface, which is deeply clothed by muscles. In addition, this muscle mass conceals and protects the neuromuscular bundle to the forearm and hand. Hence the flexor approach is rarely utilized for routine exposure of the elbow.

Bone prominences present the most constant and readily palpable periarticular landmarks. The medial and lateral humeral epicondyles with the olecranon process and the subcutaneous crest of the ulna form the salient skeletal points of reference. The radial head is palpable through the skin and annular ligament distal to the lateral epicondyle, at the skin dimple.

At level of humeral epicondyles. Posteriorly, the triceps tendon, on its medial margin has a constant relationship with the ulnar nerve, which passes behind the medial epicondyle. The subcutaneous and superficial position of the humeral epicondyles and ulnar nerve is apparent (Fig. 2-9). Anteriorly, under the deep fascia in the antecubital fossa, the median nerve, brachial artery, and biceps tendon overlie the brachialis muscle. The anterior aspects of the medial and lateral epicondyles are covered, respectively, by the flexor-pronator and the extensor-supinator groups of muscles. The ulnar nerve, resting directly on the back of the medial epicondyle and on the tubercle of the coronoid process, is often exposed to injury. The radial nerve is separated from the capitellum by the brachialis muscle. The posterior interosseous branch of the radial nerve passes lateral to the radial neck in the substance of the supinator.

At level of radial tuberosity. The anatomic relationship has undergone considerable alteration at this level. The biceps tendon between its medial and lateral bursas attaches to the radial tuberosity. Under cover of the pronator teres, the median nerve branches in a medial direction only to the flexor-pronator muscles. The ulnar nerve, passing between the humeral and ulnar heads of the flexor carpi ulnaris, rests on the tubercle of the ulnar coronoid process. Although the triceps is commonly said to insert into the olecranon process, it also gains a firm aponeurotic attachment to the deep extensor fascia of the forearm. The additional attachment is essential for full elbow extension.

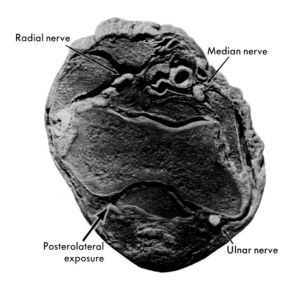

Radial nerve

Median nerve

Posterolateral
exposure

Ulnar nerve

Fig. 2-9. Epicondylar level of left elbow. Note site of larger nerves. (From Harty, M., and Joyce, J.J.: Orthop. Clin. North Am. 6(2):553-564, 1975.)

Surgical exposures of elbow joint

The posterolateral, the posteromedial, the lateral, the medial, and the anterior exposures of the elbow are more commonly used. Because each approach offers only limited access to the elbow joint, the surgeon must evaluate carefully the requirements and limitations of each procedure. Occasionally a combination of incisions is necessary to complete an operation.

Posterolateral approach to elbow. This provides a versatile and relatively safe exposure for a large area of the elbow joint and the adjacent bone structures (Fig. 2-9).

Indications. The exposure is used to reach distal humeral fractures and elbow dislocations that require open reduction. The route may also be employed for arthroplasty or arthrodesis, triceps lengthening, and the removal of loose or foreign bodies from the posterior part of the joint.

Limitations. Unless the elbow is dislocated (osteotomy of the olecranon or not), the posterior route does not allow easy visualization of the anterior joint cavity or its allied structures. Those specific fractures of the epicondyle or of the radial head that require open reduction are more readily approached through other incisions.

Landmarks. The landmarks for the posterolateral approach are the lateral epicondyle of the humerus with its lateral supracondylar ridge, the medial epicondyle, the olecranon process, and the subcutaneous border of the ulna. At a deeper level, the attachment of the lateral margin of the triceps tendon to the lateral supracondylar ridge is easily identified. The olecranon process and its fossa are obvious points that aid in orientation at the joint level.

Danger points. Although few vital structures are imperiled in the posterolateral approach, the ulnar nerve, hidden by the medial margin of the triceps, and, proximally, the radial nerve, lying in the spiral groove, are vulnerable. If the incision is extended distally to the proximal part of the radius, the posterior interosseous branch of the radial nerve may be injured.

Technique. A longitudinal skin incision parallels the lateral margin of the triceps tendon and the olecranon process to expose the deep fascia, and skin flaps are fashioned as needed. The deep fascia is opened, and the triceps tendon is displaced medially from the lateral supracondylar ridge to expose the posterolateral aspect of the distal portion of the humerus, the olecranon, and the posterior joint capsule. To reflect the periosteum and expose the bone, one needs sharp dissection. An inverted V-shaped division of the distal triceps tendon allows wide exposure of the lower end of the humerus, but the anatomic position of the ulnar nerve must be recalled (Fig. 2-9). The posterolateral route is versatile, is relatively safe, and affords excellent access to the area.

Lateral approach. The lateral approach is one of the most frequently used exposures at the elbow region. Not only does it provide good visualization of the capitellum, radial head, and lateral aspect of the elbow, but also the anterior fossa is seen.

Indications. The exposure is used to reach the radial head and capitellum for fractures and osteochondritic lesions.

Limitations. Only a limited view of the posterior joint is available. The medial compartment is not visualized until after resection of the radial head.

Landmarks. The subcutaneous lateral epicondyle, the olecranon, and the radial head constitute easily recognizable prominences in most patients. The common extensor mass, which lies anteriorly, further aids in anatomic orientation. At a deeper level, the annular ligament is partially hidden by the lateral ligament of the elbow joint, which fans distally from the lateral epicondyle.

Danger points. The radial nerve and its branches are the most vulnerable structures encountered in the lateral exposure of the elbow region. The main trunk of the nerve is concealed between the brachioradialis and brachialis muscles, both of which are directly anterior to the capitellum and the radial head. The posterior interosseous branch, which winds around the lateral aspect of the radial neck passes between the two layers of the supinator muscle.

Technique. The skin incisions is from 10 to 15 cm long and is centered over the lateral epicondyle. Distally it passes behind the extensor mass. The deep fascia is opened to expose the interval between the anconeus and extensor carpi ulnaris. This interval is further developed by partial detachment of the origins of the anconeus and the extensor carpi ulnaris. Reflection of these structures reveals the lateral joint capsule and the annular ligament. Division of the ligaments exposes the radiohumeral joint with the radial head and neck.

Anterior approach. Of limited usefulness, but it has a definite place in elbow exposures.

Indications. It is used in exploration of the brachial vessels and median nerve with or without associated supracondylar fractures. Removal of foreign or loose bodies from the anterior compartment, reattachment of an avulsed biceps or brachialis tendon, and excision of exostoses or other masses constitute additional indications. It is the exposure of choice in treating those fracture dislocations of the elbow joint that require excision of loose radial-head fragments from the anterior capsular region.

Limitations. Although the anteromedial aspect of the elbow can be viewed through the anterior exposure, the radial side of the joint is more readily accessible. Forceful retraction may traumatize the neurovascular bundle and produce paralysis or ischemia by causing spasm of the brachial vessels.

Danger points. The lower part of the brachial artery and the median and radial nerves are the major vulnerable structures during the anterior approach. Subcutaneous veins and deeper musculotendinous structures may pose problems.

Technique. A Z-shaped incision is used, with the transverse segment parallel to the flexor crease. Skin flaps are developed as required. In the subcutaneous tissue, the cephalic vein and lateral cutaneous nerve of the forearm are present on the lateral side, whereas on the medial side the basilic vein and part of the medial cutaneous nerve of the forearm are less constant. The deep fascia is opened in the interval between the medial margin of the brachioradialis muscle and the biceps tendon. In the distal part of the wound, the radial artery may be encountered crossing the biceps. To facilitate distal exposure, ligation and division of the radial recurrent vessels is frequently desirable.[4] Medial displacement of the brachialis muscles exposes the capsule covering the anterior joint cavity.

CONCLUSION

In limb surgery the size and site of the incision gets the careful consideration it deserves. It will be influenced by the direction of the skin creases and by the position and course of the underlying neurovascular bundle, tendons, muscles, ligaments, and bone structures. However, during the operative procedure when extension of the incision is deemed necessary the position of these vital structures may be overlooked. If enlargement of the exposure is contemplated, exact identification of these essential components is imperative before additional cutting is performed.

The foundations of the art of surgery are based on a sound knowledge of anatomy and its variations under physiologic and pathologic conditions. The functional anatomic aspects of the shoulder and elbow joints are emphasized as they relate to the more commonly described surgical exposures.

In February 1965, Harold Ellis wrote "In spite of a vastly increasing array of basic sciences which a surgical candidate is now expected to absorb, it remains an unassailable fact that anatomy must be one of the foundations of the art to which he aspires." It is still true.

REFERENCES

1. Courtiss, E.H., Longacre, J.J., deStefano, G.A., et al.: The placement of elective skin incisions, Plast. Reconstr. Surg. **31**:31-44, 1963.
2. Harty, M., and Joyce, J.J., III: Surgical approaches to the elbow, J. Bone Joint Surg. **46A**:7, 1598-1606, 1964.
3. Harty, M., and Joyce, J.J., III: Surgical approaches to the shoulder, Orthop. Clin. North Am. **6**(2): 553-564, 1975.
4. Henry, A.K.: Extensile exposure, ed. 5, Baltimore, 1957, The Williams & Wilkins Co.
5. Holmstrand, K., Longacre, J.J., and deStefano, G.A.: The ultrastructure of collagen in skin, scars and keloids, Plast. Reconstr. Surg. **27**:597-607, 1961.
6. Joyce, J.J., III, and Harty, M.: Orthopaedic approaches: a stereoscopic manual. Section I, Lower extremity, Baltimore, 1961, The Williams & Wilkins Co.
7. Kraisal, C.J.: The selection of appropriate lines for elective surgical incisions, Plast. Reconstr. Surg. **8**:1-28, 1951.
8. Webster, J.P.: Deforming scars: their causes, prevention, and treatments, Penn. Med. J. **38**:929-938, 1935.

PART TWO

The shoulder

3. Some bioengineering considerations of prosthetic replacement for the glenohumeral joint

Peter S. Walker, Ph.D.

The glenohumeral joint and the hip joint are similar in that the articulating surfaces are closely spherical and conforming, so that as long as the surfaces are in contact, the centers of rotation are at the centers of the spheres. However, the hip joint is inherently more stable than the glenohumeral, primarily because the degree of containment of the acetabular surface is far greater than that of the glenoid, and because the motion allowed at the shoulder is greater than at the hip. Thus, to a much greater extent than in the hip, the articular surfaces of the shoulder rely for their stability on muscular forces, and on the correct balance of these forces around the joint.

In a study of the motion during abduction in the plane of the scapula,[2] it was found that from the dependent position to 24 degrees of abduction most of the motion was glenohumeral. From there up to full elevation, the ratio of glenohumeral to scapulothoracic motion was 5:4. Other authors' have quoted ratios of 3:2 or even 2:1, but the difference stems from the fact that Poppen and Walker treated the first 24 degrees separately. Thus, for the entire elevation up to 180 degrees the glenohumeral motion was about 105 degrees.

The force vectors were also calculated.[3] For small abduction angles, the resultant force vector between the humeral head and the glenoid was at the lower rim; up to 60 degrees, the vector was close to the upper rim; whereas beyond that, the vector was close to the center. The components of the force are shown in Fig. 3-1. External rotation of the humerus tended to move the vector toward the center of the glenoid, whereas internal rotation did the opposite. The maximum force was 0.9 times body weight in neutral rotation and occurred at 90 degrees of elevation.

Data on the motion and forces in the transverse plane is not yet known, but because of the narrowness of the glenoid, the balance of forces by the rotator cuff must be delicate.

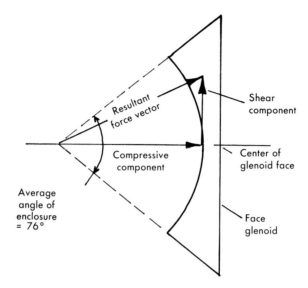

Fig. 3-1. Resultant force between the humeral head and the glenoid in the scapular plane consists of a compressive and a shear component.

FACTORS IN PROSTHESIS SELECTION

In cases of shoulder pain and joint degeneration where a prosthesis is indicated, the type of prosthesis used will depend upon various factors as follows:

1. Functional rotator cuff (especially supraspinatus) and preservation of dished shape of glenoid, with reasonable glenoid cartilage surface: humeral head replacement.
2. As above but with eroded glenoid cartilage or erosion of bony margins: humeral head and glenoid replacements.
3. Inadequate rotator cuff, usually with erosion of cartilage surfaces: linked design of prosthesis.

Different designs of the above types were reviewed by Post and others.[4] Some of the design considerations are now discussed.

DESIGN CONSIDERATIONS
Motion and force vectors

In the normal shoulder, the cartilage surface of the glenoid encloses 76 degrees and that of the humerus 155 degrees.[6] Accounting for the relative angulations in the dependent position, the humeral excursion in abduction is 79 degrees, which corresponds to a total abduction angle of 120 degrees. At or before that elevation, external rotation of the humerus occurs to avoid acromial impingement and to provide additional cartilage surface of the humeral head for further elevation.

A surface replacement design that reproduced normal geometry would ob-

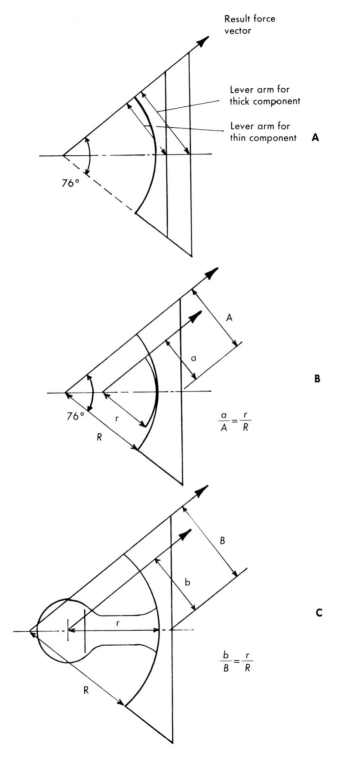

Result force vector

Lever arm for thick component

Lever arm for thin component **A**

76°

76°

$\dfrac{a}{A} = \dfrac{r}{R}$

B

$\dfrac{b}{B} = \dfrac{r}{R}$

C

Fig. 3-2. Effect of geometry on the lever arm of the force vector about the centrode of fixation. **A,** Effect of component thickness. **B,** Effect of radius of curvature of the bearing surface. **C,** Comparison between surface replacement and ball-in-socket types.

viously be satisfactory for motion. The maximum stress on the plastic surface of a glenoid component would be between one fifth and one tenth of that in a Charnley Total Hip.

However, if it is required to provide additional stability, especially to the shear-force component up the face of the glenoid, one would need to increase the angle of enclosure of the glenoid component superiorly. The likely effect of this is impingement of the plastic on the superior humerus, impacting the fixation. This can be counteracted by increasing the angle of enclosure of the humeral head, the approach used by Gristina in the Monospherical design.

Some of the design variables for the surface replacement type of prosthesis are shown in Fig. 3-2. The resultant force vector is shown at 38 degrees to the horizontal. This is the line action for the maximum shear-to-compression ratio calculated by Poppen and Walker.[3] This condition occurred at 60 degrees of abduction.

An important geometric point is the center of the glenoid component at the implant-bone interface. This will be regarded (somewhat arbitrarily) as the center of fixation, or the center or rocking of the component.

For an anatomically designed glenoid component enclosing 76 degrees and with a radius of 46 mm (Fig. 3-2, *A*), the lever arm of the force vector from the center of the glenoid face increases with the component thickness. This increase is 5% for each millimeter of additional thickness. Decreasing the radius of the glenoid component and the humeral head (Fig. 3-2, *B*) reduces the lever arm of the resultant force about the center of the glenoid face, in proportion to the radius itself.

It follows therefore that the thinner the glenoid component, and the smaller the radius of curvature, the less is the moment of the force vector about the center of the glenoid face. Such design considerations will be particularly important if the superior aspect of the glenoid component is extended for greater functional stability.

So far the anatomic surface replacement type of prosthesis has been considered. It is generally assumed that the ball-in-socket type of prosthesis will transmit greater "rocking" forces to the components. For the same resultant humeral head–to–glenoid force vector, this need not be the case however (Fig. 3-2, *C*). Whether the ball protrudes from the humerus[4] or a reversed geometry is used,[5] if the center of the ball is closer to the face of the glenoid than the center of curvature of the surface replacement, the rocking moment will be less. However, an obvious potential disadvantage of a ball-in-socket arrangement, particularly if the ball is captured, is that the limit of motion is reached, producing an impingement force. Another disadvantage to the captured type is that tension forces will be transmitted. Furthermore, in the type of shoulders where these prostheses are generally indicated, the stabilizing force components of the rotator cuff will be lost, and the resultant force vector will be more vertical. The restriction of motion aspect has apparently been solved by a double ball-in-socket arrangement (Gristina, Chapter 5). This device has a total motion of about 150 degrees.

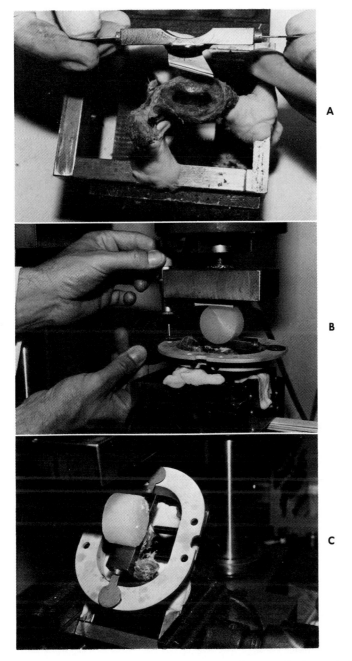

Fig. 3-3. Measurement of tilting of the glenoid component relative to the bone. **A,** Mounting the glenoid, preparing the face, the fixation fin, the metal bar, and the two targets. **B,** Loading perpendicular to the glenoid face. Target-to-ring distance was measured by micrometer. **C,** Loading at 45 degrees. The elliptical ring is shown with its set screws for clamping to the rim of the glenoid.

Fixation of glenoid component

Several different designs have been used, using spikes, screws, and a fin or a blade protruding from the back of the component. The preparation of the bone can be removal of the face of the glenoid, or retention except for an access slot. The cement can be introduced into a cavity just large enough for the device or into a scalloped-out cavity including the lateral border and the base of the coracoid.

Experiments were designed to investigate two variables, the cement technique and the quality of the bone. The cement technique is believed to play a significant role, as in femoral stems. Other variables were kept constant, namely, the design of the component (similar to the Trispherical; Gristina, Chapter 5), the retention of the glenoid face except for a slot, and the scalloping out of the cancellous bone inside (Fig. 3-3, *A*).

A formalized glenoid specimen was cemented securely to a metal frame. An elliptical metal ring was placed around the glenoid and held tightly to the rim by four pointed screws (Fig. 3-3, *B* and *C*), and the glenoid component was then cemented in place. The component was attached to a metal bar, at the ends of which were circular targets. These targets were arranged to lie about 1 mm above the metal ring.

To apply a load to the component, a plastic cylinder was placed in a groove in the bar (Fig. 3-3, *B*), a rubber sheet placed over the plastic to spread the load evenly, and the load applied by an MTS test machine (MTS Corp., Minneapolis). Progressive loads were applied perpendicular to the glenoid face (Fig. 3-3, *B*) and at 45 degrees to produce an inferosuperior shear component (Fig. 3-3, *C*).

Rocking or tilting of the component relative to the bone was measured with a micrometer to a reproducibility of 0.05 mm (Fig. 3-3, *B*). The rationale is that the greater the amount of tilting, the greater the implied cement-bone stresses and tensile distraction. This was the same principle as the experiments to measure tilting of tibial components using electronic displacement transducers.[7]

Three tests were carried out on separate specimens as follows:
1. *Good technique, medium bone.* A slot was made on the glenoid face. The cancellous bone was undercut. The bone surfaces were cleaned with an air jet. The cement was applied soft and pressurized.
2. *Medium technique, poor bone.* A slot was made on the glenoid face. The cancellous bone was only slightly undercut. The surfaces were cleaned with an air jet. The cement was applied in a dough form and only moderately pressurized.
3. *Poor technique, good bone.* The bony face of the glenoid was removed. All the cancellous bone was removed, but there was minimal undercutting. There was no surface cleaning. The cement was applied doughy.

Results

When direct compressive loading was applied, the component compressed more or less uniformly into the bone. However, when the force was applied at 45 de-

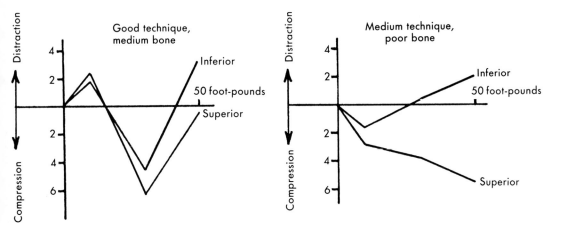

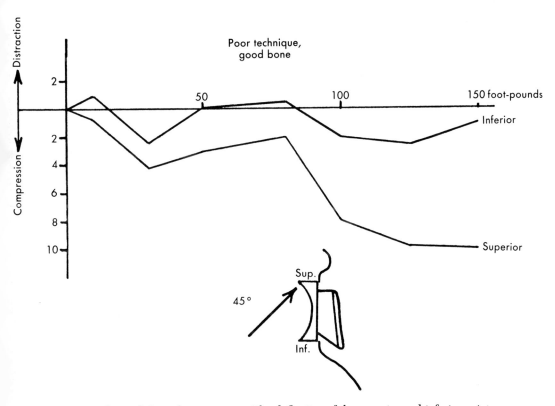

Fig. 3-4. Tilting of glenoid components. The deflection of the superior and inferior points on the glenoid component relative to the bone (vertical-axis units, 0.001 inch) plotted against load (horizontal axis, foot-pounds.)

grees, the relative deflection was nonuniform as expected (Fig. 3-4). For all three tests, the superior tended to compress inwards, and the inferior to remain level or distract slightly.

At a load of 50 pounds, the compression was greatest with the soft bone, at 0.006 inch (0.15 mm). There was inferior distraction with the medium and poor bone of 0.002 inch (0.05 mm) but not with the hard bone. When the load was carried to 150 pounds with the third specimen, there was still about zero deflection at the inferior and 0.010 inch (0.25 mm) compression superiorly. It is difficult to make any positive conclusions from these few tests about technique and bone quality. However, the indication is that, even for these three different conditions, distraction did not seem to be significant, but that high compressive stresses might be generated superiorly. A postulation of a loosening mechanism is that the high compression leads to bone resorption and replacement by a fibrous tissue, allowing increased rocking and the generation of tensile stresses inferiorly. In any case, careful attention to technique, and the design itself, are likely to be important.

REFERENCES

1. Doody, S.G., Freedman, L., and Waterland, J.C.: Shoulder movements during abduction in the scapular plane, Arch. Phys. Med. Rehab. **51:**595, 1970.
2. Poppen, N.K., and Walker, P.S.: Normal and abnormal motion of the shoulder, J. Bone Joint Surg. **58A:**195, 1976.
3. Poppen, N.K., and Walker, P.S.: Forces at the glenhumeral joint in abduction, Clin. Orthop. **135:**165, 1978.
4. Post, M., Jablon, M., Miller, H., and Singh, M.: Constrained total shoulder joint replacement: a critical review, Clin. Orthop. **144:**135, 1979.
5. Reeves, B., Jobbins, B., and Flowers, M.: Biomechanical problems in the development of a total shoulder endoprosthesis, J. Bone Joint Surg. **54B:**193, 1972.
6. Walker, P.S.: Human joints and their artificial replacements, Springfield, Ill., 1977, Charles C Thomas, Publisher.
7. Walker, P.S., Greene, D., Reilly, D., Thatcher, J., Ben-Dov, M., and Ewald, F.C.: Fixation of tibial components of knee prostheses, J. Bone Joint Surg. **63A:**258, 1981.

4. Indications for shoulder replacement and surgical technique for shoulder replacement

Allan E. Inglis, M.D.

No two surgeons will have the same indications for surgical therapy for the painful shoulder. The differences in the patient populations combined with differences in the surgeons' experience and skills will dictate a balanced therapeutic approach to the painful shoulder. It is the purpose of this paper to explore some of the priorities in the surgical approach to shoulder problems. Additionally, the surgical alternatives, the indications, contraindications, and special problems should be reviewed. The surgical technology employing both the anterior and the posterior approach to the shoulder joint are reviewed.

The pectoral girdle is the pivotal system for a functional upper extremity. Although the shoulder forms the foundation upon which the upper extremity functions, it is ultimately the *hand* that is the essence of a functional upper extremity. Therefore attention should be directed first toward obtaining a functional hand. This should include a stable wrist combined with a hand with a good grasp and release pattern, a good pinch pattern, and a good sensation. Secondarily, a functional elbow is essential. A painful elbow will retard the use of a good hand. Also, a painful elbow will aggravate and inhibit the rehabilitation of a shoulder replacement arthroplasty. Similarly, an elbow fixed in extension or retaining only 45-degree flexion will detract from the benefits of a mobile shoulder. Therefore, a functional hand, wrist, and elbow are needed before a shoulder replacement is considered. Usually the patients will volunteer their own priorities in terms of hand, wrist, elbow, and shoulder function and will assist the reconstructive surgeon in selecting the areas that require attention first.

Alternative, more conservative surgical procedures should always be considered before replacement arthroplasty. The hemiarthroplasty of Neer has enjoyed success with many surgeons after trauma or in traumatic arthritis of the shoulder. Repair or reconstruction of a ruptured external rotator cuff will restore many shoulders to full function. The impingement syndromes will respond to coracoplasties or acro-

33

mioplasties or resection arthroplasties of the acromioclavicular joint. Certain patients will respond to a synovectomy of the glenohumeral joint. This is particularly useful in pigmented villonodular synovitis and osteochondromatosis and in certain young patients with rheumatoid arthritis of the shoulder. These and perhaps other alternative procedures should be considered before any total joint replacement arthroplasty is considered for the shoulder joint.

INDICATIONS

The major indication for surgery is *pain* emanating from the glenohumeral joint. Although patients may complain of reduced mobility, is the pain that ultimately limits the function of the shoulder and ultimately use of the hand. Osteonecrosis is a common source of severe glenohumeral pain (Fig. 4-1). In our series this was most commonly attributable to either systemic lupus erythematosus or was induced by corticosteroids. The steroids usually had been given in high dosages for life-threatening diseases such as hepatitis or lupus nephritis. The shoulder pain in these patients was usually refractory to any form of therapy other than replacement ar-

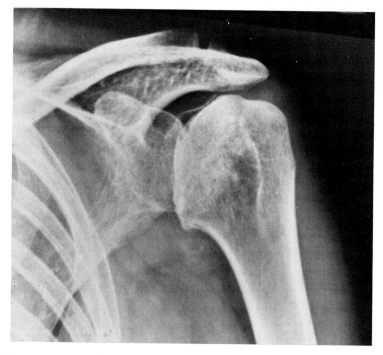

Fig. 4-1. Roentgenogram of a patient's shoulder with osteonecrosis. This patient has severe systemic lupus erythematosus. Because of pain and synovitis the patient had a secondary adhesive capsulitis. The tightness of the capsule made the surgical exposure difficult at the time of the arthroplasty. Sufficient damage had occurred to the glenoid process to make total shoulder replacement the procedure of choice.

throplasty. Although degenerative arthritis of the shoulder (Fig. 4-2) is common, it rarely produces pain sufficient that surgical therapy is required. However, when degenerative arthritis is of sufficient degree that painful glenohumeral function occurs, surgery is usually required to correct this problem. These shoulders usually have a considerable restriction in motion and chronic synovitis with pain. Chondrocalcinosis is common in these patients. Traumatic arthritis (Fig. 4-3) of the shoulder produces pain through distortion of the joint but more important distortion and ossifications within the capsule of the glenohumeral joint. Frequently there is osseous fragmentation or loose bodies, which produce chronic synovitis and pain. This group also may require replacement arthroplasty, particularly if there is damage to the glenoid. Rheumatoid arthritis (Fig. 4-4) and similar disorders frequently require replacement arthroplasty. Synovectomy has been recommended in the past. However, not uncommonly, the patient will have a recurrence attributable to retained synovium either within the subscapularis bursa or in the infraglenoid recess or within the tendon sheaths of the long head of the biceps. Not infrequently

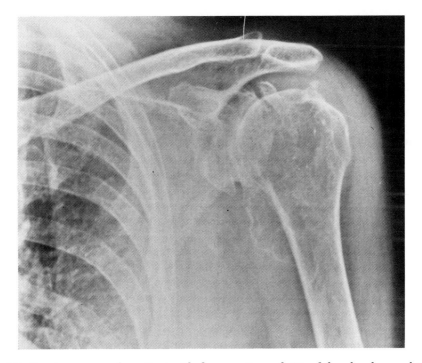

Fig. 4-2. Roentgenogram of a patient with degenerative arthritis of the glenohumeral joint. Note narrowing of the joint with subchondral sclerosis. The marginal osteophytes have infiltrated the capsule and musculotendinous cuff producing stiffness and pain. Adequate surgical exposure was difficult because of these osteophytes. Extreme care was necessary to protect the insertion of the muscles into the greater tuberosity sufficient that the stability of the shoulder is assured at completion of the arthroplasty.

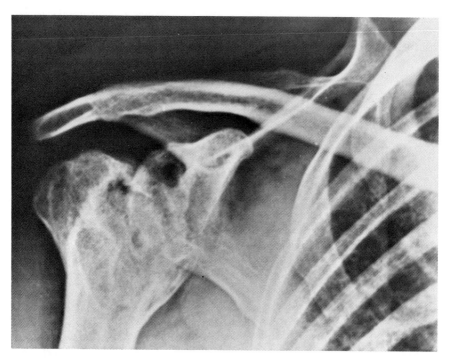

Fig. 4-3. Roentgenograms of a patient with painful traumatic arthritis. Segmental osteonecrosis has occurred with secondary damage to the humeral head and glenoid process. The musculotendinous cuff was intact, and an excellent result was obtained.

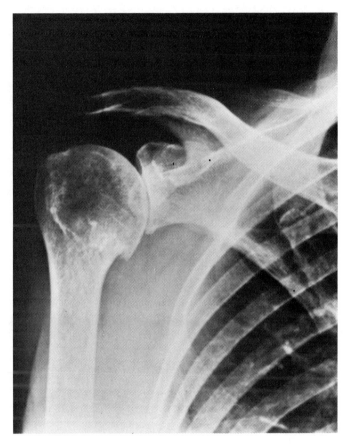

Fig. 4-4. Roentgenograms of a patient with severe rheumatoid arthritis of the shoulder. She could not use her hand for anything but the simplest functions. Grooming, feeding, and hygienic care were not possible. Note subchondral sclerosis, joint narrowing, and minimal osteophyte formation. During surgery it was noted that the musculotendinous cuff was normal, and as predicted, the patient obtained an excellent surgical result.

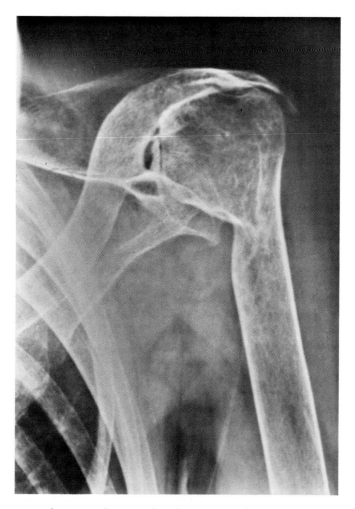

Fig. 4-5. Patient with severe rheumatoid arthritis. Note thin, worn glenoid process with minimal bone stock in glenoid neck. A secure fixation of the glenoid implant with methyl methacrylate cement is difficult to achieve in this deformed scapula.

the patients with rheumatoid arthritis will have damage to the external rotator cuff. It has been our experience as well as that of others that a functioning rotator cuff is key for success, particularly if motion is required. In certain patients with rheumatoid arthritis in which there has been severe synovitis with joint destruction, there will be insufficient glenoid for attachment of the glenoid prosthetic component (Fig. 4-5). At times one can consider a joint replacement for tumors that have been locally resected from the proximal humerus. These implants usually must be custom designed and fabricated for these patients. The manufacturers are usually very cooperative and helpful in the production of these special components.

CONTRAINDICATIONS

There are certain conditions in which shoulder replacement is contraindicated and should be avoided. The glenoid at times is insufficient to support the glenoid component (Fig. 4-5). There may be inadequate borders of the glenoid, or it may be simply lacking with fragmentation of the neck of the glenoid as well as fragmentation of the coracoid and axillary borders of the scapula. Seating the glenoid component in the neck without satisfactory support along the sides of the implant will result in loosening. Total shoulder replacements should not be used in acute fractures. If the patient has a history of failed total joint replacements in other areas such as the hip and knee, the shoulder should be approached with caution. There is no reason to believe that the shoulder implant arthroplasty will be less vulnerable to failure than these other joints will be. If the patient has had a recent bout of sepsis or has concurrent sites of infection, arthroplasty should be deferred until the patient clearly is free of other infections. Although it is not an absolute contraindication, vasculitis with secondary neurologic and vascular deficiencies may mitigate against replacement arthroplasty. Gangrene of a finger or neurologic loss in the upper extremity after implant arthroplasty, even though the patient was aware of the risks, would place the surgeon in a highly vulnerable position.

DIAGNOSTIC EVALUATION

Once the decision has been made for a replacement arthroplasty there are a number of preparations that will greatly assist the procedure. At times certain special diagnostic procedures should be considered before surgery. Radionuclide scans are particularly useful in patients with suspected osteonecrosis. Aspiration of the shoulder along with arthrography (Fig. 4-6) may provide valuable information regarding the synovial fluid, the state of the external rotator cuff, and the tightness of the capsule. Preoperative photographs showing the range of motion are extremely useful. If there are any unusual aspects to the surgical technique or if the patient possesses certain anatomic problems, such as the need for bone grafting, a telephone call to a more experienced reconstructive surgeon of the shoulder may be extremely helpful. At times there are new simplified surgical techniques known only to or recently developed by the more experienced surgeon. A careful review of the intraoperative surgical equipment is essential. A full assortment of implants

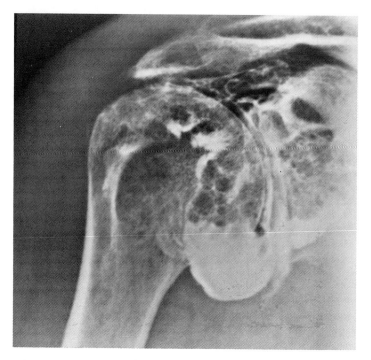

Fig. 4-6. Preoperative arthrogram of shoulder showing complete rupture of external rotator cuff. Note that the air and radiopaque dye fills the area posteriorly where the external rotator cuff normally attaches to the greater tuberosity. It was anticipated that this long-standing cuff rupture would be difficult to repair at the time of shoulder arthroplasty through an anterior surgical approach. Therefore a posterior approach was planned so that the entire external rotator cuff could be mobilized and restored to its normal insertion into the greater tuberosity at the time of the joint replacement.

and dummies should be available. There should be a full assortment of retractors, especially those that are used to retract the head of the humerus and to expose the glenoid. Oscillating saws with small blades are particularly helpful for removal of the humeral head. The high-velocity Hall or Stryker burrs are essential for the preparation of the glenoid surface and for the small keel of the glenoid implant. A full assortment of osteotomes including an osteotome with a curve on its flat side and angled curettes to reach up into the coracoid process and down along the axillary border of the scapula are required.

SURGICAL TECHNIQUES

There are two surgical approaches for implant arthroplasty of the shoulder joint. The anterior approach is more familiar and therefore easier for the average orthopaedic surgeon. It is useful when the external rotator cuff is intact or when there is only a small defect in the external rotator cuff to be repaired. The posterior approach should be reserved for those patients usually with rheumatoid arthritis in which the external rotator cuff is grossly torn or deficient. The arthroplasty is not more difficult; however, mobilization and repair of the entire external rotator cuff is necessarily more time consuming. The anterior approach is as follows: The patient is placed on the operating table so that the shoulder is just free of the operating room table surface. The patient is flexed at the hip approximately 20 degrees. A small sterilely draped movable Mayo stand is used to support the arm. The incision should begin at the border of the clavicle over the infraclavicular fossa and extend distally to the anterior edge of the midpoint of the anterior axillary fold (Fig. 4-7, *A*). The cephalic vein is identified, the interval between the pectoralis major and the deltoid muscles is developed, and these two muscles are separated from one another. Usually there is a small tendinous origin of the deltoid muscle that can be released from the clavicle. This released portion of the deltoid muscle is about $1/2$ inch and does not involve the muscle itself. The white clavipectoral fascia is now in view (Fig. 4-7, *B*). The interval between the conjoined tendon of the short head of the biceps and the coracobrachialis and the deeper subscapularis muscle is developed. Distally the tendinous insertion of the thoracic head of the pectoralis major muscle will be noted. Approximately one-half inch of this insertion is released to provide greater exposure for the arthroplasty. If the coracoid process is small, a tenotomy of the lateral two thirds of the conjoined tendon of the short head of the biceps and the coracobrachialis is used. If the coracoid process is large and extends over the glenohumeral joint, an osteotomy of the coracoid process is helpful (Fig. 4-7, *C*). Usually the osteotomy is required for good exposure. The lesser tuberosity to which the subscapularis attaches is carefully identified and then the subscapularis and the capsule of the shoulder joint are incised as a single flap. The anterior capsule of the shoulder joint is extremely strong, and combining this capsule with the subscapularis as a single unit for closure permits early movement during the postoperative convalescence period. This combined release of the capsule and the subscapularis proceeds forward to the top of the lesser tuberosity (Fig. 4-7, *D*). The release is then continued inferiorly until the shoulder can be easily externally rotated. At this point the coracohumeral ligament, which normally forms the roof for the intertubercular groove, is identified and incised. The tendon of the supraspinatus muscle is protected. At this point the head of the humerus can be easily dislocated and delivered into the wound. Meticulous planning of the humeral head resection by use of the dummy implant is now carried out (Fig. 4-7, *E*). Three separate planes must be observed in the removal of the humeral head for accurate seating of the humeral component. Retroversion of the humeral component of 30 to 45 degrees is essential for proper seating of the humeral component into the glenoid unit. The oscillating saw is then used for incision of the head of the humerus. The deeper portion of the resection is carried out with narrow osteotomes, with great care being taken to prevent injury to the external rotator cuff.

After the humeral head has been removed, the remaining greater tuberosity and rotator cuff can be retracted posteriorly for preparation of the glenoid. The

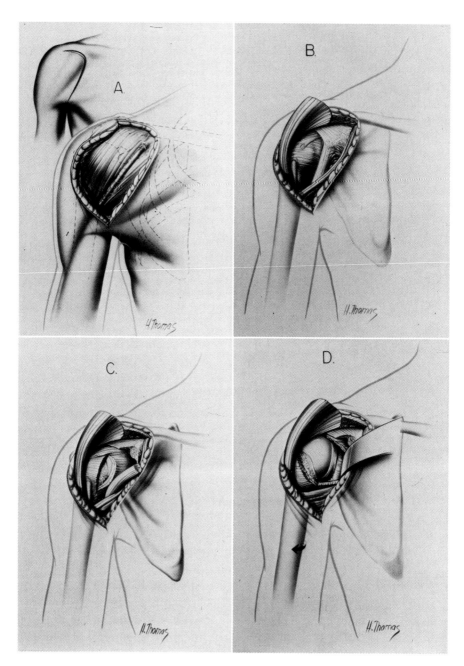

Fig. 4-7. Serial illustrations of the anterior surgical approach to the shoulder joint as required for a total shoulder replacement. **A,** Incision over the deltopectoral groove. It should be curved proximally toward the acromion in the event that it is necessary to detach a portion of the deltoid muscle. **B,** Interval between the deltoid and pectoralis major is developed and the clavipectoral fascia incised. **C,** Coracoid process is drilled, for subsequent reattachment, and then osteotomized to facilitate insertion of the humeral prosthesis. The coracoacromial ligament is incised. **D,** Subscapularis muscle and capsule including the coracohumeral ligament are incised and retracted medially.

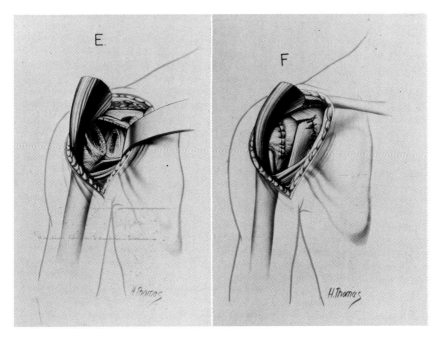

Fig. 4-7, cont'd. E, Anatomic humeral head is excised. The glenoid is prepared to receive the glenoid implant. **F,** Capsule and subscapularis muscle are secured to the lesser tuberosity. And the wound is closed.

labrum should not be excised at this time. The labrum can be trimmed at the time of the final fitting and seating of the glenoid implant. The surface of the glenoid is carefully burred away with the high-velocity burrs. The surface of the glenoid is extremely dense; therefore care must be taken not to remove too much of the surface while one is looking for cancellous bone. After the surface has been prepared, a longitudinal cut is made in the center of the glenoid with the burr. The neck of the glenoid will be apparent. Further curetting with the angle curettes up into the coracoid process and down into the axillary border of the scapula will allow for better filling of cement and more secure fixation of the implant. Frequently it is necessary to cut the tip from the glenoid component to allow for firm fitting of the implant against the glenoid process. The labrum can be trimmed away for an exact tight fit of the implant. It should not be removed. The humeral shaft is carefully reamed in the diaphyseal area. The proximal or metaphyseal end is shaped with the high-velocity burrs and curettes to conform to the shape of the humeral component. After the humeral component is seated, both implants should be inserted and the arm tested through a range of motion. The glenoid implant is cemented first, followed by the humeral unit. The shoulder is then reduced. The capsule and the subscapularis are then closed with multiple fine sutures (Fig. 4-7, *D*). The arm is then placed in a sling and swathe. Pendulum exercises are started in 3 days and active exercises in 5 days.

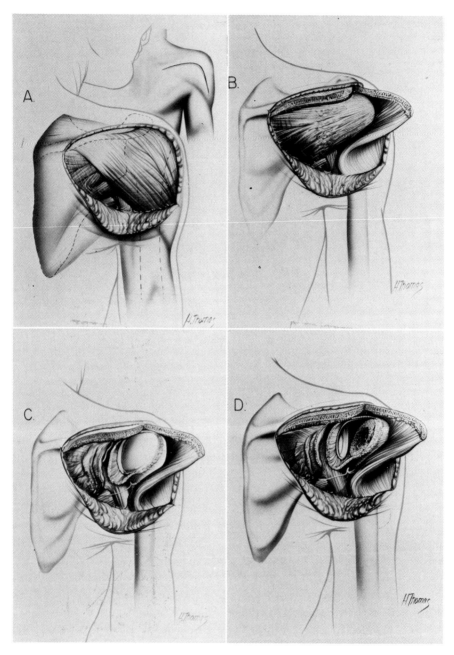

Fig. 4-8. Serial illustrations of the posterior surgical approach to the shoulder joint as required for a total shoulder replacement with a massive rotator cuff tear. **A,** The skin incision should be ample. **B,** The posterior deltoid is detached with a sliver of bone from the spine of the scapula. **C,** The capsule and attenuated portions of the rotator cuff are incised along the border of the greater tuberosity. **D,** The anatomic head of the humerus is excised.

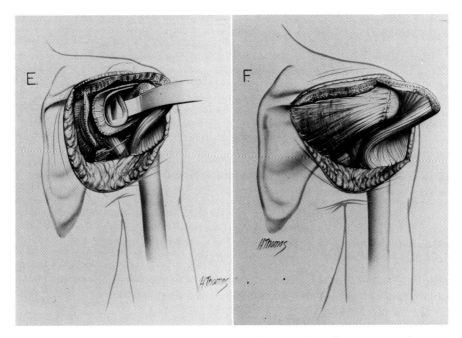

Fig. 4-8, cont'd. E, The glenoid process is prepared for the glenoid implant. **F,** The external rotator cuff is mobilized and restored with the capsule to the greater tuberosity.

The posterior approach to the shoulder is reserved for those patients with large tears in the external rotator cuff. It is through this approach that these tears can be accurately repaired. The patient is placed in the lateral decubitus position on the operating room table. The entire extremity and shoulder area are prepared and draped free. The incision is carried just superior to the spine of the scapula to the tip of the acromion process and then downward approximately 2½ inches parallel-ing the shaft of the humerus (Fig. 4-8, *A*). The flap superiorly and laterally is undermined approximately 1 inch and the flap medially is similarly undermined approximately 1 inch. The spine of the scapula is identified, along with the origin of the posterior head of the deltoid muscle. The deltoid muscle is then released from the spine of the scapula with an osteotome (Fig. 4-8, *B*). Only a small sliver of bone is removed to facilitate suturing of the deltoid muscle back to the spine at the completion of the arthroplasty. The deltoid muscle is removed as far forward as the lateral edge of the acromion process. Posteriorly the acromion process has a flared area. Approximately ¼ inch of this flared area posteriorly is removed with a bone biter. As the deltoid muscle is retracted, the entire posterior aspect of the external rotator cuff can be observed. A large fascial covering, the infraspinous fascia, will be noted; this must be incised along the scapula and along the greater tuberosity. The quadrilateral space is easily noted just beneath the edge of the infraspinatus muscle. The torn portion of the external rotator cuff is incised with the capsule (Fig. 4-8, *C*). This torn portion usually includes the teres minor, the infraspinatus and portions of the supraspinatus. The capsule and the torn portions of these muscles are then retracted medially. The humerus is then rotated internally so that the humeral head is brought into view. The anatomic neck of the humerus is carefully identified. The osteotomy site is then planned (Fig. 4-8, *D*). Again the humeral component must be retroverted 30 to 45 degrees. After the humeral head has been excised, the retractors are then placed across the joint so that the humerus is depressed anteriorly and the glenoid is elevated posteriorly. The high-velocity burrs are then used to prepare the surface of the glenoid (Fig. 4-8, *E*). Again, one must not remove supporting bone while looking for a cancellous bed for cement fixation. A groove is cut longitudinally in the glenoid. The neck of the glenoid is curetted as deep as possible and, by use of angled curettes the inner portion of the coracoid process and the axillary border of the scapula are deepened for cement fixation. Only enough of the labrum is removed to allow accurate seating of the glenoid component. The humerus is then reamed distally and the proximal portions prepared with high-speed burrs. A trial fit should be carried out and the shoulder put through a range of motion. The glenoid component is then cemented first, followed by the humeral unit. The shoulder is then reduced. The new attachment of the external rotator cuff requires careful attention to detail (Fig. 4-8, *F*). The muscles must be dissected free so that they may be advanced for attachment into the greater tuberosity. They should not be attached with the arm in full external rotation but in the neutral position. The deltoid muscle is then reattached to the spine of the scapula. Several small holes are made in the spine of the scapula with a small hand drill, and the deltoid is securely attached to the spine again. The arm is then placed in neutral rotation with 45-degree abduction. A double-pillow splint is satisfactory in the early postoperative period. Circumduction exercises are started at 1 week and a full physical therapy program in 3 weeks.

PROBLEM AREAS

Several potential problems and pitfalls are unique to shoulder-implant arthroplasties that can make the arthroplasty extremely difficult. Failure to fully visualize and gain access to the glenoid radiographically may prevent the surgeon from knowing that the glenoid is insufficient for seating of the glenoid component. Good, clear roentgenograms of the glenoid are essential in preparation for the arthroplasty. Correction of an old anterior or posterior dislocation with an implant arthroplasty can be difficult. There may be either extensive damage to the glenoid or to the tuberosities, making it difficult to seat the implant and to adjust the soft-tissue tension about the shoulder at the completion of the procedure. A prominent coracoid process overlapping the glenohumeral joint can make seating of the humeral component quite difficult and also can interfere with reduction of the shoulder after cementing of the prosthesis. The coracoid process should be osteomized to provide good access to the shoulder when it is prominent. Another serious problem is a stiff

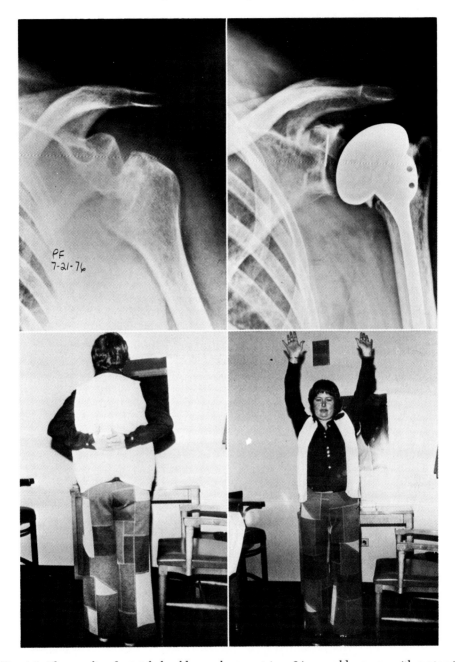

Fig. 4-9. The results of a total shoulder replacement in a 34-year-old woman with systemic lupus erythematosus. **A,** Roentgenograms showing complete loss of the humeral head secondary to osteonecrosis with damage to the glenoid. **B,** Roentgenogram showing result 2 years after her shoulder replacement (1977). **C,** Internal rotation of the shoulders observed when she was seen in follow-up for bilateral total hip replacements in 1979. **D,** Extension and abduction in 1979. Patient has returned to work and cares for a young family. She is currently pain free and functions satisfactorily.

shoulder, or a shoulder with adhesive capsulitis. These shoulders require extensive capsular release before the arthroplasty can be carried out. Even after a careful capsular release it can be difficult to seat the implant and reduce the shoulder. Another troublesome problem is the presence of extensive osteophytes about the greater and lesser tuberosities or calcifications within the capsule or tendons of the shoulder. It is desirable to remove the osteophytes from the edges of the tuberosities because they will impinge upon the glenoid component at the extremes of motion and may be a potential source of glenoid loosening. Removal of these osteophytes can be tedious. However, it is worth the effort to be certain that the capsule and tendons are free of any excrescences that can interfere with the movement of the shoulder.

COMMENT

Although the glenohumeral joint is a nonweightbearing articulation, great forces are normally transmitted across the surfaces. To achieve a quality arthroplasty, the surgeon must accurately align the implant surfaces and restore the normal stabilizing musculature. Preoperative assessment of remaining anatomic resources through detailed physical examination and special roentgenographic studies are essential. With this information at hand the surgical approach can be selected and a meticulous arthroplasty performed. Excellent results (Fig. 4-9), as observed in the hip, knee, and elbow, can be achieved. The relief of pain and restoration of motion is dramatic and long lasting.

5. The Trispherical Total Shoulder prosthesis

Anthony G. Gristina, M.D.
Lawrence Webb, M.D.

STRUCTURE AND DESIGN

The glenohumeral joint is surprisingly complex and unique in its requirements for prosthetic replacement: it has a greater range of motion than any other joint, it is nonweightbearing, and the limitations of its capsule and ligamentous attachments make it vulnerable to dislocation. Those were factors that we considered when we designed the Trispherical Total Shoulder prosthesis.

The Trispherical Total Shoulder prosthesis (Fig. 5-1) is basically composed of three elements: a scapular component, a humeral component, and a central polyethylene sphere, which captures the two lateral components. The polyethylene sphere is then encapsulated with a Vitallium shell for extra strength. The trispherical concept is a three-bar linkage, which allows a greater than anatomic range of motion. Stress of mechanical components on the bone-cement interface is thereby reduced, since soft tissues can absorb the stress forces. Fig. 5-2 shows the trispherical prosthesis in cross section positioned in the bony elements of the scapula and humerus. The cross-hatched areas represent polymethylmethacrylate cement. The prosthesis may be made with (constrained) or without (nonconstrained) the Vitallium capsule, but the constrained version has increased resistance to dislocation. The initial nonconstrained prosthesis was designed for dislocation at 150 inch-pounds, the Vitallium constrained prosthesis, for dislocation at 500 inch-pounds. These factors were engineered into the prosthesis to prevent fracture of the osseous anchorages.

When one designs a prosthesis of this sort, there is a trade-off between equatorial overlap and the size of various parts of the prosthesis, such as the size of the neck component. This trade-off results in decreased motion as these areas are strengthened, as can be seen in Fig. 5-3. When one uses a simple ball and socket, as on the left, the amount of motion is limited, even though the head size has been increased. On the right, the trispherical three-bar linkage allows for essentially

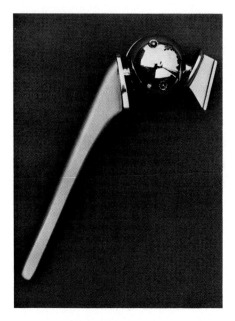

Fig. 5-1. Trispherical Total Shoulder prosthesis.

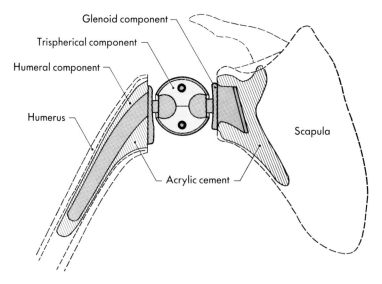

Fig. 5-2. Schematic drawing of Trispherical Total Shoulder prosthesis in relation to humerus and scapula.

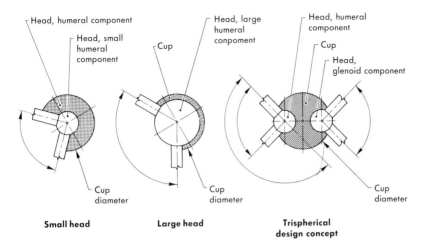

Fig. 5-3. Correlation of equatorial overlap, range of motion, and size of parts of the various shoulder prostheses.

twice as much motion in the same amount of shoulder space. The initial noncon-strained prosthesis was designed for 175 degrees of motion, the encapsulated ver-sion for 160 degrees of motion.

OPERATIVE INSERTION PROCEDURES

Briefly, the operative insertion of the Trispherical Total Shoulder prosthesis is as follows: Prophylactic antibiotics are started intravenously on the morning of the operation and continued for 3 days. The approach is deltopectoral, with the skin incision beginning just superior and medial to the coracoacromial joint, curving over the coracoid process and distally along the anterior surface of the deltoid in the deltopectoral groove to end in the interval between the lateral margin of the biceps and the medial margin of the deltoid. The deltopectoral interval is separated and the medial 1 to 3 cm of the origin of the deltoid, the periosteum, and small flecks of bone are removed from the anterior edge of the clavicle. After the coracoid process has been identified and exposed, the conjoined tendon containing the short head of the biceps and coracobrachialis and a small flake of bone are detached from the tip of the coracoid; the conjoined tendon is gently retracted. The pectoralis minor is left intact. These steps simplify reattachment of the deltoid and conjoined tendon during closure.

When the humeral head is fixed posteriorly in internal rotation contracture, the joint space is best entered through a longitudinal incision made just medial to the bicipital groove. When the capsule adheres to the humeral head, as it does in many patients with severe rheumatoid arthritis, a true joint space cannot always be de-veloped until extensive and careful dissection is carried out.

Once the humeral head is exposed, it is removed with a power saw, the proxi-

mal humerus is retracted, and attention is turned to the glenoid. Any fibrohemor-
rhagic redundant synovial tissue is scraped off the glenoid surface, and a fenestra-
tion large enough to admit the fin of the glenoid component is made with dental
burrs. The underlying intrascapular cancellous bone is curetted beneath the surface
of the glenoid to form a cavity for anchoring the glenoid component (Fig. 5-4).
Retention of the subchondral cortical bone allows for maximum structural integrity
of the scapula. After a trial fitting and any necessary corrections, the cavity is filled
with methyl methacrylate resin under pressure and the glenoid component is inserted.

The humerus is then reamed by conventional means, and, after trial seatings
are satisfactory, the humeral component is cemented in place in 35 degrees of
retroversion (or whatever is the most appropriate retroversion for the individual
patient) and the two components are then assembled into the central sphere. The

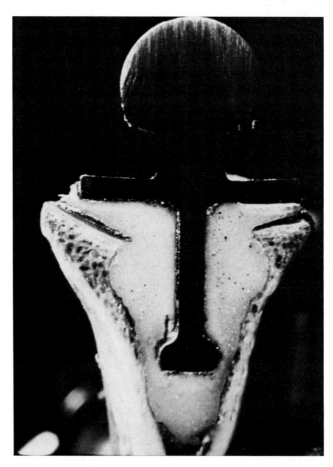

Fig. 5-4. Cross-section of scapular component embedded in scapula. Note retention of subchondral cortical bone.

success of seating the two components depends partly on use of a Water-Pik to remove all fragments of reamed-out material and placement of the cement under pressure.

If anterior capsuloplasty is required to reduce internal rotation contractures and to provide capsular and subscapular closure and joint stability, it is done, the stability of the joint is verified, and closure is completed with a Hemovac being left in place for drainage.

RESULTS

The shoulder is immobilized for 3 weeks, but early use of the hand, wrist, and elbow is encouraged. By 6 months, the range of motion has improved, but roentgenograms show that it is primarily scapulothoracic motion. However, by 1 year, roentgenographic studies show that true glenohumeral motion has been obtained (Fig. 5-5).

To date, we have inserted 17 constrained and two partially constrained Trispherical Total Shoulder prostheses. The patients chosen for this prosthesis always have the most severe degree of rheumatoid arthritis, and they are not usually considered to be candidates for placement of any other type of prosthesis. The patients have been followed up for 3 to 41 months, and their range of motion and level of pain have been used to grade the results (see box). Most patients had pain at the 4 or 5 level before operation, and at the 1 or 2 level after operation. In most also, the range of motion has improved, especially abduction and external rotation (Table 5-1).

Since the presentation of this material, we have had two cases of dislocation in the constrained prosthesis. We have not removed the two prostheses yet, but we believe they dislocated because the patients, both of whom had hips and knees severely involved with rheumatoid disease, had exceeded the design parameters during certain activities such as raising themselves from chairs or using crutches. It may be that we will need to design the prosthesis for increased resistance to dislocation by strengthening the rigidity of the central component; that can be done with a minimum sacrifice of motion. We have had one dislocation of a nonconstrained prosthesis when the patient fell on her outstretched arm, and one of fatigue fracture at 41 months in a patient with severely porotic rheumatoid arthritis who had achieved excellent use of the prosthesis up to that time.

GRADATION OF PAIN POSTOPERATIVELY

1. None
2. Slight—no compromise in activity
3. Mild—after unusual activity
4. Moderate—interfering with activity, requiring analgesics occasionally
5. Severe—with serious limitations of activity

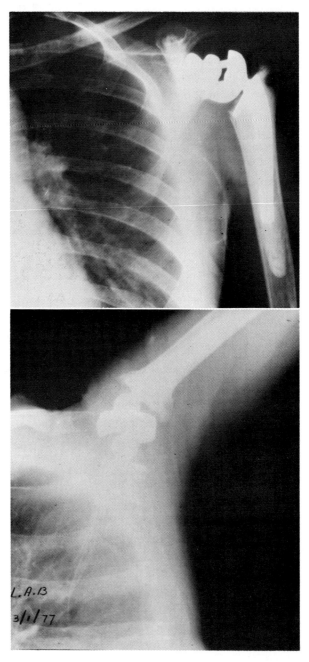

Fig. 5-5. Shoulder at rest and with arm raised (1 year after operation). Note range of motion obtained by true glenohumeral motion.

Table 5-1. Active-shoulder range of motion in degrees preoperatively and postoperatively

	Average preoperatively	Average postoperatively		
		3 months	12 months	18 months
Flexion	35	50	65	50
Extension	35	43	45	39
Abduction	40	57	67	69
Internal rotation	50	70	90	90
External rotation	20	33	39	32

Loosening of cement is a predicted problem in all prosthetic replacement and, as in total hip surgery, has been discovered in increasing percentages, especially at the 5- and 10-year points. To date, roentgenograms of four of our patients show halos measuring 2 to 3 mm about their prostheses, but those have not increased between the 6-month and 3-year points. To prevent loosening, optimum design and surgical technique are necessary. However, regardless of whether a prosthesis is constrained or nonconstrained, or articulated or nonarticulated, compressive forces transmitted to the glenoid will produce rocking moments, which will ultimately produce loosening at the cement-bone interface. Further, if a constrained prosthesis does not have more than an anatomic range of motion, additional stresses will be added directly to the prosthetic elements and the cement-bone anchorage. We believe that our design and surgical approach, which preserve as much of the structural integrity of the scapula as possible and allow for a locking of a mantle of cement beneath the cortical surfaces, will minimize this loosening tendency and maximize strength of anchorage.

CONCLUSION

We are using the Trispherical Total Shoulder prosthesis in severely diseased selected patients with a deficient rotator cuff that requires a fulcrum of this sort to compensate for extensive bone destruction and soft-tissue disease. However, total shoulder replacement, regardless of the prosthesis used, remains in a trial state of development.

6. Total shoulder replacement indications and results of the Neer Nonconstrained prosthesis

Russell F. Warren, M.D.
Chitranjan S. Ranawat, M.D.
Allan E. Inglis, M.D.

The severely painful shoulder secondary to destruction of the articular surface of the glenohumeral joint is a difficult problem for which many solutions have been sought. In an attempt to resolve the problem total shoulder replacement has evolved over the past 8 years along three basic designs. They have been termed the "nonconstrained or resurfacing prosthesis" such as those of Neer, Bechtol, and O'Leary-Walker (Figs. 6-1 and 6-2). A semiconstrained design with increased superior glenoid coverage has been designed by McNab and English. Fixed fulcrum or constrained types have been described by Fenlin,[2] Post,[4] Buechel,[1] and Gristina.[3] For full arm elevation to occur, a fulcrum must be established at the glenohumeral joint about which the deltoid will act to effect forward flexion or abduction. In the normal shoulder this fulcrum is established by the depressor action of the rotator cuff. If the cuff is severely attenuated or has a large tear, function may be partially or completely loss.

For the shoulder with a functioning cuff a resurfacing or nonconstrained device should allow recovery of satisfactory shoulder function. For the shoulder with a nonfunctional cuff increasing degrees of constraint will be required for shoulder elevation to occur. Our experience to date indicates that for most shoulders the nonconstrained prosthesis will be the procedure of choice, but there is a small group of patients in whom increasing degrees of constraint will be required because of deficiency of the rotator cuff.

The nonconstrained prosthesis has the inherent advantages of decreasing the forces at the bone-cement interface while allowing motion to be restricted by the soft tissue rather than by the prosthesis. As a result one would expect to develop fewer mechanical problems such as metal failure, dislocation of the prosthesis, fracture, and subsequent loosening, particularly of the glenoid component.

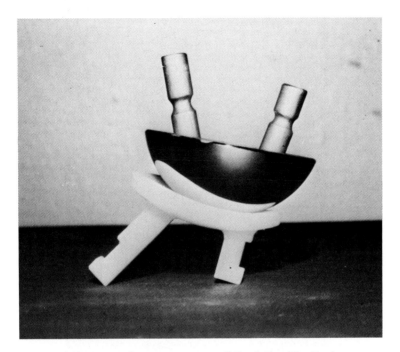

Fig. 6-1. O'Leary-Walker Nonconstrained Total Shoulder Replacement.

REQUIREMENT FOR NONCONSTRAINED PROSTHESIS

The nonconstrained prosthesis thus needs a functioning rotator cuff for reasonable shoulder elevation to be achieved. Preoperatively a double-contrast arthrogram will often give excellent visualization of the size of the rotator cuff defect, thus guiding the surgeon in the choice of surgical approach and the type of prosthesis to be utilized. In addition to a functioning cuff the deltoid must be normally innervated. At times, particularly in old trauma, the deltoid may be functioning poorly because of disuse atrophy, denervation, or detachment from the acromion. The electromyographic evaluation of both the cuff musculature and deltoid may be quite helpful when one is evaluating these difficult patients. Proper roentgenographic evaluation preoperatively is essential for a proper assessment of the adequacy of the bone stock. A true anteroposterior view of the glenohumeral joint should be obtained. Since the scapula lies at a 35- to 40-degree angle to the chest wall the x-ray beam should be angled perpendicularly to the scapula for proper evaluation of the depth of the remaining glenoid and narrowing of the glenohumeral joint. In addition an axillary view should be obtained for further evaluation of the adequacy of the remaining bone in the glenoid. Protrusio and destruction of the glenoid is not infrequent in rheumatoid arthritis and may require modification of the glenoid component of the prosthesis. Finally, patient motivation and the ability

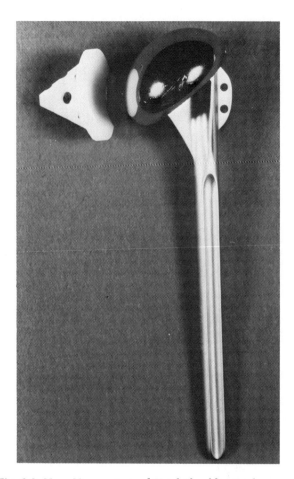

Fig. 6-2. Neer Nonconstrained Total Shoulder Replacement.

to carry out a satisfactory physical therapy program must be assessed preoperatively. Without physical therapy significant pain improvement may occur, but limited function and range of motion will be noted and the patient will continue to complain of stiffness and pain at the extremes of motion.

Contraindications

Irreparability of the rotator cuff is a relative term, but certainly in some patients it fits the description, and a nonconstrained prosthesis, though providing pain relief and functional improvement, will not improve motion significantly. Previous infection and a neuropathic joint are also believed to represent contraindications for this type of procedure. Instability of the shoulder joint with a type of pseudosubluxation may well represent a contraindication to a nonconstrained prosthesis, though this has been treated with a Neer prosthesis followed by immobilization in a shoulder spica for the first 6 weeks until soft tissue healing has been achieved. In this situation pain relief is achieved but motion is limited to about 100 degrees of forward flexion.

Indications

Candidates for a nonconstrained prosthesis include those patients with severe shoulder pain over an extended period of time without relief with the usual conservative programs of exercises and anti-inflammatory agents. Generally, there is considerable limitation of motion and functional impairment of daily activities. To date, total shoulder replacement has been carried out in 34 patients involving 40 shoulders. This has included 38 nonconstrained prosthesis. The average patient age was 59.4 years with a range of 21 to 80 years. Of these, 32 were of the Neer design and 6 of the O'Leary-Walker design (Figs. 6-1 and 6-2). Diagnostic indications for nonconstrained prosthesis have included 14 with rheumatoid arthritis, osteoarthritis in eight, degenerative arthritis secondary to trauma in seven, and avascular necrosis in nine patients. Bilateral replacements have been carried out in six, four of whom had avascular necrosis and two had rheumatoid arthritis.

SURGERY

Surgery was performed in the beach chair position utilizing a superior, or deltopectoral approach in most patients. Additional surgery at the time of replacement included acromioclavicular joint resection, frequently in those with rheumatoid arthritis, acromioplasty and biceps tenodesis as indicated. Rotator cuff repair has been required in six shoulders, comprising three patients with rheumatoid arthritis and three trauma patients. No tears of the rotator cuff were observed in patients with osteoarthritis or avascular necrosis. Rotator cuff repair was possible in four patients, but in one rheumatoid patient with bilateral rotator cuff tears the defect was described as irreparable. In addition, trimming of the base of the glenoid component in the Neer design was necessary in six patients, five of whom had protrusio of the glenoid secondary to rheumatoid arthritis.

Postoperative program

After surgery the patients have been managed either with the arm in a sling or an abduction splint for a variable period depending upon the quality of the rotator cuff and the need for a more relaxed position after cuff repair. Passive motion exercises of the shoulder are generally started about the fourth postoperative day if it was judged that the soft-tissue repair was adequate. If a large rotator cuff defect was present, an abduction splint was used for 3 to 4 weeks. Passive motion would start from the splint during the second to third week. In those patients utilizing the deltopectoral approach it has been found that active assisted motions could be started earlier and were generally instituted during the second week. Inhospital physical therapy averaged over 3 weeks. After this, patients were carefully managed on an outpatient basis with active stretching programs carried out over the next 6 months. Improving strength, function and motion could be noted up to as late as 6 months after surgery.

Complications

After surgery no early or late infections have been noted. To date, no dislocation of a nonconstrained prosthesis has occurred. A neuropraxia of the lateral cord of the brachial plexus was noted in one patient with avascular necrosis in whom a Neer prosthesis was inserted. This resolved 6 weeks after surgery. Excessive bleeding requiring 10 units of blood was noted in one patient with old trauma, and considerable shortening of the humeral neck. In patients with previous fractures the anatomic distortions about the humeral neck can be quite severe and result in

THE HOSPITAL FOR SPECIAL SURGERY
Score Sheet for Total Shoulder Replacement

DOMINANT ARM ___ INVOLVED ARM ___	Score	LEFT							RIGHT						
		PRE	6M	1Y	2Y	3Y	4Y	5Y	PRE	6M	1Y	2Y	3Y	4Y	5Y
PAIN ON MOTION (15 points - Circle one)															
None:	15														
Mild: Occasional, no compromise in activity	10														
Moderate: Tolerable makes concession, uses ASA	5														
Severe: Serious limitations, disabling, uses Codeine, etc.	0														
PAIN AT REST (15 points - Circle one)															
None: Ignores	15														
Mild: Occasional, no medication, no affect on sleep	10														
Moderate: Uses ASA, night pain	5														
Severe: Marked medication stronger than ASA	0														
FUNCTION: (20 points - Circle all appropriate)															
Comb hair	5														
Lie on shoulder	5														
Hook brassiere (back)	5														
Toilet	5														
Lift weight in pounds 1 - 10 1 point per pound - Maximum 10 points															
None															
MUSCLE STRENGTH (15 points - Rate each) (Normal = 3, Good = 2, Fair = 1, Poor = 0)															
Forward Flexion															
Abduction															
Adduction															
Internal Rotation															
External Rotation															
RANGE OF MOTION (25 points - 1 point per 20° of motion)															
Forward Flexion (Maximum 8)															
Abduction (Maximum 7)															
Adduction (Maximum 2)															
Internal Rotation (Maximum 5)															
External Rotation (Maximum 3)															
RECORD RANGE OF MOTION (NO POINTS)															
Backward Extension															
Glenohumeral Abduction (scapula fixed)															
TOTAL															

PATIENTS NAME: _____ HISTORY NUMBER: _____

Fig. 6-3. Shoulder score sheet for preoperative and postoperative evaluation.

scarring about the neurovascular structures with significant risk of injury when dissection is done at the fracture site.

Each patient was evaluated preoperatively and at follow-up on a 100-point scoring system (Fig. 6-3). This system allocates 30 points for relief of pain, 25 points for motion, 20 for functional activities, including toilet care, combing hair and feeding oneself, and 25 points for strength. Follow-up roentgenograms were obtained on each patient. Twenty-one of the first 23 Neer prostheses were seen at an average follow-up of 23 months. A second group of six O'Leary-Walker Nonconstrained prostheses had an average follow-up of 30.5 months.

POSTOPERATIVE RESULTS
Neer prosthesis total score

Those patients with a Neer prosthesis inserted improved from a preoperative average score of 25 to a follow-up average score of 73.3. No deterioration of results over time has been noted because 10 patients who were followed from 12 to 24 months had an average score of 70.4 whereas 6 patients followed more than 24 months had an average score of 71. Five patients in whom surgery was more recently carried out with a 6- to 12-month follow-up had a score of 82.6. Concerning the age of the patient, it appears that better results were noted in the younger patient. In four patients under the age of 30, follow-up scores averaged 93 points. In 11 patients with a Neer prosthesis over the age of 60 the follow-up score aver-

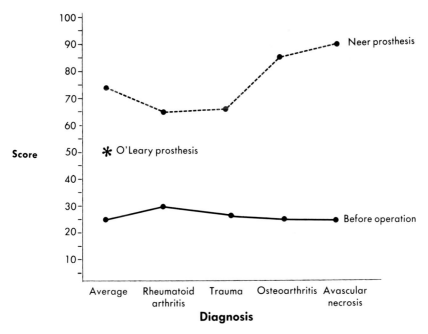

Fig. 6-4. Total preoperative and follow-up score for the Neer prosthesis.

Table 6-1. Neer prosthesis score

	Rheumatoid arthritis	Trauma	Osteoarthritis	Avascular necrosis
>85	1	1	2	4
70-85	2	—	1	1
50-70	5	1	—	—
50	2	1	—	—

aged 72 points. These results are somewhat prejudiced by the fact that the younger patients tended to have avascular necrosis with excellent soft tissues and a rotator cuff of good quality. Reviewing our results, relative to the diagnostic indications, the best results were noted in avascular necrosis and osteoarthritis (Fig. 6-4). In these patients, repair of the soft tissues were a minor problem and motion was started early after surgery. Significant, but less dramatic, results were noted in rheumatoid arthritis and degenerative arthritis secondary to trauma. Overall, three patients with a Neer prosthesis scored less than 50 points and were regarded as failures (Table 6-1).

Pain relief

Patients were evaluated subjectively as to the degree of pain and scored on a mild, moderate, and severe basis. Those with mild pain required no medication stronger than aspirin and had no night pain. They did not regard pain as a significant factor in their life. Pain was evaluated both at rest and with activity (Fig. 6-5). Pain relief was one of the prime indications for surgery and accounted for 41% of our total score improvement. Overall, 15 patients had no pain, four had mild pain requiring no medication, and two were regarded as failures of pain relief. Improvements were noted in all diagnostic groups with the best results in osteoarthritis and avascular necrosis. In those patients with rheumatoid arthritis, pain relief was noted in all but one patient.

Function

Function was evaluated as the ability to carry out certain tasks including toilet care and the combing of hair. Again, improvements were seen in all groups with the best results in those with osteoarthritis and avascular necrosis. Toilet care was possible in all but two patients at follow-up, and the ability to comb hair was limited to some degree in five of 21 patients with a Neer prosthesis.

Range of motion

Significant improvements in motion were seen in all diagnostic groups with again the most draumatic being in avascular necrosis (Table 6-2). Forward flexion, which is the most functional position to evaluate, demonstrated gains of greater

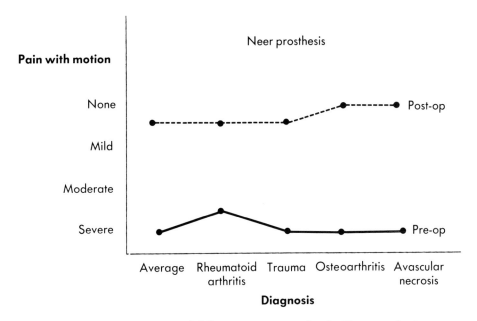

Fig. 6-5. Preoperative and follow-up pain scores for the Neer prosthesis.

Table 6-2. Active flexion of Neer prosthesis for 21 patients

Motion change	Total	Rheumatoid arthritis	Trauma	Osteoarthritis	Avascular necrosis
Gain	16	7	2	2	5
No change	1	—	—	1	—
Loss	4	3	1	—	—
Average change (in degrees)	+45	+17	+20	+48	+116

than 10 degrees in 16 of 21 patients, whereas four patients lost some motion. Three of these had rheumatoid arthritis where the loss was limited to 10 degrees. The average gain of forward flexion was 45 degrees for the Neer prosthesis. In those patients with rheumatoid arthritis gains of 17 degrees were noted, whereas those with old trauma averaged 20 degrees, osteoarthritis 48 degrees, and avascular necrosis 116 degrees. When viewed as to the type of surgical approach utilized, those patients in whom the deltoid was left attached to the clavicle with a deltopectoral approach being utilized had the best forward flexion, averaging 137 degrees in six patients versus 101 degrees in 11 patients in whom the deltoid was detached superiorly, and 89 degrees in four patients in whom a posterior approach was carried out. Considerable preselection went into the use of the deltopectoral approach,

Table 6-3. Radiolucent line noted on follow-up roentgenograms for two prostheses

Usage	Prosthesis	
	Neer	O'Leary-walker
Glenoid	21	6
Radiolucent line	16	5
<1 mm	14	3
1 to 2 mm	2	2 (loose 1)
Humeral	5	2 (loose 2)

since no rotator cuff tears were present and a disproportionate number had avascular necrosis. When viewed as to the onset of physical therapy, those patients starting motion within the first week had an average forward flexion of 115.9 degrees and scored 75 points whereas those starting motion during the second week had more limited motion averaging 83 degrees and 60.4 points. Again, those starting motion later had a disproportionate number with a rotator cuff tear.

Roentgenographic evaluation

Follow-up roentgenograms in all 21 Neer prostheses were evaluated carefully for the presence and progression of a radiolucent line about the glenoid and humeral component (Table 6-3). In 16 shoulders a radiolucent line was noted about the glenoid. This was less than 1 mm in width in 14 patients and 1 to 2 mm in width in two patients. A nonprogressive radiolucent line was noted about the humeral component in five patients. Loosening has not been documented by arthrography or surgery in any patient to date, but is suspected in two glenoid components.

FAILURE
Neer prosthesis

Three patients were believed to be failures of surgery, scoring less than 50 points at follow-up and having an unsatisfactory relief of pain in two. Two patients had rheumatoid arthritis, and one was a trauma patient who had undergone a previous hemiarthroplasty. In two patients a cuff tear was noted, with the repair described as difficult. It appeared that in the third patient a cuff tear had subsequently developed at 1 year after surgery. In the patient with previous trauma, persisting pain at the acromioclavicular joint and a partially detached deltoid were significant factors in the poor result.

Revision surgery was subsequently necessitated in one patient in whom a Neer prosthesis was inserted for avascular necrosis. At follow-up 1 year later this patient had pain in the acromioclavicular joint. Subsequent exploration was carried out with resection of the acromioclavicular joint. No loosening of the prosthesis was noted, and a dramatic relief of her pain was noted shortly later during a follow-up study.

O'Leary-Walker prosthesis

Initial experience at the Hospital for Special Surgery included the use of the O'Leary-Walker Nonconstrained prosthesis in six patients. As a result their follow-up time averaged 30.5 months, slightly longer than that of those who had a Neer prosthesis. These patients were evaluated in a similar manner preoperatively and had an average score of 25.3 points and at follow-up had improved to 52.3 points. Three of six patients were considered as failures, scoring less than 50 points, and only one patient scored over 85 points. In view of the small size of this group the results will not be broken down as to the diagnostic indications. As a group there was no improvement in their average forward flexion. Follow-up roentgenograms demonstrated a radiolucent line in five of six glenoid processes, with two in the 1 to 2 mm range (Table 6-3). One of these patients subsequently has had loosening documented at revision surgery. In addition, two of the six humeral components were found to be loose at revision surgery. In one patient with a diagnosis of avascular necrosis the humeral component had been inserted in an anteverted position. This resulted in instability of the humeral head with progressive loosening of both components. A second patient underwent revision because of persistent pain at the acromioclavicular joint. During the procedure there was noted a loose humeral component requiring replacement. A third patient had persistent pain as a result of impingement of the greater tuberosity on the acromion.

DISCUSSION

Total shoulder replacement has evolved during the past 8 years to a point at which one can obtain predictable pain relief by utilizing a nonconstrained prosthesis in a majority of patients. Function, motion, and strength improvement will be dependent on the adequacy of the soft tissue and the ability to carry out repairs of the rotator cuff. It is our impression that a nonconstrained prosthesis is the procedure of choice in the majority of patients. Careful preoperative evaluation must be carried out to select out those few patients in whom a more limited improvement should be predicted or possibly a more constrained prosthesis utilized. In those patients in whom a cuff arthropathy has developed with progressive degeneration of the glenoid and pronounced narrowing of the subacromial space, it is obvious that little or no cuff remains (Fig. 6-6). In this type of patient a more constrained prosthesis using an increased superior coverage of the glenoid may help to establish a fulcrum to allow improved motion as well as pain relief after surgery. In the less obvious patient arthrography utilizing the double-contrast technique supplimented with tomography may allow more adequate evaluation of the remaining rotator cuff tissue. Neurologic impairment, particularly in old trauma will obviously compromise the result. An electromyographic evaluation is often required. It should be emphasized that surgery in those with avascular necrosis and osteoarthritis is easier and the results more predictable than in the other conditions because the soft tissues are in their proper alignment and no rotator cuff tears have been seen. This is in contrast to those patients with rheumatoid arthritis and in particular old trauma

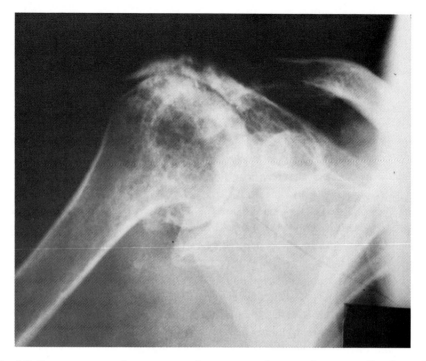

Fig. 6-6. Roentgenogram demonstrating degenerative changes of rotator cuff arthropathy.

in which there is considerable distortion of the tissues, the rotator cuff is often inadequate, and bone stock may be severely compromised. Overall pain relief has been obtainable in 90% of those patients with a Neer prosthesis. Functional and strength improvements have been significant and correlated with the degree of pain relief. Motion improvements have been dramatic in those with avascular necrosis and osteoarthritis, but significant improvements have also been seen in rheumatoid arthritis averaging 17 degrees of forward flexion and old trauma averaging 20 degrees of forward flexion. For those patients regarded as failures several points should be emphasized. The acromioclavicular joint should be carefully evaluated in all patients, particularly in those with rheumatoid arthritis and old trauma. If pain is suspected at this joint, excision of the lateral 2 cm of the clavicle should be performed at the time of surgery; often carried out in association with an acromioplasty to facilitate clearance of the rotator cuff. Tuberosity impingement can occur after prosthesis insertion if the humeral head is set too low on the anatomic neck. It can particularly occur in trauma in which the rotator cuff is left attached to a bony fragment and reattached to the prosthesis. In this situation the tuberosity must be reattached low enough to allow clearance beneath the acromion. On insertion of the glenoid component, if protrusio is present, the stem of the prosthesis may have to be trimmed to allow adequate seating of the polyethylene glenoid component. Careful cement technique with control of all bleeding and use of the

Water-Pik should decrease the incidence of lucency about the glenoid component. Upon insertion of the humeral component with the arm at the neutral position the humeral component should face directly toward the glenoid. If excessive anteversion is allowed, instability will develop, with progressive loosening of both components. When total shoulder replacement utilizing a nonconstrained prosthesis is being performed, the ability to carry out repair of the rotator cuff is critical to the result. If a large tear is present, an attempt must be made to mobilize the rotator cuff to allow adequate coverage of the humeral head if significant improvement in function and motion is to be expected. In those few patients with a large contracted rotator cuff tear precluding an adequate repair, a more constrained glenoid component should be available. Deltoid reattachment is critical to a satisfactory result because it was a significant factor in one of our poor results. Finally, the role of physical therapy in the postoperative treatment cannot be overemphasized. Inability to carry out an adequate prolonged program, inhospital and at home, along with some improvement in pain will not achieve satisfactory improvement in function and motion. From this review it appears that our results have improved with improved technique. It does not appear that the O'Leary-Walker design offers any significant advantages over the Neer design and has an increased risk of malpositioning and subsequent loosening of the humeral component.

SUMMARY

Follow-up studies have been carried out in 21 of 23 patients with Neer prostheses and six of the O'Leary-Walker design. Pain relief has been satisfactory in all but two of the Neer design, whereas there were three failures in the O'Leary-Walker group. Significant range-of-motion strength and functional improvements have been noted in all diagnostic groups, with the best results being seen in those patients with osteoarthritis and avascular necrosis.

REFERENCES

1. Buechel, F.: Personal communication.
2. Fenlin, J.M.: Total glenohumeral joint replacement, Orthop. Clin. North Am. 6(2):565-582, April 1975.
3. Gristina, A.: Personal communication, 1975, Winston-Salem, N.C.
4. Post, M., editor: The shoulder: surgical and nonsurgical management, Philadelphia, 1978, Lea & Febiger.

7. Philosophy and technique of rehabilitation of total shoulder replacement

Allan E. Inglis, M.D.
Russell F. Warren, M.D.

The philosophy of the rehabilitation of the total shoulder replacement is the development of painless function and motion in the glenohumeral articulation. This is a complex problem because of the preoperative stiffness in degenerative arthritis or muscle spasm and disuse atrophy in the patient with rheumatoid arthritis. Historically, synovectomy and at times joint débridement were the only procedures available to the patient with severe joint loss caused by arthritis. Arthrodesis was frequently the only avenue for restoration of a modicum of shoulder function. This was followed by synovectomy and hemiarthroplasty with replacement of the damaged humeral head. This achieved some success in degenerative arthritis and traumatic arthritis. However, in rheumatoid arthritis, the hemiarthroplasty with synovectomy was found to yield 70% good results in terms of pain, with motion being not much better than that of the preoperative condition. With the introduction of glenohumeral joint replacement arthroplasty, relief of pain and improved functional ranges of motion could be obtained. The preoperative anatomic resources dictate in part the type of rehabilitation program. The stiff shoulder or those patients with adhesive capsulitis present special problems in the rehabilitative programs after total shoulder replacement. It is important that the patient, the surgeon, and the therapist understand the possible level of function after surgery and rehabilitation. Additionally, it is important that the patient understand the nature and duration of the postoperative rehabilitation program. Frequently one should have a consultation, during which time an activities-of-daily-living (ADL) profile can be obtained. This will bring into view any other functional deficiencies that may require alteration in the rehabilitation program. The type of rehabilitative program will be dictated and modified in part by the status of the acromioclavicular joint. It will also depend on complete restoration of the deltoid muscle origins to the clavicle and to

68

the acromion process and to the spine of the scapula. It will also be altered by the type of surgical approach, whether it be an anterior or a posterior surgical incision.

REHABILITATION TECHNIQUE PRINCIPLES

There are several general principles in the technique for rehabilitation of a total shoulder replacement. Constant patient encouragement is required to increase patient compliance and confidence. There must be a coordinated effort by the surgeon and therapist and patient. The surgeon must not delegate his responsibilities to a nurse or a secretary but must be *directly* involved in the rehabilitation process. After surgery, the patient should be kept in hospital for at least 2 weeks, longer if necessary, to be certain that the program is well established and proceeding satisfactorily. The basic approach to rehabilitation depends in part on the type of surgical reconstruction required. Patients with an intact external rotator cuff require less protection during the postoperative period than those in which the external rotator cuff required repair or reconstruction.

TREATMENT MODIFICATIONS

There are certain treatment modifications. The first consists of the status of the external rotator cuff. If the external rotator cuff is intact, the patient is immobilized in a sling for a 3-week period. The sling is removed for exercises and bathing. The passive and assisted range-of-motion program is started on the fourth postoperative day, with active motion being added at the 3-week point. If the external rotator cuff has been damaged and requires repair, the patient may be either immobilized in a sling or in an airplane splint for approximately 3 weeks. At that time, limited, passive range of motion may be started, with assistive and active range of motion being added at approximately 6 weeks. The treatment may be modified by the surgical approach. The anterior deltopectoral type of approach, during which time the subscapularis is detached along with the capsule, will allow early external rotation and late internal rotation. Whereas, with the posterior approach, during which time the external rotator muscles will be either detached or repaired, active external rotation will be avoided whereas active internal rotation will be permitted. The overall physical and occupational therapeutic program should include an evaluation implementation of ADL. A preoperative range of motion and muscle-strength measurements are useful in management of the postoperative rehabilitation program. Assistive devices for ADL can be provided early in convalescence as well as instruction in one-hand activities that may be temporarily needed.

POSTOPERATIVE CARE

Our postoperative therapeutic protocol for total shoulder replacement is divided into two stages.

Stage 1. During this period of time passive and active assistive ranges of motion are started. These exercises are performed five times each day in 5-minute sessions. The patient is seen twice daily in the occupational therapy department and performs the other three daily sessions independently in their room. If the patient is in an airplane splint, the exercises are started at the third week when the splint is removed. On the fourth postoperative day, when the wound is quiet and dry, they begin their therapeutic program. This consists of passive flexion with the patient in the supine position. The patient is also instructed through an active, assistive, forward flexion program, again, in the supine position. They are also allowed to carry out active, assistive, external rotation to the neutral position. Pendulum or Codman exercises are begun on the fourth postoperative day with the arm still in the sling or with the elbow flexed. Isometric exercises are also initiated with emphasis on external rotation (external rotators) and abduction (deltoid). If the posterior surgical approach has been used, isometric internal rotation and deltoid function will be started. During week 2 and, specifically, on days 7 through 10, the same exercises are continued. In addition, active assistive internal rotation with the arm behind the back is started. Also, active, assistive extension and flexion in the sitting position are also started. During days 14 through 18 the same exercises are continued. However, active, assistive, horizontal, external rotation behind the head at 120 degrees is initiated. Also, active, assistive, horizontal abduction and adduction of the shoulder are started.

Stage 2. The stage 2 therapeutic program is started at approximately 2 1/2 weeks. The patient performs all the exercises in stage 1 four times a day until the sixth week or longer if necessary. The sling immobilization is gradually decreased and discontinued. The patient is discharged from the hospital at this time and followed in an outpatient facility. During the $2^{1}/_{2}$ to 3 weeks, all the previous exercises are continued, and now the patient begins active forward flexion in the supine position with the elbow flexed. The patient is also allowed to begin flexion by raising the extended arm from a table top. All exercises are increased from the supine to the upright position.

Between 3 and 6 weeks, the patient is encouraged to begin a gradual increase in the active range-or-motion exercise program. At the 3-week point, light resistive exercises are begun throughout the entire range of motion. The patient is recommended to see a therapist once or twice a week for at least a month and then weekly thereafter. All patients are encouraged to continue with the range-or-motion program for at least 6 months in an effort to regain muscle strength and tone needed for the activities of daily living.

The dowel-stick exercise program is very useful. These dowels can be purchased at a local hardware store for less than $1. The contralateral shoulder is allowed to assist the surgically reconstructed shoulder in range-of-motion and strengthening exercises. Rolling-pin exercises are also useful in obtaining coordinated flexion of the shoulder. The simple overhead pulley device is easily purchased and installed. Again, the contralateral shoulder can be used to aid in the rehabilitation of the operated shoulder. We have found that job-simulated activities are also useful. Discussion with the patient about their work requirements will frequently reveal a simple exercise routine that can return the patient to work more quickly.

CONCLUSION

It is essential that the planning of a shoulder replacement arthroplasty include the postoperative rehabilitative program. A preoperative visit by the therapist, including not only getting aquainted, but also some discussion of the postoperative program, will be helpful in obtaining the patient's confidence and cooperation. The surgeon must remain an integral part of the rehabilitation team both to encourage the patient, and at times himself, and to make alterations in the program as needed. No other joint replacement requires the skill and detailed planning and meticulous follow-through, as is required in total shoulder replacement. A successful total shoulder replacement rehabilitative program will produce delighted patients and present the surgeon with superb results for his efforts.

PART THREE

The elbow

8. History of total elbow arthroplasty

Ralph W. Coonrad, M.D.

Historically, there are four overlapping eras in the development of elbow arthroplasty, beginning with resection arthroplasty described as early as 1885 by Ollier[27] and followed by interposition arthroplasty, reported by Jones,[19] in 1885. These four eras can be defined as follows:

First	1885 to 1947	Era of resection, interposition, and anatomic arthroplasty
Second	1947 to 1970	Era of partial and occasional total (straight-hinge) joint arthroplasty
Third	1970 to 1975	Era of constrained metal-to-metal, hinge joint replacement with methacrylate fixation
Fourth	1975 to 1980	Era of semiconstrained metal-to-polyethylene hinge or snap-fitting prostheses and unconstrained metal-to-polyethylene resurfacing arthroplasty

FIRST ERA

In the initial era, Ollier described resection arthroplasty for tuberculous involvement that consisted of simple joint excision, with interposing scar tissue being relied on for stability. Later, interposition arthroplasty took the form of muscle flap, fascia, or adipose tissue interposed between the joint surfaces, and satisfactory results were reported in 60 cases by Murphy[26] in 1913, who also recommended periosteum removal to help prevent myositis ossificans. In 1895 Jones interposed gold foil, which usually extruded. Baer,[2] in 1913, referred to Chlumsky (1900), who reported on the experimental use of tin, zinc, silicone, celluloid, rubber, linoleum, decalcified bone, chromatized pig's bladder (known as Baer's membrane), and magnesium. Putti,[31] in 1921, reported 38 arthroplasties of the elbow, emphasizing the importance of a living membrane being used to cover bone ends. Campbell,[5] in 1921, analyzed 100 arthroplasties at the Campbell Clinic and indicated that although any ankylosed joint was easy to mobilize with sufficient bone resection, caution should be exercised if an unstable joint were to be prevented. Anatomic arthroplasty described by Defontaine[4] as early as 1887 consisted of an attempt by limited carpentry to maintain congruous surfaces that would move on each other, with or without interposing tissue. This form of reconstruction was reported by many authors, Knight and Van Zandt[20] in 1952, and Henri, Pulkki, and Vainio[4] in 1964. Although Knight and Van Zandt's cases included 56% good results, 20% were total failures, and as late as 1969, Dee[11] reported a small series of unsatisfactory results in 9 patients.

SECOND ERA

The limited predictability and long-term failures with interposition, resection, and anatomic elbow arthroplasty initiated the second era and stimulated efforts to totally replace one side or the other. Virgen[35] developed a metal replacement for the proximal olecranon as early as 1937, and Mellen and Phalen[24] in 1947, and later MacAusland[22] in 1954, reported hemireplacement of the lower end of the humerus with acrylic-stemmed prostheses. In 1965, Barr and Eaton[3] reported an intramedullary stemmed metal prosthetic replacement of the distal humerus that had two transfixing cortical screws to prevent rotation and had a 4-year satisfactory result. However, longer term follow-up studies on sleeve or stem replacements, with or without screw fixation, reported failures, and after removal, fusion was difficult and flail elbows were difficult to accept. Carr,[6] in 1951, and Cherry,[8] in 1953, reported the successful use of a radial-head prosthetic replacement from Vitallium and acrylic cement, respectively. Street and Stevens,[32] in 1974, reported the use of a metal cuff replacement for the trochlea and capitellum in 9 patients over a period of 7 years and with better results in the posttraumatic cases. Satisfactory use of silicone-implant replacement of the radial head was reported by Swanson[33] in 1968, with long-term, satisfactory follow-up studies in 1978.

The use of custom metal-to-metal hinge prostheses was occasionally reported throughout the 1950s and 1960s. The Austenal Company had a straight-stem metal-hinged total-replacement prosthesis available in the early 1950s, but it lacked an anatomic center of rotation, and, as a result, flexion was limited and skin and tendon breakdown over the extensor surface led to early failures. Chatzidakis[7] reported the use of a hinged Vitallium prosthesis in 1970, and Driessen[14] in 1972, reported a satisfactory 30-year follow-up study of a flat steel-hinged plate, wired through multiple drill holes to the humerus and ulna.

THIRD ERA

The third era in the development of elbow arthroplasty was initiated by Dee,[12] in 1972, with the use of a metal-to-metal hinge prosthesis cemented with polymethylmethacrylate. However, biomechanical information on the major forces and motion of the elbow joint was not available, and early satisfactory results were followed by reports of a high incidence of failure in 2 to 3 years, primarily because of prosthetic loosening. The need for design changes based on developing biomechanical and biomaterial information gradually became evident but not before rather large numbers of metal-to-metal prostheses were implanted. Many early designs of totally constrained metal-to-metal prostheses reported varying results on short-term follow-up including those by Dee, McKee, Stanmore, Shiers, GSB, and Mazas. During this same period, Swanson and Niebauer designed double-stemmed flexible silicone implants; however, the breakage factor was great even with extraordinary ligamentous reinforcement, and the results are not discussed here.

FOURTH ERA

The fourth era of elbow arthroplasty, beginning about 1975, has virtually been limited to two primary types of implants: semiconstrained metal-to-polyethylene hinge types, and snap-fitting prostheses, or totally unconstrained metal-to-polyethylene resurfacing implants. Some examples of the semiconstrained types of prostheses with varying degrees of side-to-side laxity, include the Mayo, Pritchard-Walker, Tri-Axial, Coonrad, and Schlein. Examples of resurfacing and totally unconstrained prostheses are the Ewald, London, and Stevens-Street distal humeral cuff replacement for the trochlea and capitellum. A partial list of elbow implants being used in this fourth period in the development of joint replacement and some of the characteristics and results of those implants are as follows.

Types of elbow implants

Semiconstrained types

Mayo Clinic design (Howmedica, 1972). This is a three-part semiconstrained but loose snap-fitting design of the ulnohumeral component and a separate varying-sized component replacing the radial head. The radial and ulnar components are polyethylene, and the humeral portion is metal, with the trochlea being replaced by two metal cones and the capitellum by a cylinder of variable height to permit loading. The humeral and ulnar stems utilize methacrylate for fixation.

The first Mayo implant was carried out in October 1972, with a 5-year follow-up period reported[9] in February 1980 on 53 prostheses. There was an overall 80% satisfactory level of results with the Mayo prosthesis, with a complication of loosening in 12%. The prosthesis requires good bone stock and was used almost exclusively in patients with rheumatoid arthritis (Fig. 8-1).

Pritchard-Walker design (DePuy, 1974). This is a hinged metal-to-polyethylene prosthesis with 5 to 7 degrees of mediolateral and rotary laxity. The Mark I design has a polyethylene humeral stem component, and a second model, Mark II, has the polyethylene humeral component replaced with a metal stem, incorporating a polyethylene condylar component for use in elbows with poor bone stock.

A 5-year follow-up study of 48 patients over a mean of 29 months was reported[29] in May 1979 with 21 Mark I and 27 Mark II prostheses. There were 30 patients with rheumatoid arthritis, three with posttraumatic arthritis, and seven from other failed implants. Results were classified as satisfactory in 39, with 3 poor results, and complications included no loosening but breakage of 2 polyethylene stems (Fig. 8-2).

Coonrad design (Zimmer, 1973). This semiconstrained metal-to-polyethylene hinged prosthesis was first implanted at the Mayo Clinic in May 1973. Laxity in the joint in side-to-side and rotary direction was increased from 2 or 3 degrees to 7 degrees in the period 1978 and 1979 (Coonrad II model). The prosthesis is of

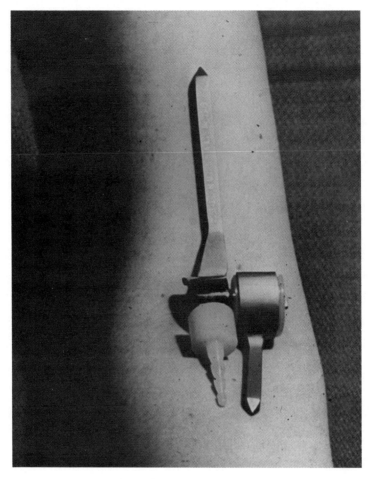

Fig. 8-1. Mayo Clinic Design—three-part semiconstrained but loose snap-fitting design of the ulnohumeral component and a separate varying-sized component replacing the radial head.

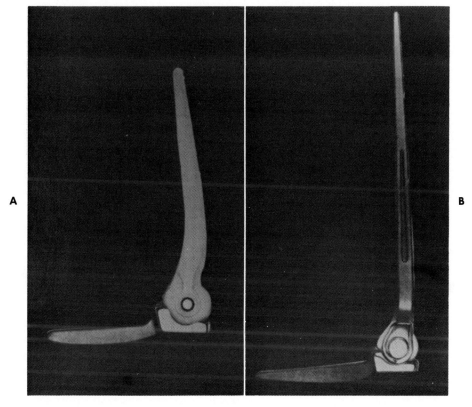

Fig. 8-2. Pritchard-Walker Design—hinged metal-to-polyethylene prosthesis with 7 degrees of mediolateral and rotary laxity. **A,** Pritchard Elbow. **B,** Pritchard Elbow II.

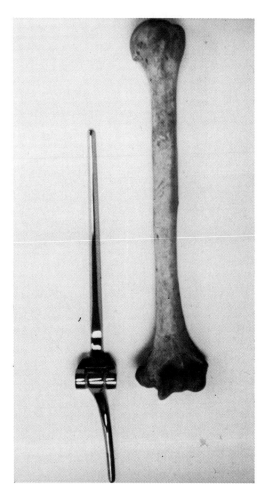

Fig. 8-3. Coonrad Design—semiconstrained metal-to-polyethylene hinged prosthesis, in relation to humerus of average length.

polyethylene and titanium metal with a near anatomic center of rotation in line with the anterior cortex of the humerus and ulna. A long-stemmed model was added in 1977. The most important features of its design are the *large size, length,* and *contour* of the stems, requiring patient cabinetry for implantation. However, once implanted, the long-stemmed prosthesis is usually stable in the humerus, even before cementing. Although methacrylate has been used in all but one of the patients in the initial protocol series, one patient without methacrylate usage has a satisfactory result at 5 years (Fig. 8-3).

A prospective protocol series of 150 elbows was initiated in 1973, including 39 elbows[10] from the Mayo Clinic series. (No Coonrad II implants with laxity added

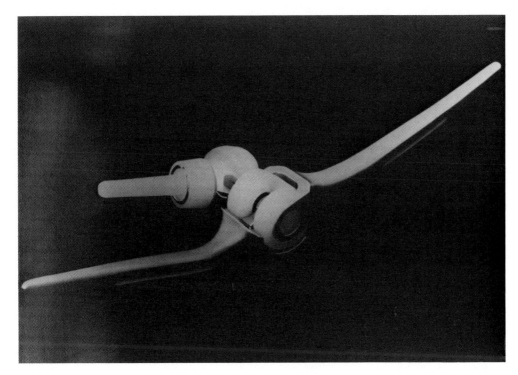

Fig. 8-4. Voltz Design—three-component, semiconstrained metal-to-polyethylene hinged prosthesis.

to the prosthesis of 7 degrees are included.) With a follow-up of 3 to 7 years, 87 rheumatoid elbows with good bone stock had 66 good, 19 fair, one poor result, and one failure, or a *satisfactory rating of 95%*. Loosening occurred in two patients insufficient for removal. In 60 posttraumatic elbows, results with poor bone stock were not so successful, with 35 being rated good, 16 fair, 2 poor, 6 failed, and 1 person who fell and fractured the elbow, giving a *satisfactory rating of 84%*. Documented loosening occurred in 7 posttraumatic elbows with lucent lines in 10 or an overall incidence in this group of 13%. It is anticipated that laxity added to the prosthesis will significantly diminish the incidence of loosening when used in elbows having poor bone stock.

Volz design (Zimmer, 1975). This is a three-component, semiconstrained metal-to-polyethylene hinged prosthesis with 15 degrees of laxity and with a load-bearing radial-head replacement component. This prosthesis was first implanted in 1980, with 24 prostheses inserted by this writing.[36] A current follow-up of 1 to 4 years reveals a satisfactory result in 23 of the 24 implants. One failure occurred with loosening of all three components and was removed. Eighteen of the 24 patients had rheumatoid arthritis (Fig. 8-4).

Tri-Axial–Hospital For Special Surgery design (Codman, 1974). This is a semi-constrained hinged metal-to-polyethylene prosthesis with a very loose fit; an original polyethylene humeral stem has been replaced with a metal stem (Fig. 8-5).

A 4-year follow-up study[17] of 33 elbows in 1978 revealed satisfactory results in 95% of the elbows with good bone stock having rheumatoid arthritis, and 70% satisfactory results in the elbows with degenerative arthrosis and traumatic arthritis.

Schlein design (Howmedica, 1974). This is a small loose snap-fitting hinged semiconstrained implant of metal with polyethylene bushing. Over 400 implants have been reported; however, a follow-up study on these has not been accurately documented[31] (Fig. 8-6).

Unconstrained types

Ewald design (Codman, 1974). A nonconstrained two-component essentially articular resurfacing type of implant with a stemmed metal humeral component and an articulating polyethylene ulnar shoe, both requiring methacrylate fixation. The design requires good bone stock and intact collateral ligaments.

This prosthesis was first implanted in July 1974, and 69 cases were reported[15] in 1978 and updated at this time with a 2- to 5-year follow-up having 87% satisfactory results. Loosening has occurred in one ulnar component, and there have been four dislocations. (Fig. 8-7.)

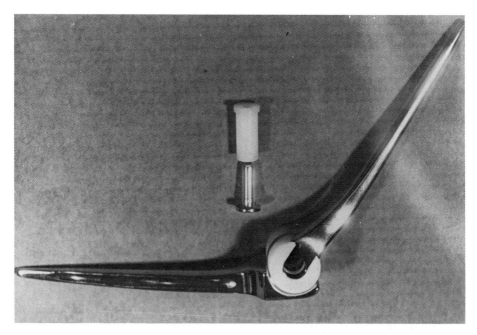

Fig. 8-5. Tri-Axial–Hospital for Special Surgery Design—semiconstrained hinged metal-to-polyethylene prosthesis.

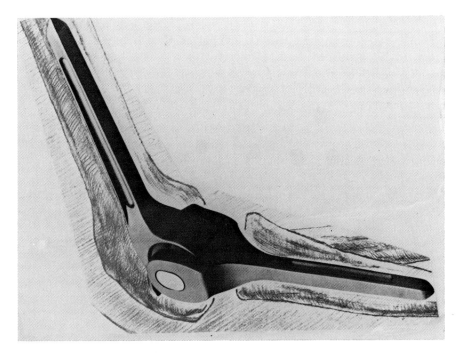

Fig. 8-6. Schlein Design—small loose snap-fitting hinged semiconstrained implant of metal with polyethylene bushing.

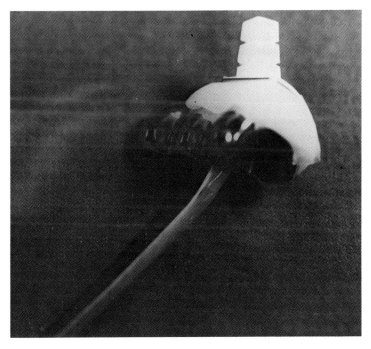

Fig. 8-7. Ewald Design—nonconstrained two-component essentially articular resurfacing type of implant.

London design (Wright-Dow Corning, 1976). This is a resurfacing, totally un-constrained, two-part implant of metal and polyethylene with use restricted to in-tact bone stock situations.

An average 15-month follow-up study of 16 elbows in 1978[21] revealed satisfac-tory early results in 14 with complications of a loose ulnar component in one and unexplained pain in one (Fig. 8-8).

Stevens-Street design (Zimmer, 1974). A slotted metal cylinder with capitellar and trochlear contours was designed to replace the lower humerus in a cufflike manner, requiring intact lower humeral bone stock at the epicondylar level and joint stability with intact collateral ligaments and olecranon.

Twenty-two cases were reported in 1978[32] with generally satisfactory results with one dislocation and three subluxations (Fig. 8-9).

Allograft replacement

A small series of glycerin-frozen allograft replacements of the elbow involving two lower humeri and a composite of two lower humeri with proximal ulnas has been carried out by Urbaniak[34] at Duke University and has been followed 1 to 3 years with a range of motion averaging 60 to 90 degrees. Bone grafting for non-union was necessary in one patient and degenerative arthrosis may be anticipated in the future, but all replacements were done for massive bone stock loss in young people, for tumor or trauma, and will make total elbow replacement easier at a later date.

Total elbow arthroplasty

Indications. Some pathologic indications for consideration of replacement elbow arthroplasty can be listed as follows:

1. *Rheumatoid arthritis,* where good medical treatment has failed and joint destruction precludes lesser procedures such as synovectomy and radial head excision.
2. *Degenerative arthrosis* that has progressed with joint destruction beyond the value of single or repeated débridements.
3. *Traumatic arthrosis,* from such problems as persistent subluxation or dislo-cation.
4. *Bone stock loss,* from tumor or trauma with ankylosis, pain, or instability that is unacceptable. An ankylosed elbow in functional position with a nor-mal opposite extremity is probably not an indication for the risk of replace-ment arthroplasty.
5. *Failed arthroplasties,* of any type that become unacceptably painful or un-stable.

Contraindications. The basic contraindications to joint replacement arthroplasty at the elbow are the following:

1. Infection
2. A demand or need for other than sedentary activity with the elbow

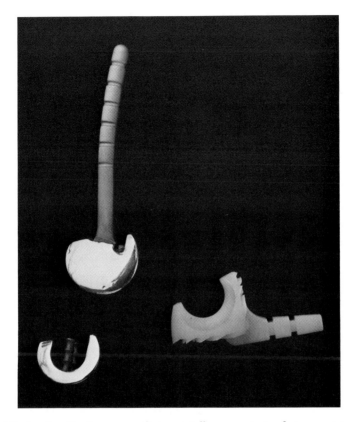

Fig. 8-8. London Design—resurfacing, totally unconstrained, two-part implant.

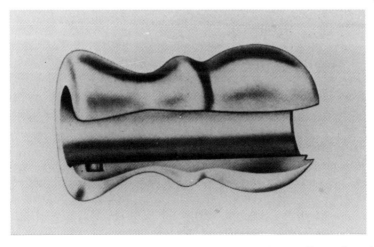

Fig. 8-9. Stevens-Street Design—slotted metal cylinder with capitellar and trochlear contours designed to replace the lower humerus in a cufflike manner.

3. Ankylosis of the shoulder on the same side, and particularly with internal rotation deformities such as in rheumatoid disease
4. Neurotrophic joints

There are two prime functions of the elbow: first, to place the hand, a precision instrument, at any point in space and, second, to act as a fulcrum for the forearm in lifting. In the instance of crutch-walking, gymnastics, and certain sports, it becomes a weight-bearing joint. The three major goal requirements of elbow arthroplasty are to relieve pain, restore or maintain mobility, and restore or retain stability.

A stable elbow that is painless, but with limited motion in midrange, does not ordinarily warrant the risk or extent of joint replacement. Probably the most significant complication noted in a review of many arthroplasties is that of *improper selection*. An example is the ununited childhood medial or lateral epicondylar epiphyseal bone fragment with instability that becomes symptomatic in adult life and can be readily treated by the lesser procedure of bone grafting rather than arthroplasty. In rheumatoid arthritic patients with stable joints and before extensive bone destruction occurs, synovectomy and radial head excision can offer satisfactory results. Cofield et al.,[9] in combining the results of Petersen and Janes,[28] Dickson et al.,[13] Marmor,[23] Inglis et al.,[18] and Taylor,[37] reported satisfactory results in 75% of 161 patients after an average of 4.5 years from surgery.

Design and biomechanics. The ideal replacement arthroplasty should be pain free, stable, durable, mobile, retrievable, and reproducible in the hands of most surgeons.

The initial failures and experience of 25% loosening in the early 1970s with totally constrained metal-to-metal prostheses stimulated an interest in the biomechanical factors singular to the elbow joint. Asher,[1] in 1973, brought about some basic understanding of the magnitude of forces crossing the joint with the finding that nearly 2.6 times body weight can be transmitted across the elbow during lifting. Hui and others[16] demonstrated that forces across the joint are greater in extension than in flexion and that large shearing and torsional moments occur. Walker,[37] Hui, and Pearson have all shown that the greatest force component at the distal humerus is in a posterior direction, and Bryan[9] pointed out that this tends to cause an anterior tilt of the proximal stem of a humeral component with bony resorption of the anterior humeral cortex. Murrey and Chao[25] showed that the locus of the instant axis of rotation of the elbow joint is located in the center of the trochlea, in line with the anterior cortex of the humerus, but is constantly changing with rotation of the long axis of the ulna during passive motion.

Of particular concern in the design of an elbow prosthesis is the relation of the reactive joint forces when the elbow lever arm is the longest at 90 degrees of flexion. Torque force is greatest at this point and calculations, according to Volz and others,[36] have indicated that an object lifted by hand at 90 degrees of flexion produces reactive forces of eight to ten times at the elbow-joint level. Since 60% of the transmitted force across the elbow joint from the hand passes across the capitellar-radial portion of the joint, Volz and the Mayo Clinic have each designed prostheses that incorporate a capitellar-radial load-bearing component.

In an attempt to reduce angular and, to some extent, torque force the Coonrad design is significantly large with contoured ulnar and humeral stems and has been modified with a much longer humeral-stem length with the rationale that resistance to torque force is directly proportional to the surface area of the stem or methacrylate interface.

There are more than 20 total elbow prostheses available on the market at the time of this writing. They can be basically differentiated into two groups by the degree of constraint, and only the totally unconstrained or semiconstrained metal to high molecular weight polyethylene types are essentially in current use. *Both resurfacing and hinge types have been employed with about equal success in situations with good bone stock where the collateral ligaments and soft tissues provide for the prime dissipation of stresses at the joint interface, as with rheumatoid disease.* Results have not been as good where bone stock has been lost. Resurfacing implants have an inherent tendency for instability and dislocation, whereas hinged implants have a tendency to loosen because of increased stress at the bone-methacrylate interface. Laxity designed into the hinged prosthesis then appears important, though the ideal degree of laxity or toggle is unknown. The Pritchard-Walker has 7 degrees, the Tri-Axial is described as a "floppy joint," the Coonrad originally had 2 degrees, increased to 7 degrees, and the Volz has 15 degrees. The increased wear factors on polyethylene and the impact force from fixed limits of side-to-side and rotary movement of hinged joints is also yet unknown.

Technique considerations. A midline posterior longitudinal incision has apparently diminished, in some reports, the number of problems with wound healing when compared with curvilinear incisions. Ewald and Pritchard utilize the classic technique of a V-resection, taking down the triceps, and with the Ewald prosthesis, a T-capsulotomy is necessary as an important part of the technique of preparation of the humerus and ulna for resurfacing. Bryan[9] described an exposure of the elbow joint in which the triceps tendon is dissected subperiosteally from the olecranon in continuity with the proximal ulnar periosteum, and shifted either to one side or the other. This virtually eliminates the problem of triceps rupture. An alternative method is longitudinal splitting of the triceps mechanism with the proximal ulnar periosteum, and a portion is separated to each side of the olecranon for total exposure.

Poor technique and inexperience in the early use of methyl methacrylate with inadequate fixation is undoubtedly one of the important causes of the early poor results reported with many types of prostheses. The use of cement in liquid form with a syringe or gun and a clean dry canal with careful impaction of the cement have unquestionably significantly improved results during the last few years.

Regardless of the type of prosthesis used, a minimal amount of bone should be excised from the humerus and extreme care taken to preserve both medial and lateral epicondyles and collateral ligaments in all cases where possible. Even the retention of one epicondyle as a buttress is important. The use of a Hemovac drain, compression dressing, elevation and mobilization of the elbow after initial edema has subsided, and isotonic exercises at 2 to 3 months postoperatively are important features of the postoperative regimen in virtually all total elbow replacement routines.

Complications. The major complications of total elbow replacement include the following:

1. Loosening
2. Dislocation
3. Breakage
4. Triceps rupture
5. Nerve palsy
6. Fracture
7. Infection
8. Improper selection.

Dislocations have occurred with snap-fitting prostheses and with resurfacing implants. Dislocations with the Schlein prosthesis have occurred, though the incidence is unknown. The Ewald prosthesis followed for 2 to 5 years has a 5% incidence of dislocation. Breakage is rare but occurred in one of the Hospital for Special Surgery implants when an axle broke early, but others have not been reported. Fractures of the polyethylene stem in the Pritchard-Walker and early Hospital for Special Surgery implants occurred, but a change of design in the latter to a metal humeral component and also with the Mark II Pritchard prosthesis has eliminated this problem. Triceps rupture, attenuation, or deficiency from scarring, is probably more common than we think and is disabling. Thin tissue over the posterior elbow makes subsequent reinforcement by tendon transfers difficult and fascia lata grafting has not been routinely successful. Ulnar nerve palsy or neuropathy should not occur if routine identification, protection, or transfer is carried out. Fractures at operation, particularly with revisions, can only be prevented where adequate exposure and extreme care is taken. Postoperative infection does not always make prosthesis removal mandatory. One Coonrad prosthesis exposed for over a month was ultimately covered with a local pedicle skin graft and has a functional range of elbow motion after 6 years.

SUMMARY

Total elbow joint replacement is still a salvage procedure. Our increasing knowledge of the biomechanics and kinematics of the elbow joint, and of biomaterials, has produced a significant transition in the 30-year history of total elbow arthroplasty. Compared to the earlier choice between the limitations imposed by fusion or the instability of joint resection, most patients at this point in time can expect to achieve a stable, painless joint for sedentary use with only a small percentage of failures, most of which can be salvaged by revision. Improvement in the technique of methacrylate insertion, improvement in the design of implants with greater laxity in metal-to-polyethylene components, restoration of a near-anatomic center of rotation, longer stems to distribute torque-resistant forces, and the preservation of all bone stock and ligamentous structures possible have lessened many problems of the past. The major hazard of loosening has been significantly reduced, and in the rheumatoid or patient with good bone stock, satisfactory results have been demonstrated over a 3- to 7-year period with the Pritchard, Tri-Axial, Coonrad, and Ewald prostheses almost equally above a 90% level. The Mayo prosthesis has had 80% satisfactory results in this category. Where humeral epicondyles are absent, long-term results with many prostheses have not been as reliable.

REFERENCES

1. Asher, M.A., and Zilber, S.: Biomechanics of the elbow and forearm, presented at the American Academy of Surgeons Postgraduate Course in the Elbow, Wrist and Forearm, Kansas City, Mo., Oct. 13, 1973.
2. Baer, W.S.: Cited in McGehee, F.O.: Elbow arthroplasty. Thesis submitted to American Orthopaedic Association, Jan. 1959.
3. Barr, J.S., and Eaton, R.G.: Elbow reconstruction with a new prosthesis to replace the distal end of the humerus, J. Bone Joint Surg. 47:1408, 1956.
4. Bryan, R.S., Linscheid, R.L., Dobyns, J.H., and Peterson, L.F.: A total elbow arthroplasty sound slide series, Rochester, Minn., 1976, The Mayo Foundation.
5. Campbell, W.C.: Arthroplasties, J. Orthop. Surg. 19:430, 1921.
6. Carr, C.R., and Howard, J.W. Metallic cap replacement of the radial head following fracture, West. J. Surg. Ob. Gyn. 59:539-546, 1951.
7. Chatzidakis, C.: Arthroplasty of the elbow joint using a Vitallium prosthesis, Int. Surg. 53:119-122, 1970.
8. Cherry, J.C.: Use of acrylic prosthesis in the treatment of fracture of the head of the radius, J. Bone Joint Surg. 35B:70-71, 1953.
9. Cofield, R.H., Morrey, B.F., and Bryan, R.S.: Total shoulder and total elbow arthroplasties: the current state of development, J. Contin. Educ. Orthop., part II, pp. 17-25, Jan. 1979.
10. Coonrad, R.: Coonrad Total Elbow replacement, American Orthopaedic Association Presentation, Homestead, Va., June 1978.
11. Dee, R.: Elbow arthroplasty, Proc. R. Soc. Med. 62:1031-1035, 1969.
12. Dee, R.: Total replacement arthroplasty of the elbow for rheumatoid arthritis, J. Bone Joint Surg. (Br.) 54:88-95, 1972.
13. Dickson, R.A., Stein, H., and Bentley, G.: Excision arthroplasty of the elbow in rheumatoid disease, J. Bone Joint Surg. (Br.) 58:227-229, 1976.
14. Driessen, A.P.P.M.: Thirty years with a complete elbow prosthesis, Arch. Chir. Neerl. 24-II:87-92, 1972.
15. Ewald, F.C.: American Academy of Orthopaedic Surgeons Continuing Education Course in Upper Extremity Joint Replacement, New York, Sept. 27, 1979.
16. Hui, F.C., Chao, E.Y., and An, K.N.: Muscle and joint forces at the elbow during isometric lifting (Abstract), Orthop. Trans. 2:169-170, 1978.
17. Inglis, A.E.: American Academy of Orthopaedic Surgeons Continuing Education Course in Upper Extremity Joint Replacement, New York, Sept. 27, 1979.
18. Inglis, A.E., Ranawat, C.S., and Straub, L.R.: Synovectomy and débridement of the elbow in rheumatoid arthritis, J. Bone Joint Surg. (Am.) 53:652-662, 1971.
19. Jones, R.: Cited in McGehee, F.O.: Elbow arthroplasty. Thesis submitted to American Orthopaedic Association, Jan. 1959.
20. Knight, R.A., and Van Zandt, I.L., Arthroplasty of the elbow: an end-result study, J. Bone Joint Surg. (Am.) 34:610-617, 1952.
21. London, J.T.: Resurfacing total elbow arthroplasty, Presented at the 45th Annual Meeting of the American Academy of Orthopaedic Surgeons, Dallas, Texas, Feb. 23-28, 1978.

22. MacAusland, A.R.: Replacement of the lower end of the humerus with a prosthesis: a report of four cases, West. J. Surg. Ob. Gyn. **62:**557-566, 1954.
23. Marmor, L.: Surgery of the rheumatoid elbow: follow-up study on synovectomy combined with radial head excision, J. Bone Joint Surg. (Am.) **54:**573-578, 1972.
24. Mellen, R.H., and Phalen, G.S.: Arthroplasty of the elbow by replacement of the distal portion of the humerus with an acrylic prosthesis, J. Bone Joint Surg. **29:**348-353, 1947.
25. Morrey, B.F., and Chao, E.Y.S.: Passive motion of the elbow joint: a biomechanical analysis, J. Bone Joint Surg. (Am.) **58:**501-508, 1976.
26. Murphy, J.B.: Arthroplasty, Ann. Surg. **57:**593-647, 1913.
27. Ollier, L.: Traité des résections et des opérations conservatrices qu'on peut pratiquer sur le système osseux, Paris, 1885-1889, G. Masson.
28. Peterson, L.F.A., and Janes, J.M.: Surgery of the rheumatoid elbow, Orthop. Clin. North Am. **2:**667-677, 1971.
29. Pritchard, R.W.: Semiconstrained elbow prosthesis: a clinical review of five years of experience, Orthop. Rev. 8(5):33-43, May 1979.
30. Putti, V.: Arthroplasty, J. Orthop. Surg. 19:419, 1921.
31. Schlein, A.P.: Semiconstrained total elbow arthroplasty, Clin. Orthop., no. 121, p. 222, Nov.-Dec. 1976.
32. Street, D.N., and Stevens, P.S.: A humeral replacement prosthesis for the elbow: results in 10 elbows, J. Bone Joint Surg. 56A:1147, 1974.
33. Swanson, A.B., Percinel, A., and Herndon, J.H.: Long-term follow-up of implant arthroplasty following radial head excision in rheumatoid arthritis, Presented at the 45th Annual Meeting of the American Academy of Orthopaedic Surgeons, Dallas, Texas, Feb. 23-28, 1978.
34. Urbaniak, J.R.: Personal communication, 1980, Durham, N.C.
35. Virgen, 1937, cited in Schlein, A.P.: Semiconstrained total elbow arthroplasty, Clin. Orthop., no. 121, p. 223, Nov.-Dec. 1976.
36. Voltz, R.G.: Personal communication, 1980, Tucson, Ariz.
37. Walker, P.S.: Human joints and their artificial replacements, Springfield, Ill., 1977, Charles C Thomas, Publisher, pp. 190-195.

9. Seven-year follow-up of Coonrad Total Elbow replacement

Ralph W. Coonrad, M.D.

The evolution of total elbow arthroplasty has followed an unpredictable course from the early unacceptable instability of resections[10] in the latter 1800s, interposition[9] and anatomic[3] arthroplasty in the early half of the 1900s, through the failures of semiconstrained[2] and then totally constrained metal-to-metal hinge[6] replacement in the early 1970s. Probably the greatest contribution to total elbow replacement in this century has been the basic research contributions in biomechanical and biomaterial principles related to the elbow since 1974 by Asher,[1] Walker,[12] Inglis,[7] Volz,[11] Morrey and Chao,[8] and others. With the incorporation of these design principles and better surgical and cement techniques, results reported through the last half of the 1970s have predictably improved. Compared with the functional limitation of elbow fusion or resection arthroplasty, total elbow replacement, when successful, can give stability, mobility, and dramatic relief from pain to the extent that in the stable rheumatoid joint, a 90%, or better, chance of a satisfactory result can now be anticipated.

HISTORICAL BACKGROUND

Initial development of the Coonrad Total Elbow prosthesis was initiated in 1967, with the assistance of the engineering staff of Zimmer USA (Warsaw, Indiana). The Coonrad Total Elbow prosthesis is of semiconstrained, hinged design, with high molecular weight polyethylene plastic bushings, which prevent metal-to-metal contact between stems and a metal axle. The metal parts are manufactured from an alloy of titanium that is believed to possess a strength and durability superior to stainless steel or chrome-cobalt alloys now in common use. The early degree of laxity in the hinge joint was 2 to 3 degrees, and in 1978 it was increased to 7 degrees of both rotary and side-to-side toggle motion. The implant has been machine stressed in the laboratory 6 million times without significant component wear.

The humeral and ulnar stems are designed in the shape of their respective medullary canals, and loosening of the quadrangular ulnar stem, because of its contour fit in the average curved ulnar medullary canal, is almost nonexistent. The humeral stem is triangular but flattened at the base to contour fit the lower flattened and wider portion of the humeral medullary canal, and both stems of the prosthesis were designed of large enough size so that rigid fixation can usually be achieved, even before the addition of methacrylate at the operating table. Careful cabinetry for a tight fit in the intercondylar area of the humerus is necessary. The prosthesis is articulated by the manufacturer and is inserted in the articulated form with the elbow in total flexion. However, disarticulation of the prosthesis is possible with simple extrusion of the axle. The prosthesis is supplied in right or left configurations in both regular and small sizes, with provisional prostheses being available (Fig. 9-1). The two most important features in the design of this pros-

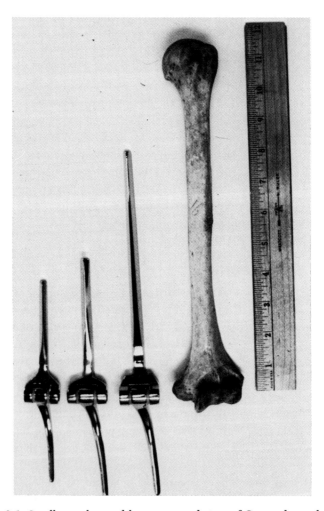

Fig. 9-1. Small, regular, and long-stemmed sizes of Coonrad prosthesis.

thesis are the near-anatomic center of the axis of rotation when properly implanted, and its relatively large size and stem length and contour, which inherently tend to increase torque resistance. A much longer humeral stem design (see Fig. 8-3) was added in the period 1978 and 1979 and, it is believed, should always be used whenever possible rather than the shorter stemmed models. Here again, the proportionate surface area for torque resistance compares to the long-stemmed prostheses used in the femoral canal with total hip replacement.

INDICATIONS AND CONTRAINDICATIONS

The three major goal requirements of elbow arthroplasty are to relieve pain, restore or maintain mobility, and assure stability. A stable elbow that is painless, but with limited motion in a midfunctional range, does not ordinarily warrant the risk or extent of total joint replacement. An ankylosed elbow, in functional position with a normal opposite extremity, is probably not an indication for the risk of replacement arthroplasty. The primary indications for total joint replacement include pain, instability, and bilateral elbow ankylosis.

The pathologic indications for consideration of total elbow arthroplasty can be listed as follows: rheumatoid arthritis where good medical treatment has failed and joint destruction precludes lesser procedures, degenerative arthrosis that has not responded to single or repeated débridement, traumatic arthrosis from such problems as persistent subluxation or dislocation, bone stock loss from tumor or trauma, and failed arthroplasties of any type that are unacceptably painful or unstable.

The basic contraindications to total joint replacement arthroplasty at the elbow are infection, a demand or need for other than sedentary activity with the elbow, ankylosis of the shoulder on the ipsilateral side, and neurotrophic joints.

Comments on biomechanical principles and joint motion are included in a separate history of total joint replacement and are not repeated here.

TECHNIQUE

The technique used closely follows that previously described by Coonrad and Bryan.[5] The patient is placed in a supine position with the arm across the front of the chest and a sandbag placed beneath the shoulder. Prepping and draping must be accomplished so that the entire elbow area and lower arm are readily visualized for proper alignment and anatomic localization. A tourniquet is used and blood is evacuated only by elevation for several minutes before tourniquet application. A relatively straight midline posterior or posteromedial, or lateral, incision is made with the ulnar nerve being initially identified, mobilized, transferred, and protected during the entire operative procedure. Where this has been carried out, ulnar nerve problems have been rare. The triceps mechanism, in continuity and together with the periosteum over the proximal ulna and olecranon, is elevated as a single intact structure and carried either to the ulnar or radial side of the olecranon as desired, for complete visualization of the proximal ulna (Fig. 9-2). The intact extensor mechanism, when replaced, has virtually eliminated rupture or poor triceps function postoperatively.

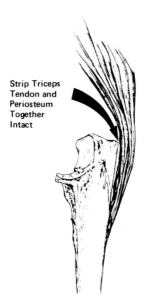

Strip Triceps Tendon and Periosteum Together Intact

Fig. 9-2. *Arrow,* Intact stripping of triceps tendon and periosteum. (Courtesy Zimmer USA, Inc., Warsaw, Ind.)

Where there is good bone stock, the collateral ligaments are always carefully preserved along with the epicondyles and, where possible, very little olecranon is removed except to gain exposure. Results seem to be the same with or without retention of the proximal inch of the olecranon to the coronoid process, which is always preserved. Implantation of the ulnar stem, with simple removal of the articular surface of the olecranon, serves as appropriately.

Bone removal from the distal humerus should be just precisely sufficient to permit insertion of the prosthesis and should be accomplished with careful cabinetry, using a trial prosthesis for repeated insertion until the level of the prosthesis is exactly level with the epicondylar articular surface margins at the capitellar and trochlear sides. Great care should be taken to hollow out the flattened area of the lower humerus to precisely fit the shoulders of the humeral stem of the prosthesis with additional curettage of cancellous bone from both the epicondylar and lower flaring portions of the humerus for good methacrylate cement fixation.

Special rasps, with instrumentation for the prosthesis, are provided for opening and contouring the humeral and ulnar intramedullary canals before insertion of the prosthesis. Right and left ulnar rasps correspond to the ulnar-stem configuration and a triangular humeral rasp is provided for preparation of the humeral stem.

After preparation of both the proximal ulna and proximal humerus, a trial prosthesis is inserted and a complete range of flexion and extension should be possible at this point. A long-stemmed variety of the prosthesis should always be used where possible and should be no more difficult to insert than the regular-stemmed prosthesis. A regular-sized prosthesis is always preferable to a small-sized pros-thesis, where careful cabinetry can permit its insertion.

The medullary canals of the ulna and humerus should be carefully brushed and dried and cement inserted in a liquid form with the use of a gun or syringe, by use of a small-calibered plastic catheter with suction just below the tip end of the level of the prosthesis to ensure methacrylate insertion to that level. The implant-able prosthesis is then inserted simultaneously, with the elbow flexed, into both the humeral and ulnar medullary canals, the joint extended fully while the cement hardens, and care taken to prevent any excess cement from being retained anteri-orly or posteriorly. Removal of the superfluous cement should be carried out by an assistant while the cement is hardening. Recesses in the distal lateral and medial flares of the lower humerus and humeral epicondyles should be carefully filled and packed snugly with cement.

In unusual circumstances, it might become necessary to disassemble the pros-thesis either to permit insertion or for replacement, and a C-clamp is provided to very simply force the axis out of the humeral stems for disassembly. Repeated assembly and disassembly is not recommended because the retention power of the bushings may become compromised. Use of the provisional prosthesis would ordi-narily indicate whether the implantable prosthesis must be disassembled for sepa-rate insertion.

After initial trial insertion of the provisional prosthesis, it is important to deter-mine whether the radial head impinges in any way on the prosthesis, and it should remain undisturbed unless impingement occurs.

The triceps tendon and proximal ulnar periosteum are replaced and sutured to the fascial structures on each side, with the ulnar nerve being left subcutaneously. The wound is closed in anatomic layers, with closed suction drainage being in-serted both into the subcutaneous tissue and adjacent to the prosthesis. A large, bulky compression dressing of sheet cotton is applied with the elbow in 90 degrees of flexion and with a posterior shell of plaster applied to maintain position.

Suction drainage is continued for 24 to 48 hours postoperatively, or until drain-age essentially ceases. Mobilization of the elbow is initiated intermittently with the continued use of a posterior shell splint beginning at 5 to 14 days, depending on the rapidity of subsidence of postoperative edema, swelling, and pain. *The elbow is elevated continuously after surgery at a level higher than the heart or, if the patient is sitting, higher than the shoulder.*

MATERIAL AND RESULTS

After 5 years of development, in 1972, a prospective protocol for 150 elbows was developed and has been monitored more than 7 years throughout the country, in-cluding several university centers. The initial implant was carried out at the Mayo Clinic in May 1973. The protocol includes 39 elbows implanted at the Mayo Clinic previously reported[4] in a 5-year follow-up study. The protocol series includes 90 fe-

Table 9-1. Coonrad total elbow replacement in patients with rheumatoid arthritis at 3- to 7-year follow-up (includes Mayo Clinic Series of 35 elbows with a total of 87 elbows in the protocol series)

Good	66	(75%)
Fair	19	(22%)
Poor	1	
Failed	1	

Table 9-2. Coonrad Total Elbow replacement in posttraumatic patients at 3- to 7-year follow-up study (60 elbows in protocol series)

Good	35	(58%)
Fair	16	(26%)
Poor	2	(3%)
Failed	6	(10%)
Fell, fractured arm	1	

males and 60 males with an age distribution predominantly in the fifth and sixth decades, particularly in those with rheumatoid arthritis. There were 150 elbows in 146 patients with 4 rheumatoid arthritic patients having bilateral implants.

From a pathologic diagnosis distribution, there were 87 elbows with rheumatoid arthritis, 60 patients with posttraumatic elbows, 2 with degenerative arthrosis, and 1 with an old juvenile pyarthrosis with limited motion and pain. The latter two categories are excluded from comparison figures below.

The entire series of 150 protocol elbows was initially reported at the 1978 meeting of the American Orthopaedic Association, has been updated in 1980, and is rated according to a classification by Bryan[3] as follows:

Good   90 degrees of motion, insignificant pain
Fair   45 to 90 degrees of motion, insignificant pain
Poor   Less than 45 degrees of motion, significant pain

It is well to remember, however, that 40 degrees of painless motion, in the midposition and with stability, can be a very satisfactory elbow, operated or unoperated, and yet, under this rating, it would be rated at a poor level.

Using this rating for the 87 rheumatoid elbows alone in the series (Table 9-1), there were 66 *good*, 19 *fair*, and 1 *poor* result, which was attributable to infection in a Mayo Clinic patient, and 1 *failure*. Since this series was reported in 1978, there is one loosening of an implant in a rheumatoid patient, with the implant still in the patient. This gives a satisfactory elbow rating, if we combine good and fair results, at about a 95% level in rheumatoid arthritis, with one instance of loosening seen on a roentgenogram.

There were 60 patients with traumatic arthritis, or severe traumatic elbow changes (Table 9-2), who had total replacement arthroplasty, and the results in

Table 9-3. Coonrad Total Elbow replacement combined series of trauma and rheumatoid patients at 3- to 7-year follow-up study (147 elbows)

Good	101	(68%)
Fair	35	(24%)
Poor	4	(3%)
Failed	7	(4+%)
Fell, fractured arm	1	

Table 9-4. Complications in 150 elbows

Triceps rupture	2
Radial nerve palsy, transient	1
Ulnar nerve palsy, transient	3
Superficial infection	2
Deep infection (2 removed)	3
Perforated cortex	3
Loose ulnar stem	1
Loose humeral stem	7
Loose humeral stem (suspected)	11
Fracture prosthesis	0

these were not so good and these patients generally had poor bone stock. Thirty-five rated *good* and 16 *fair*; 2 had *poor* results, with 6 having *failures*; and one patient fell and fractured the elbow. This gives a satisfactory, or acceptable, elbow rating in 84%, if we combine the *good* and *fair* ratings. *Failed* elbows in the traumatic group were caused by loosening in 4 and infection in 2.

If we combine the rating figures for the rheumatoid and posttraumatic patients followed from 3 to 7 years, we find that the series (Table 9-3) includes 14 *satisfactory* and 1 *unsatisfactory* at 6 years, 45 *satisfactory* and 4 *unsatisfatory* at 5 years, 45 *satisfactory* and 4 *unsatisfactory* at 4 years, and 31 *satisfactory* and 3 *unsatisfactory* at 3 years.

Looking at the rheumatoid-trauma series by percentage from 3 to 7 years, one can see that satisfactory results of *good* and *fair* were 89% and unsatisfactory were 11%.

In this series, 14 patients had prior surgery and 7 had failed implants of other types replaced with a Coonrad prosthesis.

The range of motion in the series was from 90 to 135 degrees in 110 elbows, and 60 to 90 degrees in 20 elbows. Twenty elbows had less than 60 degrees.

COMPLICATIONS

The initial protocol series of 150 elbows had implants by more than 25 surgeons, with the largest number being carried out at the Mayo Clinic, University of Iowa, and Duke University. The complications (Table 9-4) included loosening in 8

(7 of the humeral stem and 1 of the ulnar stem) surgically documented. Many of these, on review of the initial roentgenograms, showed inadequate cement insertion technically, and all occurred in posttraumatic elbow problems. There are an additional 11 that have lucent lines on the roentgenogram, with 3 being symptomatic and who may ultimately come to revision. Thus there is an overall incidence of suspected and proved humeral loosening in the series, of 13%. Additional complications included triceps rupture in 2, radial palsy in 1, ulnar palsy in 3, superficial infection in 2, and deep infection in 3. There was asymptomatic perforation of the cortex of the humerus in 3.

Of the 7 implant loosenings documented at surgery, most had long stems implanted at the time of revision, and 2 were reoperated at 1 year, followed up and satisfactory at 4 years; 2 were reoperated at 2 years, followed up and satisfactory at 3 years; 2 were reoperated at 3 years and satisfactory at 3 years; and 1 was removed at 1 year and has a flail elbow as she did before her original implant.

Of the 3 patients in the series who had deep infection, 2 prostheses were removed immediately and have not been replaced. One patient, an 18-year-old boy, who developed a gonococcal infection a year after surgery with subsequent secondary infection with coagulase-positive *Staphylococcus aureus*, had open drainage, with the implant being left in place and exposed for a period of more than a month. He ultimately responded to pHisoHex and Whirlpool therapy daily and had a late, local skin flap closure over the prosthesis. He is now asymptomatic at 6 years with 50 degrees of painless stable motion. A recent film shows lucent lines in the humerus, however.

DISCUSSION

This prosthesis, as with several other implants in use at the current time including the Tri-Axial, the Pritchard-Walker, and the Mayo Clinic designs, have had significant improvement in results during the past 3 years with improvement in methacrylate insertion, retention of good bone stock, and increased laxity in the prosthetic devices. Although all the prostheses in this protocol series of 150 patients were of the more constrained metal-to-polyethylene type with 2- to 3-degree laxity, the difference in results compared to the original totally constrained metal-to-metal hinge designs can probably best be explained on the large size and long stems of the implant together with the design contour of the implant itself, which makes it significantly torque resistant, even when implanted without methacrylate. One patient in the protocol series has a 5-year satisfactory result with a painless, stable elbow without methacrylate fixation. Although neither the ideal degree of laxity in an implant at the elbow is known, nor the long-term results of impact force from fixed limits of side-to-side and rotary movement of a hinged joint, undoubtedly the increased degree of toggle in most prostheses during the latter part of the 1970s has had a large bearing on the diminished degree of loosening.

I believe that longer stemmed and contoured implants with some degree of joint laxity, retention of bone stock and collateral ligaments, and a near-anatomic center of axis of rotation with semiconstrained implants have all contributed to the improving results in recent years.

SUMMARY

Elbow-joint replacement is still a salvage procedure. Our increasing knowledge of the kinematics and biomechanics of the elbow joint have contributed to changes in the development of the Coonrad elbow, which has performed acceptably over a 7-year period, with satisfactory results in 95% of patients with good bone stock and collateral ligaments in rheumatoid patients, and poorer with 84% satisfactory results in posttraumatic elbow problems. Increased laxity from 2 to 7 degrees has been added to this prosthesis since the period 1978 and 1979, and a longer stemmed humeral component was added in the period 1977 and 1978. It is believed that these two changes in design will further improve the results with this prosthesis in posttraumatic elbow replacement. No prosthesis with these two newer design changes was included in the protocol series of patients reported in this 5- to 7-year follow-up study. A subsequent report of an additional series with those patients will be forthcoming.

REFERENCES

1. Asher, M.A., and Zilber, S.: Biomechanics of the elbow and forearm, Presented at the American Academy of Orthopaedic Surgeons Postgraduate Course in the Elbow, Wrist and Forearm, Kansas City, Oct. 13, 1973.
2. Barr, J.S., and Eaton, R.G.: Elbow reconstruction with a new prosthesis to replace the distal end of the humerus, J. Bone Joint Surg. **47:**1408, 1956.
3. Bryan, R.S., Linscheid, R.L., Dobyns, J.H., and Peterson, L.F.: A total elbow arthroplasty sound slide series, Rochester, Minn., 1976, The Mayo Foundation.
4. Cofield, R.H., Morrey, B.F., and Bryan, R.S.: Total shoulder and total elbow arthroplasties: the current state of development, J. Contin. Educ. Orthop., part II, pp. 17-25, Jan. 1979.
5. Coonrad, R.W., and Bryan, R.S.: Technique of Coonrad elbow arthroplasty, Warsaw, Ind., 1974, Zimmer USA.
6. Dee, R.: Total replacement arthroplasty of the elbow for rheumatoid arthritis, J. Bone Joint Surg. (Br.) **54:**88-95, 1972.
7. Inglis, A.E.: American Academy of Orthopaedic Surgeons Continuing Education Course in Upper Extremity Joint Replacement, New York, Sept. 27, 1979.
8. Morrey, B.F., and Chao, E.Y.S.: Passive motion of the elbow joint: a biomechanical analysis, J. Bone Joint Surg. (Am.) **58:**501-508, 1976.
9. Murphy, J.B.: Arthroplasty, Ann. Surg. **57:**593-647, 1913.
10. Ollier, L.: Traité des résections et des opérations conservatrices qu'on peut pratiquer sur le système osseux, Paris, 1885-1889, G. Masson.
11. Volz, R.G.: Personal communication, 1980, Tucson, Ariz.
12. Walker, P.A.: Human joints and their artificial replacements, Springfield, Ill., 1977, Charles C Thomas, Publisher, pp. 190-195.

10. Tri-Axial Total Elbow replacement: indications, surgical technique, and results

Allan E. Inglis, M.D.

ANATOMY

The hand is the major organ for prehension and tactile sensation. To use the hand for grasp and for touch, we must first posture our hand in space. This requires a functional shoulder, elbow, and wrist. The elbow serves not only to rotate the hand through a 180-degree arch, but also to extend the hand from the body. A painful elbow therefore restricts rotatory movements of the hand, but it also compels us to move our entire body to and from objects upon which the hand must work. A painless functional elbow articulation is essential for activities of the hand.

The elbow joint is not a single joint but possesses three separate articulations: the ulnohumeral, the radiohumeral, and the superior radioulnar joint. The ulnohumeral joint is the major force transmitting articulation and is a pure hinge joint. The radiohumeral joint provides modest force transmissions between the radial head and the capitulum humeri. It mainly serves the upper extremity in the control of rotation of the forearm. The superior radioulnar joint allows precise stable rotation of the radius on the ulnar for pronation and supination. Anatomic stability of the elbow joint is achieved through the trochlea of the humerus and the semilunar notch of the ulna. These two surfaces fit precisely allowing an eccentric arch of motion during flexion and extension. The forearm normally assumes a 10- to 25-degree valgus attitude in extension and then flexes to a neutral position in full elbow flexion. This camlike movement is provided by the joint surfaces. The major ligamentous support to the elbow joint is through the medial collateral ligament. The anteromedial ligament of the elbow begins on the sublime tubercle of the ulna and passes proximally to the edge of the trochlea. This ligament is tight in all positions because of the true hinge design ulnohumeral joint. The orbicular or annular ligament is the other major ligament stabilizing the superior radioulnar joint. This substantial structure prevents displacement of the proximal radius by the biceps brachii muscle during biceps contraction. The lateral collateral ligament

100

is less supportive to the elbow joint. It serves mainly as the origin of the extensor carpi radialis brevis muscle. The muscles taking origin from the lateral epicondyle are the major lateral supporting structures of the elbow joint. Surgery upon the elbow joint, whether it be arthrotomy or arthroplasty, must consider preservation or correction of these anatomic structures.

INDICATIONS FOR SURGERY

Functional disability emanating from the elbow joint can occur in four situations: pain, reduced motion, weakness, and instability. Of these four problems, pain is the major factor in disabilities of the elbow. Patients may compensate with increased shoulder or body movements for reduced motion. Weakness and instability can be reduced by greater or more precise utilization of the opposite extremity. Frequently, the pain produces a reduction in motion and sense of weakness. The reduction of pain is the major goal of elbow surgery.

SURGICAL PROCEDURES

There are a number of useful surgical procedures available for disabilities of the elbow joint. Removal of the radial head and joint débridement is a useful surgical procedure in traumatic arthritis of the elbow joint. Lateral collateral ligament release and capsular release with joint débridement is also useful in old traumatic arthritis when there is preservation of the articular surfaces. It is usually necessary to approach the elbow joint through two incisions: the lateral incision for the anterior compartment, and the medial incision for the posterior aspect of the elbow joint. Fascial arthroplasty is also useful in certain ankylosed elbows and in those in which there has been prior infection. It is essential in the fascial arthroplasty to accurately prepare and align the trochlear and ulnar surfaces and, in additional, to accurately and perfectly cover these surfaces with fascia lata. Synovectomy and débridement of the elbow joint is useful in those patients with rheumatoid arthritis or diseases of the synovium in which there has been preservation of the articular surfaces. If the articular surfaces are badly damaged, the patient may require replacement arthroplasty. The last consideration for elbow surgery should be elbow joint replacement arthroplasty. The major deterrent to replacement arthroplasty, as it is in most joint replacement arthroplasties, is the limited choice of alternatives should this operation fail. The major indication for implant arthroplasty of the elbow is rheumatoid arthritis. When there has been cartilage or bone loss, synovectomy or débridement will not produce a satisfactory result with any degree of predictability. It is also indicated in patients with rheumatoid arthritis who have ankylosis of the elbow joints. This is particularly useful in those young patients with rheumatoid arthritis in whom there is a tendency for fibroarthrosis. Implant arthroplasty can also be considered in certain patients with traumatic or degenerative arthritis if their physical requirements are low. It is contraindicated in patients in which there have been prior infections or there are high-loading requirements by the patient. It is also not indicated in patients with major psychologic or emotional problems who are not able to cooperate with or follow the directions of their physicians.

During the evolutionary development of the elbow implant there have been many problems. Initially, it was not possible to secure the implant to the humerus and to the ulna. These implants failed within a short period of time when the components moved away from the adjacent bony support. This problem was in part solved by the use of polymethylmethacrylate cement. The next phase of development included implants with fixed-hinge support. These devices tended either to pull away at the cement-bone bond or to break at the hinge. The next phase involved semiconstrained implants. Thus far, these implants seem to hold the most promise. It is important that the implant be as small as possible and covered by bone. Ideally, the epicondyles should be preserved and the olecranon process retained. The implant should also have a carrying angle. The carrying angle prevents the hand from striking the hip or leg during ambulation. The implant should also be able to withstand the forces applied across the elbow joint. Isometric forces are applied to the joint in flexion and in extension by the elbow flexors and extensors and, additionally, by those muscles activating the wrist and hand that take origin from the humerus. It must also be able to withstand the rotational forces applied by the internal and external rotators of the shoulder. With forced internal rotation of the hand there is the subscapularis, the pectoralis major, the latissimus dorsi, and the teres major, all applying a force across the implant. Similarly, there are forces in pronation and supination. These forces are applied to the ulnar component. The first implant we used was designed by Rowland Pritchard and Peter Walker of The Hospital for Special Surgery. This was a constrained implant with a loose, "floppy" articulation. The next implant employed a metallic humeral and ulnar component, with a high-density polyethylene hinge and a two-piece axle. The final model was designed to provide a metallic ulnar and humeral component with a high-density hinge and a snap-fitting articulation.

The Tri-Axial elbow implant (Fig. 10-1) has been tested for its capacity to withstand varying loads. The implant has approximately 7 degrees of varus laxity and 8 degrees of valgus laxity. If the implant is loaded to 65 Newtons (kilogram-force) the varus laxity is 5 degrees and the valgus laxity is 6 degrees. Similar testing for laxity was carried out in pronation and supination, and again the implant still remained flexible with loading. Distraction loading was also carried out. It required 49.5 N to pull the implant apart. Prior studies had revealed that the major loading in a living elbow was compressive and that only under extraordinary circumstances could the elbow be distracted in a living subject.

This report is on 39 patients upon whom 44 elbow replacements were performed. The surgery was carried out at The Hospital for Special Surgery during the period between 1974 and 1978. The average follow-up period was $3^{1}/_{2}$ years. Thirty-one of the elbows have been followed for 3 years or longer. Twenty-four of the patients had rheumatoid arthritis. Four of the patients had juvenile rheumatoid arthritis and 11 patients had traumatic arthritis. Twenty-five of the patients were females, and 14 were males. The average age was 54 years.

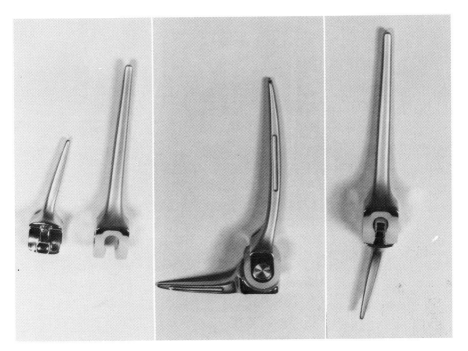

Fig. 10-1. Tri-Axial implant allows a few degrees of freedom in the mediolateral plane and the rotational plane, and full flexion and extension. A snap-fitting connection is provided for articulation of the implant during surgery.

SURGICAL TECHNIQUE

The patients are usually operated on under general anesthesia. A tourniquet is used. The patients are supine and the arm draped free and positioned over the chest. The incision is placed directly over the portion of the ulna and humerus (Fig 10-2, *A*). It is extended approximately 10 cm down the ulna and 8 cm over the humerus. The subcutaneous borders are separated away from the fascia of the triceps muscle (Fig. 10-2, *B*). The ulnar nerve is carefully dissected away from the cubital canal and elevated away from the ulna to a point just beyond the sublime tubercle. The triceps muscle is partially detached as recommended by Bryan. An incision is made in the fascia of the flexor carpi ulnaris. Between the ulna and humerus the incision is placed about 1 cm away from the ulna. The entire triceps is then mobilized laterally. The fascia is carefully elevated subperiostally from the ulna as a sling. The portion of the triceps that attaches to the tip of the olecranon process is incised close to the bone. Care is taken to avoid making any holes in the large triceps sling. The medial head of the triceps is elevated from the posterior portion of the capitellum. When this large sling is mobilized, the radiocapitellar joint is exposed. The interval between the radius and the ulna is then incised so that the extensor carpi ulnaris muscle is elevated from its origin on the ulnar bone. The head of the radius is then exposed. An oscillating saw is used to incise the

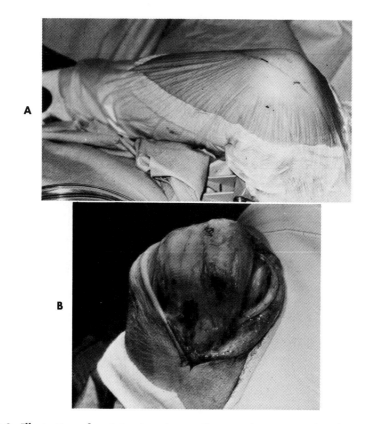

Fig. 10-2. Illustration of certain steps in an elbow replacement arthroplasty. **A,** Incision should be longitudinal and along the ulnar border of the olecranon process. **B,** Ulnar nerve should be isolated and moved out of cubital tunnel. The nerve should then be elevated away from the sublime tubercles of the ulna to prevent possible injury during the excision of the diseased semilunar notch of the ulna.

radial head. The radial head is slowly rotated as the saw is applied to the neck of the radius. The orbicular ligament is carefully protected. The capsule between the trochlea and the semilunar notch is then incised. The anterior medial ligament is incised, and after this ligament is cut, the entire ulna can be easily lifted forward exposing the distal ulna and the coronoid process. The semilunar notch is then excised with an oscillating saw (Fig. 10-2, *C*). The proximal ulna is then prepared with a Hall burr exposing the proximal ulna and coronoid process. The cancellous bone is removed sufficient that the metaphyseal area of the ulna is in view. This is then carefully reamed until the ulnar component can be inserted to fit snugly against the coronoid process (Fig. 10-2, *D*). It is important to burr out an elliptic area within the ulna to provide a wedge-shaped cement column to protect against rotatory loosening of the cement-bone bond. The humeral component is then placed on the trochlea and the area for resection marked. The oscillating saw is

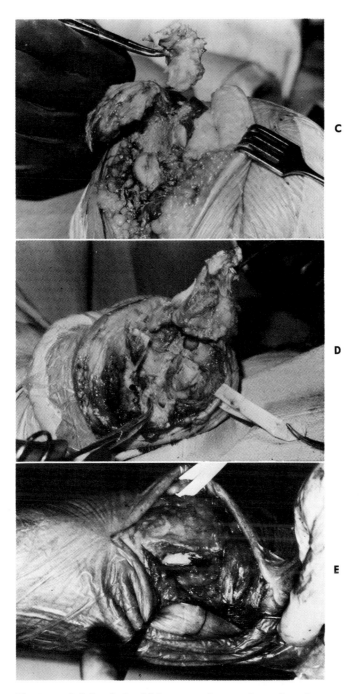

Fig. 10-2, cont'd. C, Radial head should be excised enough so that there is no further contact with the ulnar portion of the radioulnar articulation. Then the semilunar notch is excised as a single piece with a small reciprocating saw. **D,** The ulna is then carefully reamed to accept the ulnar component of the implant. The trochlea is excised so that the epicondyles are left intact. The bone in the coronoid and olecranon fossae is carefully removed with rongeurs and the humeral shaft reamed to accept the humeral component. **E,** The prostheses are inserted, and a trial reduction is checked. The implants are then cemented separated. Note little of the prostheses is exposed at the completion of the arthroplasty.

then used to remove the central portion of the trochlea. Care is taken not to cut too deeply thereby weakening the epicondyles. In the center of the cut notch will be the thin layer of bone between the coronoid and olecranon fossae. This thin layer of bone is removed with a large double-action rongeur. This is continued until the metaphyseal area of the humerus is opened. The high-speed Hall burr is then employed to open up the shaft of the humerus as well as to burr into the side of the epicondyles for subsequent cement fixation. When the opening into the humerus is large enough, circular reamers can be employed. When the humerus has been reamed enough, the humeral component will fit snugly down between the two epicondyles. At this point, both ulnar and humeral components should be inserted and articulated. The joint should be brought through a range of motion to be certain that full flexion and full extension has been achieved. The components are then removed, and the shaft of the ulna and humerus are carefully cleansed with a Water-Pik. The implants are then cemented into place, first the ulnar component and then the humeral component. Excessive cement is removed from around the implant. The two implants are then articulated. The tourniquet is released at this point, and any remaining vessels either ligated or electrocoagulated. The triceps is then repaired. Two holes are then made in the tip of the olecranon process. The entire triceps sling is then pulled back over the olecranon process. This is facilitated when the elbow is extended. A heavy, double, nonabsorbable suture is then passed through the thickened portion of the triceps tendon and through the two holes in the olecranon process and then on through the remaining portions of the triceps sling. When the triceps sling is pulled completely into position, the two, heavy, nonabsorbable sutures can be snugged up and tied. The fascia of the triceps and epimysium of the extensor carpi ulnaris are closed with interrupted sutures (Fig. 10-2, *E*). A negative-pressure drain is placed into the subcutaneous tissues. The subcutaneous tissues are then closed. The patient's arm is then placed in 45 degrees of extension, and a compression dressing applied.

The dressings are removed on the fifth day after surgery, and if the wounds are dry and there is no evidence of a hematoma, active occupational therapy is started. This therapeutic program consists of active elbow flexion and *passive* elbow extension. Rotational exercises are also started. The elbow is placed in a splint when the patient is not exercising. The splint is so fabricated that the patient is maintained in maximum extension one night and flexion another night. If the wounds drain, all exercises are stopped until the wound is dry. The splint is maintained for approximately 4 weeks or until the triceps muscle is secure. The patients are advised to avoid shock loading of their elbow and to use the usual precautions of any implant arthroplasty.

RESULTS

On a prospective basis the patients were assessed initially at 6 months and then at yearly intervals. Three major perameters were evaluated with points assigned to each parameter. These parameters included pain, function, and arch of motion.

Ninety-five percent of patients with juvenile arthritis and 92% of patients with adult type of rheumatoid arthritis had complete relief of pain. Eighty-one percent of patients with traumatic or osteoarthritis were completely relieved of pain. The remaining patients had some pain either musculotendinous or capsular or related to the proximal radioulnar joint. Three patients in the traumatic arthritis group were unimproved. The remaining were partially improved. Functional improvement in patients with rheumatoid arthritis was 92% in both the juvenile and the adult patients (Fig. 10-3). The remaining patients were improved but had disability at adjacent joints, such that their result was compromised. The patients with osteoarthritis and posttraumatic arthritis had 79% functional improvement. The remaining patients were improved, but not to the degree observed in patients with rheumatoid arthritis. Range of motion was 91% in patients with juvenile and adult

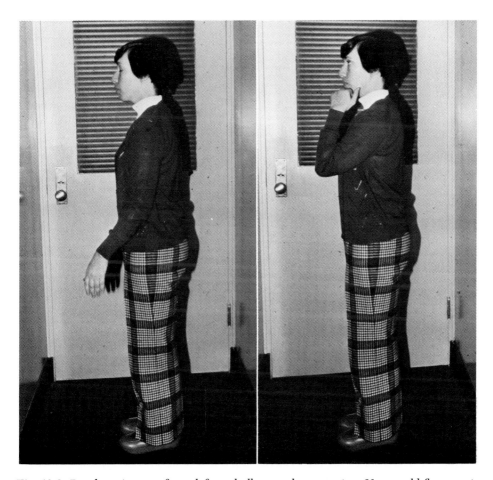

Fig. 10-3. Result at 4 years after a left total elbow replacement in a 31-year-old flute music teacher. She extends her elbow to 30 degrees and flexes to 153 degrees to show that she has normal rotation. The quality of her arthroplasty has not changed.

rheumatoid arthritis. No patient in this group has less motion after arthroplasty than before. Patients with traumatic or degenerative arthritis had less motion after arthroplasty than before. Patients with traumatic or degenerative arthritis achieved a 67% range of motion. Sixty-seven percent required an arch of flexion extension of 62 degrees. Pronation and supination in the patients with both rheumatoid arthritis and degenerative arthritis was variable. Eighty percent of patients achieved pronation of 45 degrees and supination of 45 degrees. Disabilities at the inferior radioulnar joint appeared to be the mitigating factor.

COMPLICATIONS

Two infections were observed in the series. One occurred in a patient with traumatic arthritis who had undergone three previous surgical procedures. The other occurred in a patient after reopening of the joint during triceps repair. Both of these patients had removal of the implant and application of an external fixation device, and now they have painless elbows that are functional but weak. Three

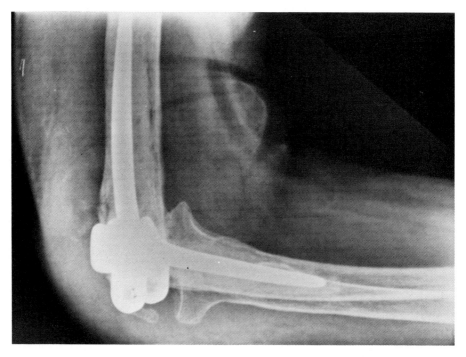

Fig. 10-4. Disarticulated implant. This individual was extremely vigorous. The dislocation could not be relocated by closed means. At reoperation the axle hubs had been disengaged and the polyethylene bearing damaged. These were replaced and reinforced. Patient has had no further problems with the arthroplasty.

patients had skin sloughs after their arthroplasty. Two healed secondarily; a third required a split-thickness skin graft. These did not compromise the final result. Implant breakage occurred in three patients. In one patient the axle gave way in an extremely vigorous individual (Fig. 10-4). The others involved disarticulation of the implant with damage to the high-density polyethylene bushing. An additional patient broke the high-density polyethylene stem. Four patients have triceps weakness secondary to either rupture or attenuation of the repair. Two of these have been repaired, one successfully, the other resulting in an infected implant. No further difficulty has been observed since we began using the triceps sling method of detachment. Two patients have complained of ulna neuropathy after their arthroplasty. One patient had gradual relief of ulnar dysesthesias; the other continues to have pain over the ulnar nerve distribution. This complication has not diminished the overall result of the arthroplasty. One implant has slow loosening (Fig. 10-5). The loosening was gradual and finally required replacement of the entire prosthesis.

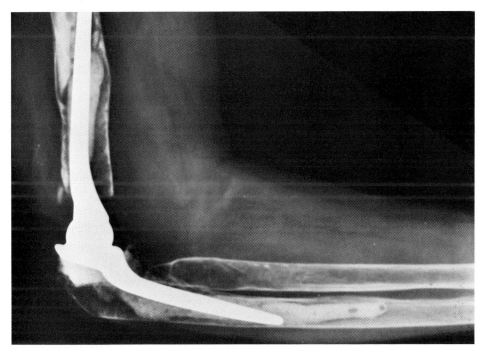

Fig. 10-5. Loosening of the cement from humeral shaft in a patient with severe osteoporosis. The patient had a nonunion of a fracture of distal humerus with comminution of the epicondyle. Fixation of the implant to the tubular osteoporotic humeral shaft proved not to be possible, hence the late loosening.

DISCUSSION

The painless, stable elbow is essential for high-level upper extremity function. If the elbow is not functional it is like answering the telephone by lifting the cord. These goals are gently achieved through a number of surgical procedures in the badly damaged elbow joint. Débridement with removal of the radial head and appropriate capsular release can restore many elbows to high-level function. Synovectomy with débridement in the elbow with good joint surfaces is also a predictable surgical procedure. Fascial arthroplasty, if correctly performed, also can provide good function with only a modest restriction in stability. Arthrodesis is the least helpful procedure. This leads to a strong, painless elbow; however, the patient will have limited capability in the placement of the hand in space. Joint replacement is a useful alternative under certain conditions.

Initially, elbow joint replacement was achieved with completely constrained implants. These implants showed some early success. However, late loosening of the implant within the humerus or ulna became apparent, and this form of arthroplasty was abandoned. Pritchard at The Hospital for Special Surgery conceptualized the solution to this problem by suggesting a semiconstrained device to reduce the shock loading across the implant. All successful implant arthroplasties today are semiconstrained or nonconstrained prostheses. The elbow joint differs from the joints in the lower extremity in a number of ways. Perhaps the most significant in terms of implant arthroplasty is the sudden acceleration-deceleration forces about the joint. Acceleration of a baseball to 90 miles an hour over an 8-foot distance is achieved by baseball pitchers. Additionally, the arm must decelerate the same speed in an even shorter distance. These torsional forces are absorbed and dissipated in part by the viscoelastic qualities of the collateral ligaments and the capsule of the joint. It is also dissipated by the stretch reflexes in the flexor and extensor muscles attaching to the epicondyles of the humerus. The capacity of the muscles to control these torsional forces is related to the square of the radius between the implant and the tip of the corresponding epicondyles. It is therefore essential to preserve the epicondyles during the arthroplasty. Indeed in some instances it may be necessary to reconstruct new epicondyles should they be absent or deficient.

The data accumulated during the first 4 years of use of the semiconstrained elbow implant suggests certain conclusions. The elbow has shown promise particularly in patients with rheumatoid arthritis. The relief of pain with increased overall function and an improved arch of motion have been substantial and sustained. The patient should have extension to at least 30 degrees and flexion to 120 degrees. The patients with degenerative arthritis or traumatic arthritis achieved less favorable results. These results can be improved with better surgical techniques and more stringent patient selection. Patients with badly comminuted fractures of the distal humerus and olecranon process or patients who will use their elbow for heavy labor are not candidates for elbow-implant arthroplasty.

11. Development and clinical analysis of a new semiconstrained total elbow prosthesis

Robert G. Volz, M.D.

When the biomechanical principles of cementable total joint replacement were applied to the elbow in the early 1970s the subsequent outcome proved to be less than satisfactory. The unacceptably high incidence of clinical loosening that soon followed after implantation promptly relegated the procedure to a questionable status.[6,10,13,16,19,22,24] Two reasonable explanations can be offered for the unacceptably high incidence of failure. One states that the skeletal features of the elbow are structurally inadequate to handle stresses associated with normal usage after implantation of a cementable prosthesis; the other explanation relates to the design of the early total elbow prostheses that were believed to be inappropriate because of their high degree of constraint, which enhanced the likelihood of mechanical loosening attributable to the transfer of considerable stress from the implant to the bone-cement interface.[12,21] Because of a personal belief that the skeletal structures of the elbow were capable of absorbing stresses associated with normal usage after total joint replacement, efforts were begun in 1975 toward the design of a semiconstrained total elbow prosthesis.

METHODS AND MATERIALS

Before any design efforts were begun, the anatomy and kinesiology of the elbow on several cadaver specimens were carefully studied.[26] Particular attention was devoted to two areas, the first being the role of the soft tissues in stabilizing and protecting the elbow joint and the second an analysis of the planes of motion occurring between the humerus, radius, and ulna.

The results of these studies disclosed that the soft tissues play an important role in stabilizing and dissipating stress about the elbows. Dissections of the posterior trochlear fossa revealed that a fat pad, located within the posterior capsule, served as an important structure in absorbing or dampening stresses associated with forceful extension of the elbows. Upon excision of this fat pad, a much more abrupt deceleration of extension movement was noted, and the elbow could be placed through an increased arc of extension by 5 to 10 degrees. Inspection of the anterior capsule identified that this structure also played an important role in limiting extension. As the elbow was brought into full extension, the thin anterior capsule became quite taut. An incision placed horizontally through this structure, however, allowed for 10 degrees of additional hyperextension. An analysis of the factors limiting acute flexion disclosed that flexion of the forearm was primarily arrested by a "wadding" effect of the soft tissues located in the antecubital fossa of the elbow. In a few specimens, mechanical contact between the coronoid process and the anterior surface of the humerus was observed.

An analysis of the relative importance of the collateral ligaments disclosed that the radial collateral ligament was smaller than its medial counterpart, an observation that can also be made for the medial and lateral ligaments of the knee and ankle. The fibers of the radial collateral ligament became taut through a very small arc of motion beginning at 45 degrees. Incision of this ligament did not appear to significantly alter the mechanical stability of the elbow. The medial collateral ligament, however, was much broader in its origin and insertion, and it remained taut through a larger arc of motion. Once incised, the elbow could easily be placed in a much greater degree of valgus deformation. Thus it can be concluded that valgus stresses predominate at the elbow and that the larger medial collateral ligament is stronger and more efficient in resisting valgus stresses when compared with the radial collateral ligament.

Although prior investigators[15] had documented the important role that the radial head played in dissipating joint reactive forces in excess of 25 kg, the relative degree in which the radial head participated in dissipating such forces was analyzed by a comparison of the surface area of the radial head and the vertical articular surface of the olecranon. A calculation of these two surface areas reveals them to be approximately equal in size. It is therefore logical that the radius and ulna would share equally in the dissipation of any compressive force placed upon the elbow whenever a weighted object is held in the hand with the elbow flexed at 90 degrees (Fig. 11-1).

Because the designs of the early elbow prostheses were based upon the concept that the humeroulnar articulation represented a simple hinge,[3-5,7-9] several freshly dissected cadaver specimens were studied to permit an analysis of the planes of motion occurring between the humerus and ulna with flexion and extension motion. After the removal of all soft-tissue structures with the exception of ligaments and capsules, the freshly dissected specimens were attached by Steinmann pins placed through the humerus to a movable rig, which permitted the humerus to be moved spatially in a plane that remained at all times 90 degrees vertical to the horizon (Fig. 11-2). The forearm and hand were allowed to rest upon a flat horizontal surface but were free to move in an encumbered manner. A single Steinmann pin was then placed in the distal ulna at a right angle to its long axis. As the humerus was flexed and extended upon the forearm, any change in position of the Steinmann pin could be

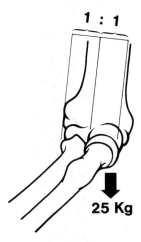

Fig. 11-1. Joint force dissipation. When an object is held in the hand with the elbow flexed to 90 degrees and the joint reactive force exceeds 25 kg, the dissipation of that stress is shared by the articular surface of the radial head. Excision of the radial head leads to an increased stress being placed upon the humeroulnar articulation.

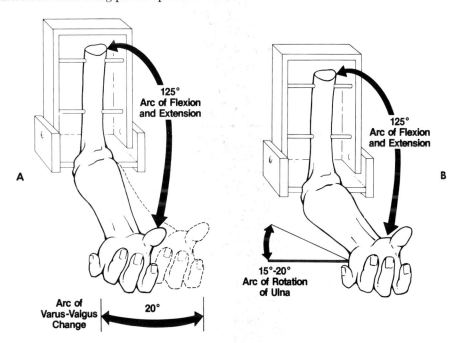

Fig. 11-2. A freshly dissected upper extremity was secured to a movable rig by several Steinmann pins. The humeral shaft was precisely positioned to permit alignment in a vertical position 90 degrees with the horizon throughout the arc of flexion and extension. As the humerus was flexed upon the unrestricted forearm, a change in the varus-valgus alignment of the forearm and the rotational alignment of the ulna upon the humerus was studied. An approximately 15- to 20-degree change in varus-valgus alignment, **A,** and ulnar rotation, **B,** was observed with the normal arc of flexion and extension of the ulna upon the humerus.

precisely determined and measured. From this study it was noted that the ulna rotated upon the humerus through an arc approaching 20 degrees as the elbow flexed and extended. A change in position of the ulna with reference to varus-valgus alignment upon the humerus was also evaluated. With flexion and extension it was observed that the ulna moved through an arc of 20 degrees of varus-valgus change; with full extension the greatest degree of valgus alignment was noted and with acute flexion the greatest arc of varus change occurred.

PROSTHETIC DESIGN

With the above background information, work was begun on the design of an artificial elbow prosthesis in 1975 at the Arizona Health Sciences Center. The design concepts were to encompass a humeroulnar interface that would allow for freedom of

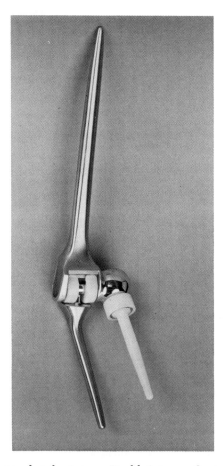

Fig. 11-3. Prosthesis designed at the Arizona Health Sciences Center and possessing a semi-constrained polyethylene interface between the ulna and humerus and the option for radial capitellar surface replacements. The snap-fitting design of the interface provides for some degree of stability when soft-tissue support is lacking.

movement in three planes. An interlocking interface mechanism was also considered advisable so that usage could be extended to situations where ligamentous soft-tissue support had been lost. A prosthetic radial head capable of articulating against a capitellar surface was also felt desirable. Stem designs were to be of sufficient length and contour to permit ease of insertion within medullary canals, especially the proximal ulna, without sacrifice of important cortical bone. Finally the dimensions of a prosthetic interface were to be kept to the smallest possible size, thereby requiring minimal removal of bone, especially at the olecranon. From these designed efforts, a cobalt-chrome prosthesis possessing a semiconstrained polyethylene interface and radiocapitellar articulation was fabricated (Fig. 11-3).

OPERATIVE TECHNIQUE

The patient is placed in a supine position on the operating table, and the involved elbow is acutely flexed across the chest. Pneumatic tourniquet hemostasis is routinely advised. A vertical posterior curvilinear incision is placed slightly radialward from the tip of the olecranon. Identification and retraction of the ulnar nerve is optional. In the absence of deformity to the olecranon, the triceps is either detached subperiosteally or sectioned more proximally at its musculotendinous junction. The posterior capsule is exised, and the tip of the olecranon removed (Fig. 11-4) by use of a reciprocating saw to improve visualization of the trochlear notch. Dissection is now carried laterally

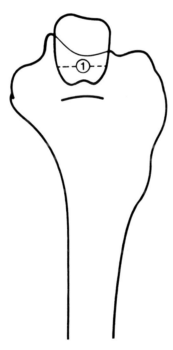

Fig. 11-4. If exposure to the posterior aspect of the elbow is gained by detachment of the triceps muscle near the olecranon in its musculotendinous junction, additional exposure to the trochlear notch can be gained by excision of the tip of the olecranon, *1*.

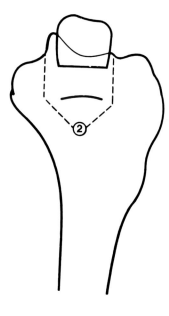

Fig. 11-5. Once the trochlear notch has been adequately visualized, its articular surface is removed by use of a reciprocating saw. Care is taken not to violate the important and lateral condylar bone, which represents the main support for the condylar structures. Resection of the trochlear bone is continued in an angular fashion to the junction of the medial and lateral condylar bony ridges, 2.

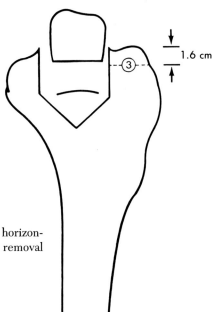

Fig. 11-6. After resection of the trochlear bone, a horizontal cut, 3, is made through the capitellum, with removal of approximately 1.6 cm of bone.

where reflection of the capsular-ligamentous-tendinous complex from the condyle is completed, thereby facilitating exposure of the anterior surface of the capitulum and radial head. By use of a reciprocating saw, the trochlear articular surface is excised (Fig. 11-5), with care being taken to preserve the important medial and lateral condylar bone masses. Next approximately 1.6 cm of the capitulum is removed in its horizontal plane (Fig. 11-6) followed by the removal of the anterior surface of the capitulum in a plane parallel with the anterior humeral cortex (Fig. 11-7). The radial head is now identified and excised through its neck (Fig. 11-8). Lastly, the articular plate of the olecranon is removed, with first a horizontal and then a vertical cut

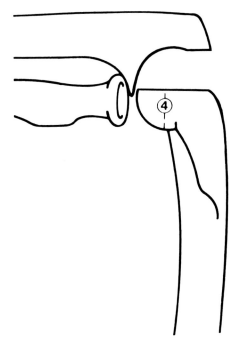

Fig. 11-7. After a horizontal cut is placed through the capitellum, the anterior surface of the capitellum is next removed by placement of a vertical cut, *4*, parallel with the anterior surface of the humeral shaft.

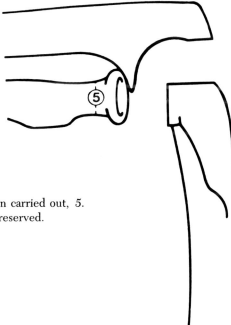

Fig. 11-8. Removal of the radial head is then carried out, *5*. As much radial neck as possible should be preserved.

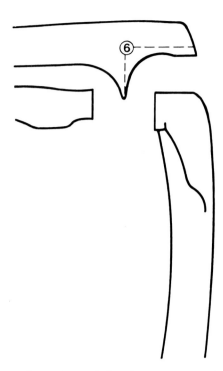

Fig. 11-9. Lastly, the articular surface of the olecranon is carefully excised, 6. As much olecranon bone as possible should be preserved. Cuts are made parallel to the long axis of the ulna and vertically at a point commencing with the prominence of the coronoid process.

each at 90 degrees to the other (Fig. 11-9). Care should be taken to preserve as much olecranon bone as possible so as to assure an adequate bone mass for the insertion of the triceps.

In cases of severe dishing of the olecranon as seen in rheumatoid patients, the olecranon can be shortened by the segmental resection of bone. Reattachment of the olecranon tip with its intact triceps tendon is later achieved by wire fixation (Fig. 11-10). By use of drills, curettes, and broaches, the humeral, ulnar, and radial canals are reamed until all cancellous bone has been removed and prosthetic stem insertion can be performed easily. A trial fit of all prosthetic components without the plastic interface is carried out.

If full extension cannot be easily achieved, it may be necessary to remove the anterior capsule or shorten the humerus. Before cementing the component parts, one should copiously irrigate all bony beds to remove blood, fat, and bone debris and then dry the beds. Plugging of the humeral canals followed by cement injection by syringe technique is highly recommended. Usually the ulnar and radial components are cemented together before the humeral component. The radial head must be precisely positioned in relationship to the ulnar component because

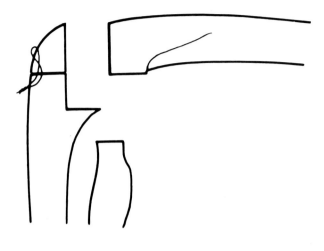

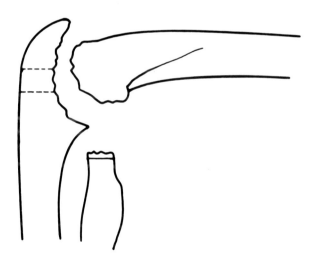

Fig. 11-10. When pronounced dishing to the olecranon process has occurred generally secondary to inflammatory arthritic changes, the olecranon process should be shortened. This is achieved by wedge resection of a segment of the olecranon. This resection should only be performed when the insertion of the triceps mechanism to the olecranon process has been undisturbed. The foreshortened olecranon process is then reattached by a figure-of-eight wire to serve as a secure means of reattachment of the triceps mechanism.

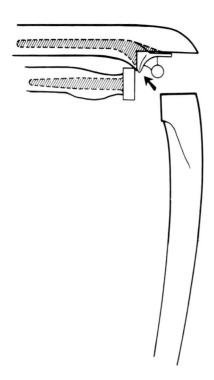

Fig. 11-11. A critical relationship exists between the precise placement of the olecranon and radial prostheses. The articulating surface of the radial head must be located at a point precisely even with the articulating surface of the ulnar component as shown.

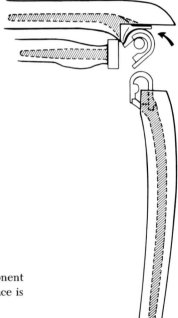

Fig. 11-12. After the secure fixation of all three component parts the ultrahigh molecular weight polyethylene interface is snapped over the olecranon trundle.

this relationship will affect the eventual articulation of the humeral component to each of these components. The articulating surface of the radial head must be exactly located at a level flush with the concave articulating surface of the ulnar component (Fig. 11-11). After removal of all excess cement, the plastic interface is pressed over the olecranon trundle (Fig. 11-12) and the elbow is then acutely flexed and the plastic component seated into the humeral groove, which then allows a snap fit (Fig. 11-13). The elbow is now placed through an arc of motion to assess alignment and stability. A layered surgical closure follows insertion of a sin-

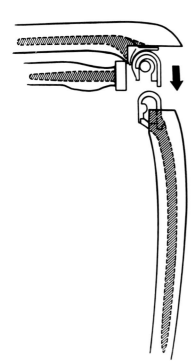

Fig. 11-13. A polyethylene interface is then securely seated in a snap-fitting fashion within the well provided by the humeral component.

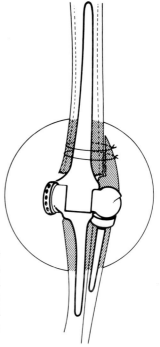

Fig. 11-14. When condylar bone is lacking, support for the capitellum must be created by use of bone graft material. This figure depicts an iliac bone graft wired to the distal humeral shaft. The incorporation of graft material in this fashion tends to minimize the likelihood of loosening because of rotational movement forces about the humeral component when objects are lifted against gravity.

gle vacuum-suction type of drain. Dressings and a posterior splint are applied and maintained for 5 to 10 days depending upon the progression of wound healing.

When the lateral condyle of the humerus is absent (Fig. 11-14), an iliac crest bone graft may be substituted, thus providing support to the capitellar surface of the humeral component. The secure fixation of the capitellar component is critical because this tends to minimize the possibility of loosening attributable to a rotational moment arm upon the humeral stem such as might occur when objects are lifted with the elbow abducted against gravity.

Table 11-1. Range of motion

	Preoperative (in degrees)	Postoperative (in degrees)	Percentage of change
Flexion	112	135	+ 20
Extension	35	39	+ 11
Arc	77	96	+ 24
Pronation	63	73	+ 15
Supination	62	65	+ 4
Arc	125	138	+ 13

PATIENT MATERIAL AND RESULTS

Since 1976, the elbow prosthesis described has been used in a carefully controlled clinical setting. All patients undergoing this type of replacement arthroplasty were required to show by clinical and roentgenographic evaluation far-advanced destructive changes to the elbow. Twenty-one prostheses have been implanted in 20 patients, of which 15 cases provide a postoperative follow-up study extending from 6 to 36 months with an average mean of 24 months. Among this group of seven females and seven males, one patient with rheumatoid arthritis underwent bilateral replacement. Two patients were osteoarthritic, whereas 12 had rheumatoid arthritis. The patients' ages ranged from 36 to 83 years, with a mean of 58 years. Two patients presented with bony ankylosis of the humeroulnar joint, one of which also exhibited bony fusion of the proximal and distal radioulnar joint of 19 year's duration.

All patients were evaluated preoperatively and postoperatively by the author, and pertinent statistical data recorded on a standardized computer analysis form. As with other types of cementable total joint arthroplasties, the most predictable postoperative result was relief of pain. The average rating of pain preoperatively was 3.5, and postoperatively 1.1. The ratings were (1) none, (2) occasional or mild, (3) moderate, (4) serious or severe, and (5) incapacitating.

An improvement in the arc of motion was also observed in all cases postoperatively though most patients failed to regain complete extension of the elbow. The observed changes in the preoperative and postoperative arc of motion for flexion and extension, pronation and supination are shown in Table 11-1. Improvement in pronation and supination was dependent on resection of a destroyed or ankylosed distal ulnar articulation in two patients. Thus the taking of routine roentgenographs of the distal radioulnar joint is advised when significant limitation of pronation or supination is observed preoperatively. An analysis of the improved range of motion observed in the two patients with the solid ankylosis of the elbow preoperatively is provided in Table 11-2.

Routine postoperative serial roentgenographs of the operated elbow have been obtained when possible. To date only two of 15 patients have shown any evidence

Table 11-2. Range of motion of two cases of ankylosed elbows

	Preoperative (in degrees)	Postoperative (in degrees)	Arc (in degrees)
Flexion-extension			
Patient 1	90/0	135-45	90
Patient 2	100/0	125-65	60
Pronation-supination			
Patient 1	30/0	75-20	95
Patient 2	40/0	40/0*	0

*Distal radioulnar joint not resected.

of radiolucency about the bone-cement interface. Two patients with a follow-up study of 36 months showed no evidence of radiolucency. No patients described any symptoms suggestive of clinical loosening, and all have expressed a pronounced increase in functional usage.

COMPLICATIONS

To date no patients have shown clinical, laboratory, or roentgenographic evidence of loosening or infection. All arthroplasties have remained stable with a single exception, a case where a manufacturing flaw in the ultrahigh molecular weight polyethylene interface allowed for an episode of dislocation. This represented the single incidence of reoperation for replacement of this defective interface. No patients have exhibited signs or symptoms of an ulnar neuritis, but two patients did partially avulse their reattached triceps tendon in the early postoperative period. In neither case did this prove to be a mechanical problem.

DISCUSSION

The high failure rate observed with earlier designs of cementable total elbow prostheses has cast perhaps an appropriate air of skepticism upon this type of surgery. Many reasons for those failures can now be readily identified. The elbow, as with other joints of the upper and lower extremity, is capable of generating significant joint reactive forces with activities of daily living.[13,18] Although a precise analysis is not available, it would appear reasonable that objects held in the hand with the elbow flexed against gravity are capable of being magnified ten- to twentyfold at the elbow joint. Thus joint reactive forces of 150 to 200 kg can easily be obtained at the elbow.[1,11] Implants that are incapable of absorbing and evenly distributing such stresses will certainly be prone to failure. It is a well-recognized fact that as the degree of prosthetic interface constraint increases, the incidence of loosening at the bone-cement interface also rises because of the greater transference of stresses to the supporting bone. Certainly the earlier designs of total elbow prostheses enhance the likelihood of mechanical loosening because of their high degree of constraint.[2,14,23,25] Also the recommendation that humeral condyles and the olecranon process be removed would appear to have added to their likelihood of failure because of the importance of these structures in supporting the respective component parts.[3-5,7] Additionally the random dismissal of the radial head as a structure of little importance added an additional dimension to design error. Perhaps if the original design of a cementable total hip prosthesis had been one of considerable constraint, loosening would have been of such magnitude that the biomechanical principles that we now accept for cementable total joint prostheses would have been considered as unsound.

The documentation that the elbow, like the knee, is a joint of complex planes of motion speaks for the need for an appropriately designed implant with interfaces allowing for freedom of motion.[17-20] Such a design should work in harmony with the soft-tissue structures that normally provide for the maintenance of stability and the dissipation of a significant degree of stress. The exclusion of a prosthetic radial head would also appear to enhance the likelihood of stem loosening based upon the observation that the radial head is capable of absorbing 50% or more of the stress placed upon the elbow with lifting activities. In its absence obviously such stress would then be increased with reference to the humeral and ulnar components.

Our experiences to date with a semiconstrained cementable total elbow prosthesis that allows for the replacement of the radiocapitellar articulation would lead us to believe that total elbow arthroplasty is not only possible, practical, and functional but that it also carries with it a degree of predictability similar to that observed for implants presently employed at the hip and knee. Caution should, however, be heeded in the selection of appropriate candidates since obviously experiences to date involve only a small number of patients with a limited postoperative follow-up. The importance of these preliminary results will only be known when measured against the true test of time.

REFERENCES

1. Asher, M.A., and Zieber, S.: Biomechanics of the elbow and forearm. American Academy of Orthopaedic Surgeons Postgraduate Course in Elbow, Wrist, and Forearm, Kansas City, Missouri, Oct. 1973.
2. Bryan, R.S., Dobyns, J.H., Linscheid, R.L., and Peterson, L.F.: Preliminary experiences with total elbow arthroplasty, Symposium on Osteoarthritis, St. Louis, 1976, The C.V. Mosby Co.
3. Dee, R.: Elbow arthroplasty, Proc. R. Soc. Med. 62:1031, 1969.
4. Dee, R.: Total replacement arthroplasty of the elbow for rheumatoid arthritis, J. Bone Joint Surg. **54B**(1):88, Feb. 1972.
5. Dee, R.: Total replacement of the elbow joint, Mod. Trends Orthop. 6:250, 1972.
6. Dee, R.: Total replacement of the elbow joint, Orthop. Clin. North Am. 4(2):415, April 1973.
7. Dee, R., and Sweetnam, D.R.: Total replacement arthroplasty of the elbow joint for rheumatoid arthritis: two cases, Proc. R. Soc. Med. 63(7):653, July 1970.
8. Dee, R.: Elbow replacement with the R. Dee prosthesis, Acta Orthop. Belg. 41(4):762, July-Aug. 1975.
9. Dee, R.: Total elbow replacement, Symposium on Osteoarthritis, St. Louis, 1976, The C.V. Mosby Co.
10. Dobyns, J.H., Bryan, R.S., Linscheid, R.L., and Peterson, L.F.: Special problems of total elbow arthroplasty, Geriatrics 31(4):57, April 1976.
11. Ewald, F.C.: Total elbow replacement, Orthop. Clin. North Am. 6(3):685, July 1975.

12. Freeman, M.A.: Current state of total joint replacement, Br. Med. J. 2(6047):1301, Nov. 27, 1976.
13. Garrett, J.C., Ewald, F.C., Thomas, W.H., and Sledge, C.B.: Loosening associated with G.S.B. hinge total elbow replacement in patients with rheumatoid arthritis, Clin. Orthop. (127):170-4, 1977.
14. Gschwend, N.: Our experiences of elbow arthroplasty with the B.S.B. prosthesis. Congrès de la Société Belgique de Chirurgie Orthopédique et de Traumatologie, Ghent, May 1975.
15. Halls, A.A., and Travill, A.: Transmission of pressures across the elbow joint, Anat. Rec. 150:243, 1964.
16. Harder, D.H., and Beauchamp, R.D.: Total joint replacement arthroplasty of elbow in rheumatoid arthritis, Can. J. Surg. 20(3):234, May 1977.
17. Morrey, B., and Chao, E.: Passive motion of the elbow joint, J. Bone Joint Surg. 58A(4):501, 1976.
18. Pauwels, F.: Pressure distribution in the elbow joint with basic remarks on joint pressure, Z. Anat. (Berlin) 123:643, 1963.
19. Pritchard, R.W.: Flexible elbow joint replacement. In Joint replacement in the upper limb, London, 1977, Mechanical Engineering Publications, Ltd.
20. Roy, R.D., Johnson, R.J., and Jameson, R.M.: Rotation of the forearm, an experimental study of pronation and supination, J. Bone Joint Surg. 33:993, 1951.
21. Schlein, A.P.: Semiconstrained total elbow arthroplasty, Clin. Orthop. (121):222, Nov.-Dec. 1976.
22. Souter, W.A.: Arthroplasty of the elbow, Orthop. Clin. North Am. 4:395, 1973.
23. Souter, W.A.: Total replacement arthroplasty of the elbow. In Joint replacement in the upper limb, London, 1977, Mechanical Engineering Publications, Ltd.
24. Street, D.M., and Steven, P.S.: A humeral replacement prosthesis for the elbow: results in ten elbows, J. Bone Joint Surg. 56A(6):1147, Sept. 1974.
25. Volz, R.G., and Jones, A.B.: Upper extremity total joint replacement, AORN J. 28(5):843, Nov. 1978.
26. Wild, J.: Personal data, 1976, Arizona Health Sciences Center, Tucson, Ariz.

12. Revision surgery after failed elbow endoprosthesis

Roger Dee, M.D.

The solution to the problem of the failed elbow prosthesis depends to a large extent on what kind of device has been inserted. Elbow prostheses may be generally classified into stemmed hinge joints and unstemmed surface replacements, but there are some intermediate hybrids.

REVISION AFTER SURFACE REPLACEMENT ARTHROPLASTY

Experience has shown the main cause of failure to be prosthetic loosening. In the case of a loose surface replacement (Fig. 12-1) the revision problem is less, since there has been minimal damage to the bone stock and the joint ligaments are usually preserved. The joint usually remains stable after removal of such a prosthesis, and it is perfectly permissible to remove the device and close the wound without extensive secondary procedures. A good functional result will be achieved, but it is as well additionally to notch the center of the distal humerus to give improved stability (Fig. 12-2). I also fashion a corresponding vertical crest on the ulnar articulating surface. This greatly improves lateral stability.

At the end of the procedure the result resembles a primary "anatomic" arthroplasty. The late result of anatomic arthroplasty without interposition is often erosion of the humeral epicondyle (Fig. 12-3). Interposition therefore is to be recommended in this situation. I perform a cutis interposition arthroplasty of the Vainio type.

After carefully dissecting the ulnar nerve and gently retracting it away from the bone, I drill and osteotomize the olecranon (Fig. 12-4). Excellent exposure is hereby obtained of the distal humerus. Holes are then drilled for attachment of the cutis graft, and the lower end of the humerus is notched (Fig. 12-5). The midline crest is fashioned within ulner articulating surface.

The skin graft is obtained from a hairless portion of the abdominal skin. A split-thickness skin graft approximately 0.3 mm thick is raised and left attached by its one end to the abdomen. The bleeding dermal layer is now elevated by sharp

126

Fig. 12-1. An early-design surface replacement that I implanted in 1970. The fixation to the humerus was inadequate. (From HSC Media Services, SUNY at Stony Brook, StonyBrook, N.Y.)

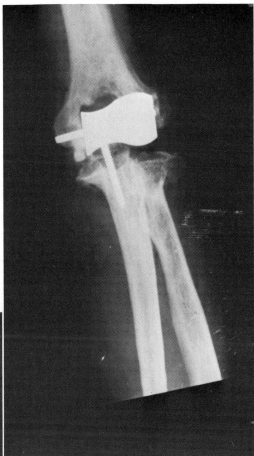

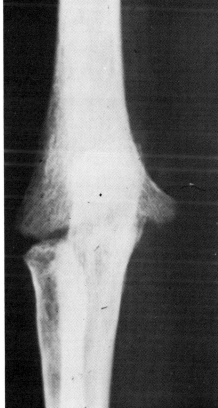

Fig. 12-2. An elbow joint immediately after anatomic arthroplasty for rheumatoid arthritis. Note the notching of the distal humerus. (From HSC Media Services, SUNY at Stony Brook, Stony Brook, N.Y.)

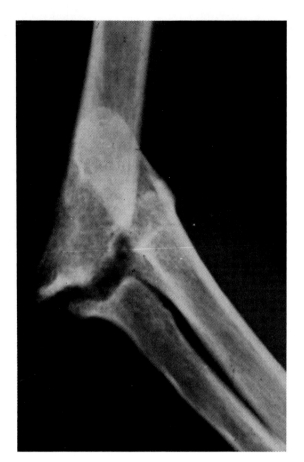

Fig. 12-3. The same joint 1 year later. It has swung greatly into varus as the medial epicondyle of the humerus has been resorbed. (From HSC Media Services, SUNY at Stony Brook, Stony Brook, N.Y.)

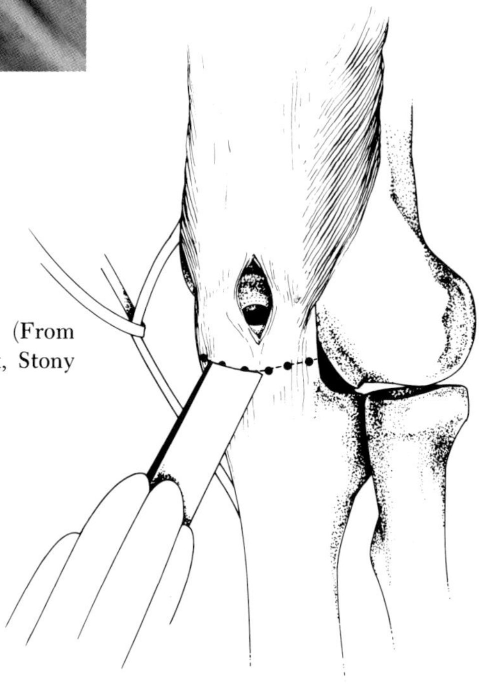

Fig. 12-4. The ulna is being osteotomized. (From HSC Media Services, SUNY at Stony Brook, Stony Brook, N.Y.)

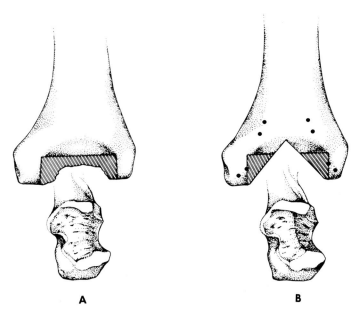

A   **B**

Fig. 12-5. This shows the manner in which the bone remaining after removal of the prosthesis, **A**, should be refashioned at arthroplasty, **B**. Note the crest fashioned on the ulna and the notch in the humerus; also the holes drilled for attachment of the skin graft. (From HSC Media Services, SUNY at Stony Brook, Stony Brook, N.Y.)

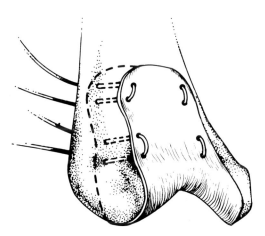

Fig. 12-6. The cutis graft is attached to the distal humerus. (From HSC Media Services, SUNY at Stony Brook, Stony Brook, N.Y.)

dissection from the subcutaneous fat and put aside to be used later as the cutis graft. After hemostasis of the underlying fat on the abdomen the split-thickness flap is sutured back down to cover the donor site on the abdomen. The free cutis graft is then attached to the lower end of the humerus with its deeper surface applied to the bone (Fig. 12-6).

When there has been gross erosion of the olecranon and there is too much laxity, which may cause instability, it is possible to pack the sigmoid notch with cancellous bone chips as recommended by Vainio to secure a snug fit. The olecranon is reattached with two parallel Kirschner wires and a figure-of-eight wire loop (Fig. 12-7).

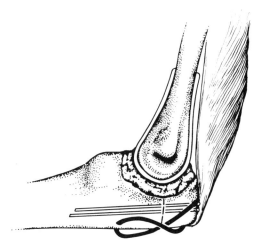

Fig. 12-7. Insertion of bone chips and reattachment of the olecranon. For explanation see text. (From HSC Media Services, SUNY at Stony Brook, Stony Brook, N.Y.)

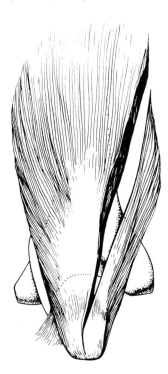

Fig. 12-8. A triceps flap is fashioned on the lateral side. (From HSC Media Services, SUNY at Stony Brook, Stony Brook, N.Y.)

If the prosthesis is removed for *infection*, it is important to remove not only components but also all the cement. One should not perform a cutis graft in such a case, since implanting devascularized material is contraindicated. On the other hand, under these circumstances one cannot leave mobile bare bone ends within a capacious joint cavity since, in this situation it will be difficult to clear up the infection. The best alternative is to perform a triceps arthroplasty.

In this operation a large flap of triceps muscle is fashioned (Fig. 12-8) and sutured to the insertion of the brachialis muscle after the muscle flap is passed through the notch in the lower end of the humerus (Fig. 12-9). This procedure obliterates the dead space and also enables one to retain motion. Obviously the usual tenets of the surgery of infection are followed. Thus all devascularized bone and obviously infected material is carefully excised under appropriate intravenous antibiotic coverage. In the two cases I have performed I have also immobilized the arm for 6 weeks after surgery using external fixation. In both cases a good arc of motion of 90 degrees was achieved, but more important this was accompanied by eradication of the infection.

In the presence of infection I am not bold enough to advise insertion of another prosthesis at revision. In the absence of infection, the use of another prosthesis is an alternative, but since the usual problem then is fixation, this usually means choosing a prosthesis that is stemmed. I prefer to avoid aggravating the local situation by broaching the medullary cavities to insert a stemmed device, since in these patients with good bone stock and ligaments good results are obtained by use of the cutis arthroplasty technique.

Arthrodesis can be considered after removal of the infected prosthesis. One can take a posterior cortical bone graft from the distal humerus, slide it distally, and

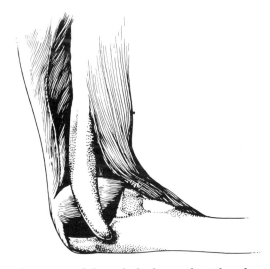

Fig. 12-9. The triceps flap is passed through the humeral notch and sutured in the region of the coronoid. (From HSC Media Services, SUNY at Stony Brook, Stony Brook, N.Y.)

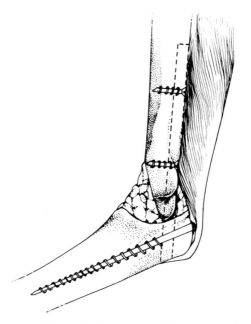

Fig. 12-10. A standard method of arthrodesis of the elbow. For explanation see text. (From HSC Media Services, SUNY at Stony Brook, Stony Brook, N.Y.)

by transfixing it with an olecranon screw obtain fusion (Fig. 12-10). This kind of technique or some method using additionally external fixation can successfully achieve arthrodesis, but it is not an acceptable option in a patient who may have restricted motion in other joints in the same limb, and I would certainly not use it on any occasion after removal of an infected joint.

REMOVAL OF A STEMMED PROSTHESIS

Much has been learned in the decade after the use of the first stemmed hinges with bone cement.[1] Rigidly constrained hinge joints are now generally regarded as unacceptable. It is important that the axis of rotation of the joint should be set into the design so that it bisects the normal carrying angle in the arm and thus reproduces the normal biomechanics of motion. In addition, a joint that has a polycentric articulation is more forgiving in that it allows for some error in placement of the axis of rotation anteroposteriorly. It goes without saying that metal-to-metal joints are obsolete.

Surface replacement alone would seem to be preferable for the architecturally good joint. In the joint that has been severely damaged by trauma or previous surgery with loss of large areas of normal bony architecture and ligaments, a semi-constrained type of linking prosthesis with stems seems a suitable compromise.

Newer prostheses are designed so that maximum bone stock is preserved when they are inserted.[2] The importance of preserving the humeral epicondyles and the

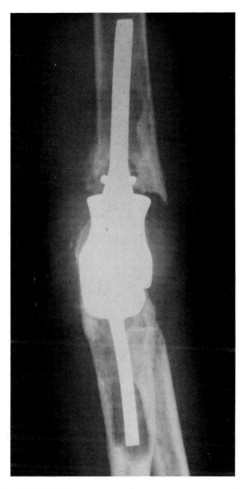

Fig. 12-11. A typical loose hinge joint. Note the gross erosion and scalloping of the inner cortex. This joint had been loose for 1 year before this roentgenogram was taken. (From HSC Media Services, SUNY at Stony Brook, Stony Brook, N.Y.)

radial head has been recognized, if these have not already been destroyed by the original injury, since their absence compounds the problem at revision.

In my own series, using an early, totally constrained metal hinge, the rate of failure attributable to loosening of the device accelerated between 3 and 5 years after sugery. Pain occurred during motion and when the arm was loaded, often well before the radiologic changes appeared. Ultimately the characteristic lucent line progressing to gross erosion of the internal cortex made the diagnosis all too obvious (Fig. 12-11). The severity of the pain is unrelated to which component is loose. Loosening of the humeral component is characteristically and accurately localized by the patient to the lower end of that bone. When the ulnar component is loose, the pain radiates down the forearm as far as the wrist.

Salvage after failure of a stemmed stabilizing type of prosthesis is technically a more difficult problem. The bony architecture is usually more severely damaged, and there remains no intrinsic stability. Also the cortex is damaged proximally and distally for a considerable distance depending on the stem length and the period the joint has been loose before revision.

A decision must be made whether the bone is too severely damaged to justify reimplantation of a further prosthesis. A lesson learned early on was that rececementing a loosened hinge component back in place, or attempting at revision to reinsert a new prosthesis of identical design, inevitably resulted in further failure. The lesson is clear: laying the blame on faulty technique or some other technical

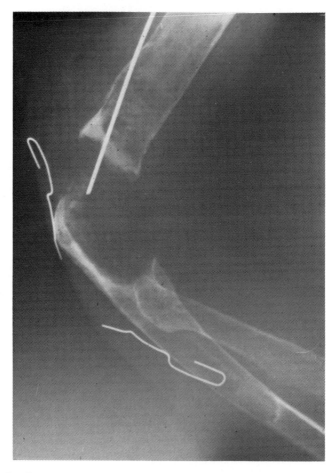

Fig. 12-12. The disastrous results after inadequate postoperative immobilization after removal of a loose hinge. The single Kirschner wire used was totally ineffective and could not hold the weight of this heavy forearm. A flail limb resulted. The paper clips are markers. (From HSC Media Services, SUNY at Stony Brook, Stony Brook, N.Y.)

error initially is a mistake. If loosening occurs, the reason is that the design is incorrect and that the stresses in that arm are such that that particular design of prosthesis will always fail. Another mistake is to believe that putting in an identical design with a longer stem will correct the situation. In my experience such a course of action usually compounds the problem, since, when loosening again occurs, the longer stem damages even more bone stock. A similar negative opinion was formed concerning the use of screws as an additional aide to cement fixation.

After removal of such a prosthesis, if one decides not to reinsert another type of endoprosthesis, something must be done to restore stability to the articulation. Leaving the arm in a cast, or without adequate fixation laterally or externally, will result in a flail limb (Fig. 12-12). My choice now is an external fixator (Fig. 12-13). If I elect to remove the prosthesis and am not going to reinsert a revision prosthesis, which is then combined with the external fixator, I usually do a local procedure designed to minimize the bone gap. Following a suggestion by Swanson, I have modified the Steindler flexorplasty.

Identifying and isolating the ulnar nerve can be the most difficult part of this revision. The nerve must be dissected well clear before one procedes to osteotomy of the olecranon. Forearm flexors are then isolated and then reattached on the humerus (Fig. 12-14). The extensors are shortened by removal of a portion of the olecranon and transferal of the attachment of this muscle a little more distally (Fig. 12-15). Occasionally one can combine this technique with some triceps interposition if the joint space is very capacious. I have performed this operation for the

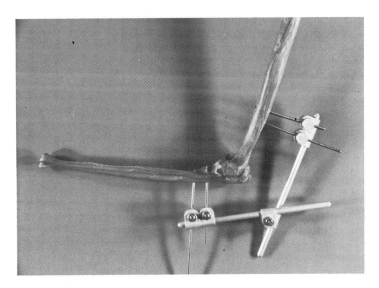

Fig. 12-13. The AO fixator may be applied to fix the elbow either for arthrodesis or as an adjunct to a postrevision arthroplasty. (From HSC Media Services, SUNY at Stony Brook, Stony Brook, N.Y.)

Fig. 12-14. First step in the revision arthroplasty—the holes are drilled in the humerus for attachment of the forearm muscle at the higher level. (The olecranon bone to be removed is shaded.) (From HSC Media Services, SUNY at Stony Brook, Stony Brook, N.Y.)

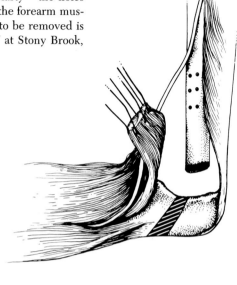

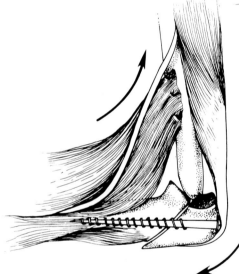

Fig. 12-15. The completed procedure. For explanation see text. (From HSC Media Services, SUNY at Stony Brook, Stony Brook, N.Y.)

infected joint, and the wound will usually remain dry. Another critical factor helping to obliterate infection is the removal of all the loose cement.

The additional surgical assault upon bone already severely eroded by loose cement may render it unsuitable for insertion of a revision prosthesis, and the modified Steindler procedure together with postoperative external fixation will then give a good functional result.

When the bone stock is good and there has been no infection, I prefer whenever possible to revise. I use for this purpose, a newly designed semiconstrained linking endoprosthesis (Figs. 12-16 and Fig. 12-17). I have used this prosthesis as

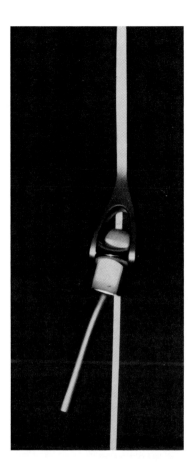

Fig. 12-16. My revision prosthesis in its original form. Note that when snap-fitted together they still have some 10 degrees of motion possible in both medial and lateral directions. The rigidity in the original hinge joint has been removed by this design. (From HSC Media Services, SUNY at Stony Brook, Stony Brook, N.Y.)

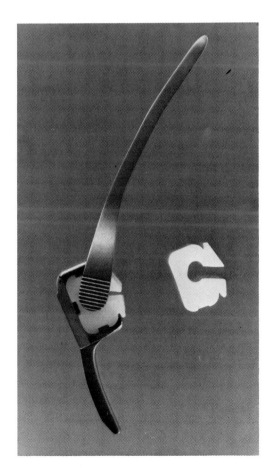

Fig. 12-17. The current design. It has the advantage of allowing replacement of worn polyethylene. (From HSC Media Services, SUNY at Stony Brook, Stony Brook, N.Y.)

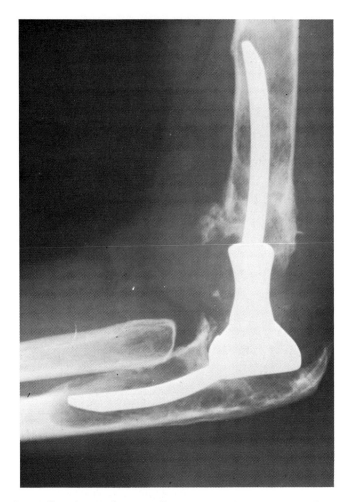

Fig. 12-18. A loose elbow hinge 2½ years after insertion. (From HSC Media Services, SUNY at Stony Brook, Stony Brook, N.Y.)

a primary prosthesis since 1975. It can be inserted without removal of the humeral epicondyles or the radial head and has thus been used as a primary prosthesis, but it is particularly useful at revision. The most recent model of this design and the one currently used has a polyethylene liner that can be replaced (Fig. 12-17).

At operation despite considerable cortical erosion (Fig. 12-18) it is possible to remove cement from both bones through the transolecranon approach and to insert this device (Fig. 12-19). The use of a headlamp, a Water-Pik, and a long-stemmed burr are recommended. It is a good plan to expose the outer cortex of the ulna for its upper 7.5 cm beyond the coronoid to avoid perforation of the shaft while the bone cement is being removed. A similar technique is followed in the humerus.

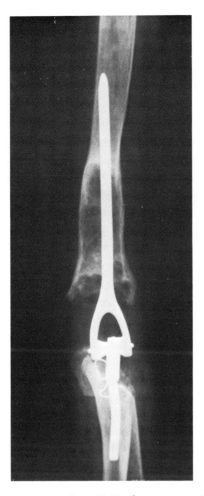

Fig. 12-19. From the same patient in Fig. 12-18 after revision. There is no barium in the new cement. (From HSC Media Services, SUNY at Stony Brook, Stony Brook, N.Y.)

Attempting to burr out cement without viewing the exterior of the cortex will frequently result in perforation.

One is occasionally left with a thin, almost translucent shell of cortex and reinsertion of more cement in such a case will certainly cause additional death of bone. Under these circumstances it is possible to insert a large iliac bone graft as a first stage in the revision process. I have successfully inserted an endoprosthesis 9 months after such a procedure and was amazed how well the bone had reconstituted itself after the grafting. The quality of the bone was much improved over that usually found in revision surgery, and it may be that a two-stage procedure will prove to be preferable. To summarize, then, for the infected case after removal of the stemmed prosthesis, I favor removal of all cement and then doing a modified Steindler arthroplasty. In the uninfected case, the Steindler method is an attractive option, but in experienced hands the revision prosthesis can give excellent results with one of the newer types of design. I have not used arthrodesis in this type of case where the bony gap is such as to make fusion difficult to obtain.

CONCLUSION

How depressing it is to give a dissertation entirely related to failure after elbow endoprostheses! The price of progress comes hard. We can be encouraged by the fact that with our increased understanding of certain of the important principles, the revision rate may fall significantly over the next decade.

ACKNOWLEDGMENTS

I am grateful to the Media Services of the Health Sciences Center of the State University of New York at Stony Brook for the illustrations, and Ms. Kathy Gebhart for the drawings.

REFERENCES

1. Dee, R.: Elbow arthroplasty, Proc. R. Soc. Med. **62**:1031, 1969.
2. Dee, R.: Elbow replacement with the R. Dee prosthesis, Acta Orthop. Belg. **41**:477-483, 1975.

13. Nonconstrained metal-to-plastic total elbow replacement

Frederick C. Ewald, M.D.

The nonconstrained total elbow replacement is a resurfacing prosthesis with components that are not linked or hinged. The humeral and ulnar components will freely distract and consequently require an adequate soft-tissue envelope to function without dislocation or instability. The loaded laxity of the nonconstrained prosthesis either in rotation or varus-valgus stress may be similar to the semiconstrained prosthesis, but any longitudinal "pistoning" of the prosthesis in vivo is possible only with the nonconstrained design. The importance of prosthetic pistoning in the elbow is unknown, and this question will only be answered by long-term follow-up studies of the clinical trials. Elsewhere in this volume the leading examples of a metal-to-plastic hinge type of prosthesis and metal-to-plastic semiconstrained prosthesis have been reported. This paper reviews the current nonconstrained prosthetic class with details of a clinical series of Capitello-Condylar implants. This is a rapidly changing area of joint replacement, and these second and third-generation prostheses may soon be outdated.

NONCONSTRAINED TOTAL ELBOW ARTHROPLASTY

The following list of prostheses is representative of the increasing activity in the concept of elbow-joint resurfacing. Other nonconstrained prostheses may be in development or in use, but these are the first ones that have come to our attention from various centers around the world. Published material in this new field is limited, and so all sources of information have been used, including conferences, meetings, and personal letters.

1. Kudo—Japan
2. Nonblocked—West Germany
3. Liverpool—England
4. Souter—Scotland
5. London—United States
6. Ishizuki—Japan
7. Capitello-Condylar—United States

Types of prostheses

The *Kudo prosthesis* (Fig. 13-1) is a metal-to-plastic resurfacing design with a plastic medullary fixation plug for the ulnar component but no stem fixation for the metal humeral component. Both articular surfaces are smooth and mediolateral sliding motion is unrestricted. In October 1978 the clinical results of 28 replacements were reviewed with follow-up of 1 to 6½ years (average 3 years, 5 months).[13] Using the elbow-rating system of Dee,[3] I rated 15 as excellent, 10 fair, and 3 poor. Complications were subluxation, one; humeral component migration, one; and ulnar nerve paresis, one.

The early results from the *nonblocked* metal-to-plastic resurfacing prosthesis without medullary-stem fixation from West Germany was reported[4] in 1977. Seven implants were performed, and one humeral component loosened and there was one dislocation. No follow-up was reported, and the authors believed the indications were limited.

The *Liverpool prosthesis* is a nonconstrained bobbin-shaped metal-to-plastic prosthesis without medullary-stem fixation. The transolecranon surgical approach is fixed with a single lag screw. The metal humeral and plastic ulnar components each have two articular facets. Maximum follow-up of 3 years has been reported[2] on 20 prostheses with good results. Two prostheses have been removed for infection and fracture.

Souter has designed a metal-to-plastic resurfacing prosthesis that articulates as

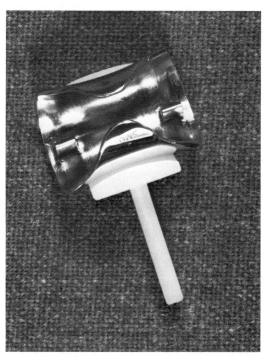

Fig. 13-1. Kudo nonconstrained metal-to-plastic elbow prosthesis showing a uniform articular surface without condylar contours.

a "rider in the saddle."[15] The ulnar plastic component has a short fixation plug, and the metal humeral component has three short fixation lugs. The first clinical review[16] of 22 implants with a follow-up of $^1/_2$ to $1^1/_2$ years showed good pain relief and flexion wih no gain in postoperative extension.

London has reported[14] on a metal-to-plastic elbow prosthesis that has an optional medullary-fixation stem for the metal humeral component (Fig. 13-2). The all-plastic ulnar piece has a fixation stem. Sixteen procedures have been performed and reviewed with follow-up of 6 to 26 months (average 15 months). Pain relief

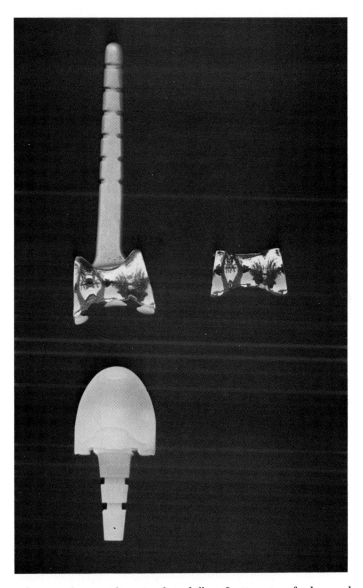

Fig. 13-2. London prosthesis with optional medullary fixation stem for humeral component. Articular surfaces are bicondylar and medullary stems are in line.

Table 13-1. Total elbow arthroplasty at the Robert Breck Brigham Division of the Brigham and Women's Hospital, 1973 to 1979

Prosthesis		Number
Capitello-Condylar		100
All plastic ulna	69	
Metal tray, ulna	31	
G.S.B. Hinge		13
Pritchard-Walker		5
Tri-Axial		3
Total		121

Table 13-2. Rotatory loaded laxity in cadaver elbow and prosthesis

Torque (N·cm)	Force (N)	Cadaver elbow (two sets)	All-plastic ulna component (degrees)	Metal-tray ulnar component (degrees)
425	620	5.3, 1.6	3.5	10.4
	1240	2.0, 0.5	0.6	3.1
85	620	16.7, 4.6	7.6	23.6
	1240	10.2, 2.0	3.6	13.9

was excellent except for one patient with continued unexplained postoperative pain and one loose ulnar component.

The *Ishizuki prosthesis* is another design from Japan that is more anatomic in configuration than the Kudo. The stemless metal humeral component articulates with a stemmed all-plastic ulnar component. Eleven prostheses have been implanted, and the maximum follow-up at review[11,10] was 2½ years. Seven were reported as excellent and four fair. Complications were dislocation, one; "technical" error, one; and intraoperative fracture, one.

The experience in total elbow arthroplasty at our institution has been mainly with the *Capitello-Condylar prosthesis* in rheumatoid arthritis. However, there has been some experience with the G.S.B., Pritchard-Walker, and Tri-Axial. The numbers are listed in Table 13-1. The first Capitello-Condylar prosthesis was implanted in June of 1974, and the first 69 implants were recently reviewed in detail with follow-up of 2 to 5 years (average 3½ years). This is a resurfacing prosthesis with three-point fixation for both the metal humeral component and the plastic ulnar component (Fig. 13-3). Bench testing has been performed in a wear simulator, which provided 50 pounds of constant joint reactive force, a flexion arc of 50 degrees, and distilled water lubrication. Three million cycles produced an estimated combined wear and cold flow of 0.4 mm. Loaded rotational laxity of the prosthesis was compared to that of fresh cadaver elbows. Both were loaded longitudinally at 30-degree flexion in an Instron apparatus. Varying normal torques were applied, and the data are seen in Table 13-2. The loaded prosthesis demonstrates more available rotational laxity than intact fresh cadaver elbows do.

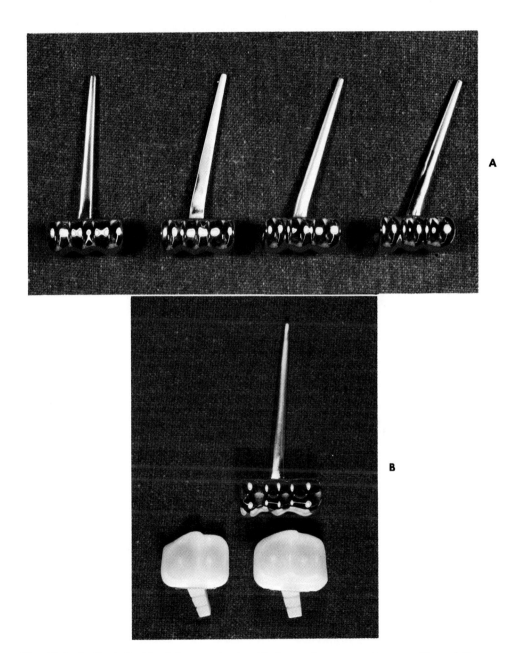

Fig. 13-3. A, Capitello-Condylar prosthesis with humeral component seen with medullary fixation stems having cubitus-valgus angles of 5, 10, 15, and 20 degrees. The condylar metal molds are designed to cap and resurface the trochlea and capitellum of the humerus. **B,** Plastic ulnar component seen with short medullary fixation plug, two undersurface fixation runners, and two thicknesses of plastic. Articular surfaces are bicondylar and mate with metal humeral component.

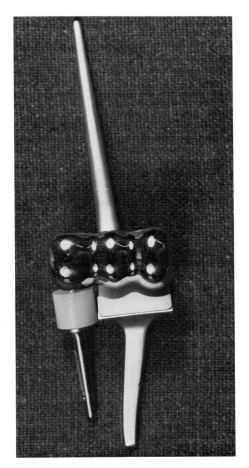

Fig. 13-4. Capitello-Condylar prosthesis with ulnar component in a metal tray with long valgus medullary fixation stem. Experimental optional radial head replacement has metal fixation stem.

The initial clinical results of the Capitello-Condylar prosthesis have been reported[5] and updated[6-7] for the all-plastic ulnar component. The 2- to 5-year follow-up recently completed has shown little deterioration of results with increasing time. The initial 69 implants represent a complete, closed series, because the all-plastic ulnar component has been placed in a metal boat with a long metal medullary fixation stem (Fig. 13-4). The metal boat or tray was added to enhance ulnar fixation and prevent excessive twisting of the plastic during torque loading.

CLINICAL RESULTS

Fifty patients with 54 implants were available for review at follow-up. However, all the complications from the entire series of 69 implants have been listed. With a prospective elbow-rating system being used,[8] 87% of the Capitello-Condy-

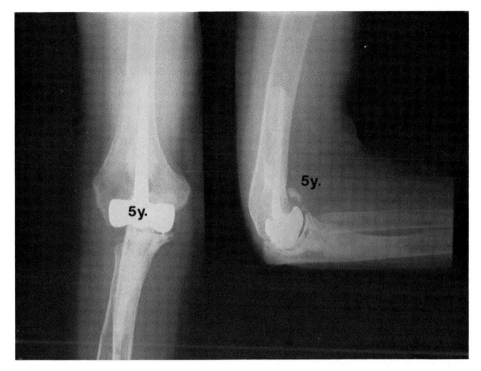

Fig. 13-5. Roentgenograms of a representative postoperative Capitello-Condylar prosthesis. Five-year follow-up shows no reaction at the bone-cement interface surrounding the medullary fixation stems on both anteroposterior and lateral views.

lar elbows were rated good to excellent, two elbows were rated fair, and five elbows rated poor or failed. Average elbow flexion improved from 122 degrees preoperatively to 136 degrees postoperatively. Pronation was 51 degrees preoperatively and 74 degrees postoperatively. These changes were statistically significant, but there was no statistical improvement in extension or supination.

COMPLICATIONS

The overall complication rate was 41%, but the complications adversely affected the final results in only three elbows. The complications include three deep wound infections, one loose ulnar component, four recurrent dislocations, six transient cases of ulnar nerve paralysis, five permanent cases of ulnar nerve paralysis, three fractures, three minor wound healing problems, and one triceps rupture. Of these complications, seven elbows required revision. Four were reoperated for dislocation, two for sepsis, and one for loosening. There was no loosening of the humeral component and no radiolucent lines at the bone-cement interface of the humeral component. Eight ulnar components had minimal radiolucent lines at the bone-cement interface in asymptomatic patients. Fig. 13-5 shows a representative roentgenogram of a 5-year postoperative prosthesis with an intact bone-cement interface and no evidence of loosening.

DISCUSSION

The surgical approach used in these first 69 procedures was posterior as described by Campbell[1] with modifications to increase exposure. This approach utilized a V incision in the triceps tendon, extensive mobilization of the ulnar nerve, and wide tissue dissection. The surgical exposure is satisfactory, but there is extensive tissue devitalization, excessive manipulation of the ulnar nerve, which may have a subclinical rheumatoid neuropathy, and creation of large tissue dead spaces. Implantation of the nonconstrained prosthesis, in my experience, requires far more exposure than one needs to implant a constrained or semiconstrained unit. For example, there were few postoperative soft-tissue problems in the G.S.B. series,[9] but in the Capitello-Condylar series, as this report indicated, postoperative soft-tissue problems were numerous. Because of these soft-tissue problems, the surgical exposure has been changed and early experience has been encouraging with elimination of the ulnar nerve paresthesias, hematomas, and dislocation. The new surgical exposure is a modification of the approach described by Kocher[12] with subperiosteal dissection of the extensor mass and lateral collateral ligament off the lateral epicondyle and the triceps mechanism from the olecranon. The elbow joint can be dislocated laterally without exposure of the ulnar nerve. In addition the collateral ligaments and the triceps tendon are not transected.

The initial goal of using nonconstraint in the design of the prosthesis to allow soft tissue to absorb as much force as possible rather than transmission to the bone-cement interface to avoid loosening of the components seems to be achieved. However, the trade-off has been increased soft-tissue problems in the form of dislocation, infection, and nerve problems. The problems appear to be solved by use of a surgical approach more suited to the nonconstrained concept for preservation of the continuity of the all-important soft-tissue sleeve.

INDICATIONS AND CONTRAINDICATIONS

The Capitello-Condylar prosthesis is currently used only in the destroyed rheumatoid elbow. If there is intractable pain refractory to adequate medical management, limitation of motion in the elbow, and radiographic evidence of joint destruction, then surgery is indicated. However, if there is a normal range of motion with preservation of the bony architecture, particularly the subchondral bone plate, a radial head resection and synovectomy should be considered. The absolute contraindications to the procedure are previous sepsis, previous fascial or other interpositional arthroplasty, and previous hinge arthroplasty. Relative contraindications to the procedure are excessive loss of bone as in giant rheumatoid cysts, deficient trochlear notch of the ulna, and posttraumatic or degenerative arthritis.

REFERENCES

1. Campbell, W.C.: Arthroplasty of the elbow, Ann. Surg. **76:**615, 1922.
2. Cavendish, M.D., and Elloy, M.D.: A single method of total elbow replacement. In Joint replacement in the upper limb, London 1977, Mechanical Engineering Publications, Ltd.
3. Dee, R.: Total replacement arthroplasty of the elbow for rheumatoid arthritis, J. Bone Joint Surg. **54B:**88, 1972.
4. Engelbrecht, E., Bucholz, H.W., Rottger, J., and Siegal, A.: Total elbow replacement with a hinge and a non-blocked system. In Joint replacement in the upper limb, London, 1978, Mechanical Engineering Publications, Ltd.
5. Ewald, F.C.: Total elbow replacement, Orthop. Clin. North Am. **6:**685, 1975.
6. Ewald, F.C.: Non-constrained metal to plastic total elbow replacement, Orthop. Trans. **1:**110, 1977.
7. Ewald, F.C.: Total elbow replacement, American Orthopedic Association Meeting, June 27, 1978.
8. Ewald, F.C., Thomas, W.H., Sledge, C.B., and Poss, R.,: Non-constrained metal to plastic elbow arthroplasty in rheumatoid arthritis. In Joint replacement in the upper limb, London, 1977, Mechanical Engineering Publications, Ltd.
9. Garrett, J.C., Ewald, F.C., Thomas, W.H., and Sledge, C.B.,: Loosening associated with G.S.B. Hinge Total Elbow replacements in patients with rheumatoid arthritis, Clin. Orthop. Rel. Res. **127:**170, 1977.
10. Ishizuki, M.: Biomechanical analysis of the elbow joint preliminary report of hingeless total elbow arthroplasty, Personal communication, Sept. 18, 1978, Tokyo, Japan.
11. Ishizuki, M., Nagatsuka, Y., Arai, T., Isobe, Y., Tanabe, K., and Fujita, T.: Preliminary experiences with hingeless total elbow arthroplasty, The Ryumachi **17:**4, 1977.
12. Kocher, T.: Textbook of operative surgery, ed. 3, London, 1911, Adam & Charles Black.
13. Kudo, H.: Total elbow replacement, Personal communication, Feb. 28, 1979, Kanagawa Prefecture, Japan.
14. London, J.T.: Resurfacing total elbow arthroplasty, Orthop. Trans. **2:**217, 1978.
15. Souter, W.A.: Total replacement arthroplasty of the elbow. In Joint replacement in the upper limb, London, 1977, Mechanical Engineering Publications, Ltd.
16. Souter, W.A.: Total replacement arthroplasty of the elbow, Personal communication, Nov. 8, 1978, Edinburgh, Scotland.

14. Biomechanics of the elbow

Peter A. Torzilli, Ph.D.

Currently, joint arthroplasty provides a viable means for the reconstruction of a damaged or diseased joint. The goal of joint reconstructive surgery is to obtain a semblance of anatomic congruity with concomitant joint stability and functional mobility. This has been achieved most successfully in the lower extremity, with less favorable results in the upper extremity.[8] Extensive biomechanical research exists for the kinematic motion and joint load characteristics of the lower limb, whereas limited information is available for the upper extremity. With the advent of new biomaterials, design criteria, and methods of analysis, an increased interest in the upper extremity joints has been nurtured. Collaborative efforts between the surgeon and engineer have provided a better understanding of upper extremity mechanical function. A determination of the muscle and joint reaction forces and of the kinematics of the joint motion will yield valuable information for the design and implantation of prosthetic joint replacements and help in the evaluation of mechanical failures.

The elbow joint plays a major role in the normal physiologic function of the upper extremity. It has long been considered a simple hinged joint, with flexion-extension motion assumed constrained to the anteroposterior plane. It was believed that since the elbow is a nonweightbearing joint the surrounding muscles exerted minor joint reaction forces during normal physiologic function. In fact, the elbow joint is characterized by complicated out-of-plane motions and subjected to forces that can be several times the body weight. This chapter presents a simplified biomechanical model of the elbow for analysis of the muscle and joint reaction forces about the normal and altered joint. In addition, an instant center analysis of the joint motion during flexion-extension and supination-pronation provides a description of the kinematics of the joint.

FORCES ABOUT THE ELBOW JOINT

Three types of joint activity are possible. *Isometric* activity requires stability of the joint under static force conditions for fixed joint positions. When the joint velocities are small or do not change abruptly between successive joint positions, the inertial effects may be ignored and a *quasistatic* or *isokinetic* analysis is per-

150

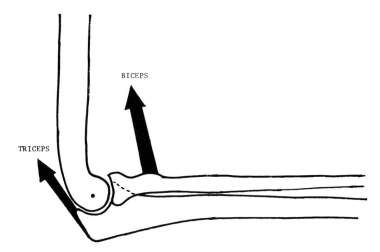

Fig. 14-1. Force of the biceps and triceps acts about an axis of joint rotation position through the center of the humeral capitulum and trochlea.

formed. However, if the accelerations or decelerations of the component masses are substantial, the *dynamic* or *inertial* forces will have a large contribution to the overall forces about the joint.

During normal physiologic function both internal muscle and joint reaction forces are necessary to balance static and dynamic external forces. These work in conjunction with the ligaments spanning the joint to provide stability throughput the entire range of motion.[10,12] External forces are usually applied at the hand and transmitted to the elbow joint through the forearm. Static external forces, such as a weight in the hand, will change the internal reaction forces significantly with joint position because of changes in the moment arm distances of each muscle pull. Dynamic forces, known as inertial or acceleration forces ($F = MA$), can contribute high joint reaction forces because of the acceleration or decleration of the limb itself. Although dynamic forces exist in both the hip and knee joint, they are significantly greater in the elbow because of the high limb accelerations possible during normal physiologic functions, as typically found in throwing a baseball or swinging a tennis racket.

Dynamic forces, though playing a major role in joint reaction forces, are at present under investigation and not fully known. An analysis of dynamic forces would require a sophisticated biomechanical formulation, which is beyond the scope of this presentation. However, they will only be significant during elbow motion in which the upper extremity is moving with a rapid motion. Therefore we will restrict ourselves to only those joint reaction forces that are developed during quasistatic function.

I describe the biomechanics of the joint forces about the elbow by including only the triceps and biceps muscles in a two-dimensional description of flexion-extension motion (Fig. 14-1). The biceps and triceps muscle forces are assumed to

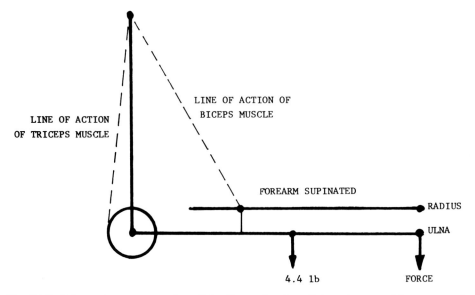

Fig. 14-2. Schematic representation of the lines of action of the triceps and biceps muscle with the forearm in supination. The weight of the forearm is approximately 4.4 pounds, and the applied force acts at the hand.

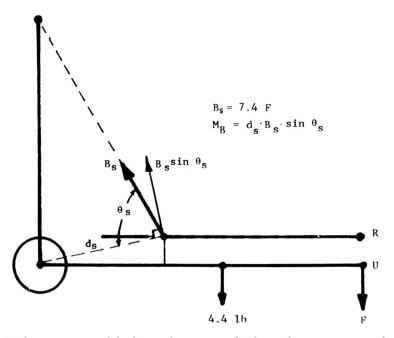

Fig. 14-3. The component of the biceps force perpendicular to the moment arm, d_s, acts to balance the forearm. *R*, Radius; *U*, ulna; *F*, force.

act about a center of joint rotation positioned at the center of humeral capitulum. A schematic representation of the elbow is shown in Fig. 14-2. The distal end of the triceps muscle line of action is attached to the olecranon process. The forearm is shown supinated with the distal end of the biceps muscle attached to the proximal radius. This radial attachment is superior to the ulna in the anteroposterior plane. During pronation this attachment site will be rotated inferiorly and becomes aligned with the ulna in the coronal plane, shown schematically in Fig. 14-8.

Two external forces will be assumed to act on the forearm: (1) the constant weight of the forearm, an average of 4.4 pounds, exerted at its center of gravity, and (2) a force, F, equal to 25 pounds, applied at the hand. This latter force will always be assumed perpendicular to the longitudinal axis of the forearm. It represents a typical physiologic load that might be experienced during the performance of a work function, that is, where a constant force is exerted against the hand during an entire flexion-extension cycle. The situation in which this force is attributable strictly to a gravitational pull (that is, a dead weight) will be treated as a minor case.

The magnitude and line of action of the biceps force at 90 degrees of flexion is shown schematically is Fig. 14-3. The biceps force, B_s, acts at a distance, d_s, from the center of rotation. Its perpendicular component about the center of rotation, $B_s \sin \theta_s$, provides a moment about the joint of $M_B = d_s B_s \sin \theta_s$. In order to achieve equilibrium and thus balance the forearm at a fixed-flexion position, this moment must equal the moment about the joint exerted by the external loads. As such, the biceps muscle force, B_s, is inversely proportional to both the moment arm, d_s, and the sine of the angle between them. For a force of $F = 25$ pounds, the biceps must exert a force of 7.4 F, or over one body weight, to achieve equilibrium.

At 20 degrees of flexion (Fig. 14-4), there is a decrease in the angle θ between the line of action of the biceps muscle and the moment arm between the center of joint rotation and the distal muscle attachment point. Thus the biceps force must increase in order to increase its perpendicular component ($B_{20} \sin \theta$). At this position a biceps force of 16.6 F is required to balance the forearm, approximately 2.3 times the muscle force necessary at 90 degrees of flexion. As the flexion angle decreases toward full extension, the advantage of the biceps muscle decreases, requiring greater muscle force to balance the applied load.

Shown in Fig. 14-5 is a graph of the biceps-triceps muscle force necessary to balance the forearm for flexion angles from 0 to 90 degrees. The biceps muscle must exert a force approximately 8 times the applied force F at 90 degrees of flexion. This increases to almost 38 times the applied force in full extension. A similar result is found for the triceps muscle. The dotted line represents the biceps muscle force required to balance the forearm when the applied force is always acting in the direction of gravity. At 90 degrees of flexion the biceps force is identical to the perpendicular force but steadily decreases during extension as the moment arm between the center of rotation and applied force decreases. In the for-

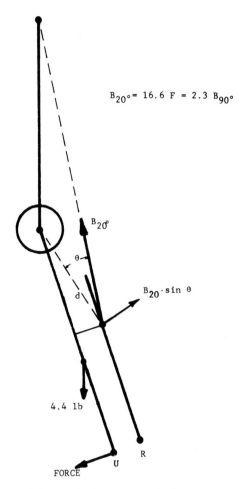

Fig. 14-4. At 20 degrees of flexion the biceps muscle force increases to exert the required moment about the joint center so that the forearm is in balance. *R*, Radius; *U*, ulna.

mer case the moment arm remained constant (length of the forearm), requiring a greater muscle force as the elbow extended. This type of constant perpendicular force is similar to that applied when one is testing isokinetic muscle response using a Cybex machine.

Because of the proximity of the muscle attachments to the joint center, the joint reaction force, *R*, attributable to each muscle pull, will be only slightly lower than the individual muscle forces themselves (Fig. 14-6). For the constant perpendicular force an extremely high joint reaction force is possible with the forearm in extension, whereas that attributable to gravity forces (*dotted line*, from biceps pull) will be lowest in extension. The direction of the joint reaction force relative to the

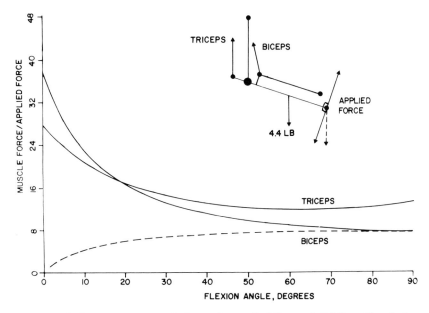

Fig. 14-5. Muscle force necessary to balance the applied force. *Solid line,* Muscle forces for an applied force always perpendicular to the forearm; *dotted line,* biceps force for a force in the direction of gravity.

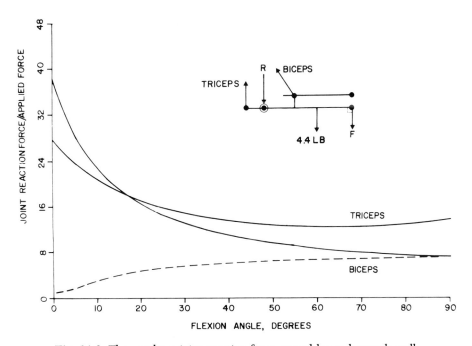

Fig. 14-6. The resultant joint reaction force caused by each muscle pull.

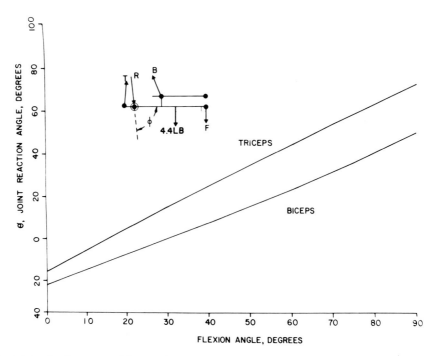

Fig. 14-7. The direction of the resultant joint reaction force, ϕ, acting at the center of elbow rotation.

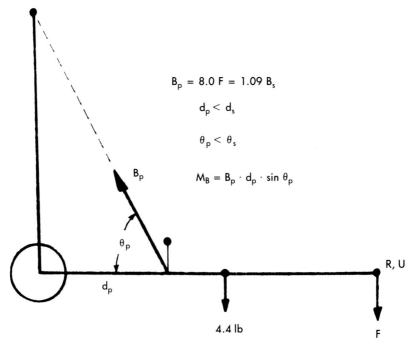

Fig. 14-8. Schematic representation of the line of action of the biceps muscle with the forearm in pronation. R, U, Radius and ulna.

forearm axis, ϕ, is shown in Fig. 14-7. At 90 degrees of flexion a large anteroposterior shear exists with a small component of axial loading. At full extension a high
axially directed force is found with a small anteroposterior shear component.

As the forearm goes into pronation, the radius rotates about the ulna such that
the radial attachment of the biceps muscle moves posteriorly until it aligns with
the ulna in the coronal plane (Fig. 14-8). This effectively decreases the moment
arm between the center of rotation and the biceps attachment point, d_p, while also
decreasing the angle between the biceps line of action and the longitudinal axis of
the forearm, θ_p. These decreases effectively reduce the moment exerted by the
biceps muscle about the joint center and require a greater biceps force to balance
the forearm (Fig. 14-9). At 90 degrees of flexion the biceps force in pronation is
approximately 9% greater than that required in supination. This increase in biceps
force in pronation as compared to supination becomes increasingly evident as the
elbow goes into extension.

During normal physiologic function the elbow joint can easily experience a force
that can be several times body weight. Both the hip and knee joints have been described as "weight-bearing" joints since they are loaded to several times body weight
during normal gait. Even though the elbow joint does not carry the body weight, it is
still a joint that experiences forces as high as those found in either the hip or knee joint.
We might term this type of joint a "force- or load-carrying joint."

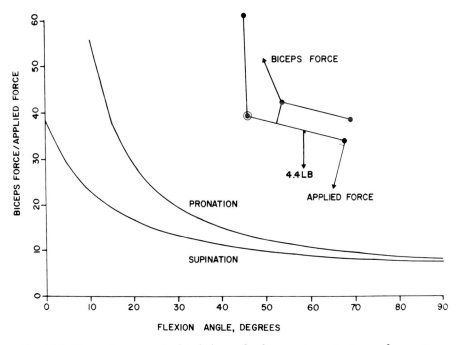

Fig. 14-9. Biceps force required to balance the forearm in supination and pronation.

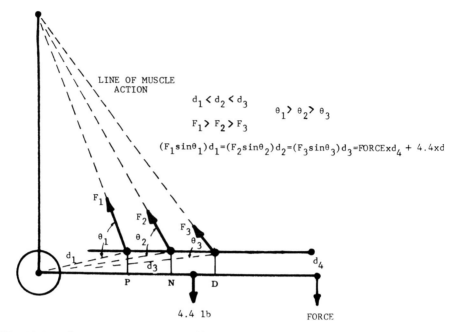

Fig. 14-10. Schematic representation of biceps muscle transfer from the normal position, N, either distally, D, or proximally, P.

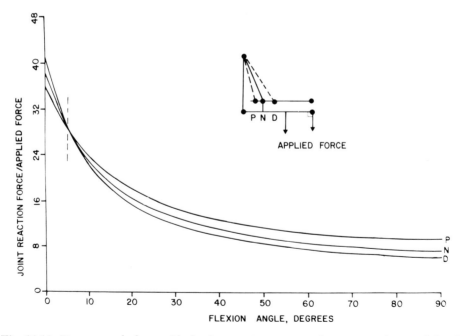

Fig. 14-11. Biceps muscle force with the forearm in supination for a proximal, P, and distal, D, transfer as compared to the normal, N, attachment site.

The position of the distal attachment point of each specific muscle and thus the distance between the center of rotation and the line of action of the muscle force play an important role in the amount of muscle and joint reaction force experienced by the elbow. This can be illustrated when one assumes the attachment point of the biceps muscle to be transferred (by $1/2$ inch) either proximally, *P*, or distally, *D*, with respect to the center of elbow joint rotation, shown schematically in Fig. 14-10. As the attachment site is moved distally from the joint center (point *N* to point *D*), the moment arm increases (from d_2 to d_3) and the angle between the moment arm and the line of muscle action decreases (from θ_2 to θ_3). A distal transfer has the result that a smaller biceps muscle force is required to balance the forearm. The opposite would occur for a proximal transfer from point *N* to *P*. Results are shown in Fig. 14-11 for various positions of elbow flexion.

At large flexion angles the proximal transfer requires greater biceps muscle force than does a distal transfer when compared to the normal attachment site. However, as the elbow joint goes into extension, an angle is reached (at approximately 5 degrees of flexion) at which this moment relation reverses. The component of the biceps force perpendicular to the moment arm in a proximal transfer, F_p', becomes greater than the perpendicular force in a distal transfer, F_d', because of the difference in the angles between the muscle line of action and the moment arm, shown schematically in Fig. 14-12. For flexion angles less than 5 degrees, the muscle force necessary to balance the forearm for the distal transfer, F_d, becomes greater than that found from the proximal transfer, F_p (Fig. 14-12).

In a similar manner, if the location of the center of joint rotation is transferred (by $1/2$ inch) while the biceps attachment site remains constant (Fig. 14-13), the biceps force for a proximal movement, *P*, is reduced as compared to a distal transfer, *D*, for large flexion angles. As the elbow goes into extension, this relationship is again found to reverse, with the distal transfer producing smaller joint reaction forces at flexion angles of 10 degrees or less. It is interesting to note that this point of load reversal occurs at a greater flexion angle for a joint transfer as compared to that found for a biceps transfer.

These illustrative examples of muscle and joint reaction force have been determined from a simplified biomechanical model. With the action of more than one muscle and the addition of inertial forces, the magnitude and direction of the resultant forces may be drastically altered. In general, however, the range of muscle and joint forces found here are consistent with those from more sophisticated studies. Hui and others[5,6] included various muscle groups in a three-dimensional biomechanical analysis of elbow forces during isometric lifting (Table 14-1). Larger joint reaction forces were found in extension as compared to the flexed elbow, and in pronation as compared to supination. Large twisting moments about the long axis of the humerus were also found. Similar results were found by Amis and others,[1] Arvikar and Seireg,[3] and Nicol and others.[10]

The role of the position of the muscle attachments and the relative position of the center of joint rotation are important considerations when elbow joint function

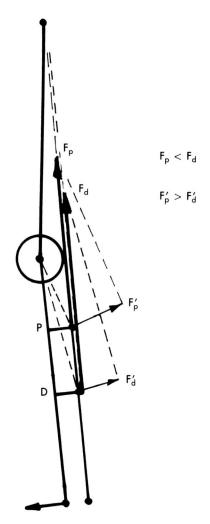

$F_p < F_d$

$F_p' > F_d'$

Fig. 14-12. Schematic representation of biceps muscle force at 5 degrees of flexion for a proximal, *P*, and distal, *D*, transfer. Here the proximal transfer exerts a greater perpendicular component, F_P', than the distal transfer, F_D'.

Table 14-1. Elbow joint forces (percentage of applied force)

	Axial	Anteroposterior shear	Mediolateral shear	Resultant
Extention-supination	12.1	8.7	0.1	14.9
Extention-pronation	16.0	5.7	4.7	17.6
Flexion-supination	2.8	5.2	1.2	6.0
Flexion-pronation	2.0	6.2	1.7	6.7

Modified from Hui, F.C., Chao, E.Y.S., and An, K.N.: Muscle and joint forces at the elbow during isometric lifting, Twenty-fourth meeting of the Orthopaedic Research Society, Dallas, Texas, 1978.

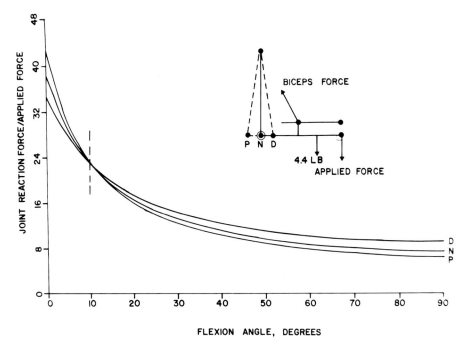

Fig. 14-13. Biceps force necessary to balance the forearm for a proximal, *P*, and distal, *D*, transfer of the normal, *N*, center of rotation in supination.

is being repaired. The complicated anatomic muscle arrangements about the joint center require a thorough knowledge of the resulting characteristics of the elbow after reconstructive surgery. When designing and choosing elbow prostheses, one must take care to utilize this information to achieve the necessary anatomic and functional relationships required for a satisfactory physiologic result.

KINEMATICS OF ELBOW MOTION

Kinematics is the branch of mechanics that involves study of the relative motion between two nondeformable rigid bodies without regard to the forces or other factors that influence the motion. When pure rotations occur, an instant center or axis of rotation can be found with respect to one of the bodies about which the other body rotates or pivots for small increments of motion. Once this axis is determined, the relative velocity between the bodies at any point of contact can be determined. Walker[13] and London[7] used a two-dimensional analysis of instant centers of rotation to determine the axis of elbow flexion-extension. A three-dimensional kinematic analysis was performed by Morrey and Chao[9] and Youm and others[14] to describe the normal range of motion of forearm pronation-supination and elbow flexion-extension.

The elbow joint is a composite of two independent uniaxial joints. The humeroulnar articulation forms a hinged or ginglymus joint. A pivot or trochoid joint exists between the humeroradial and proximal radioulnar articulations. Thus the elbow has two degrees of freedom.

Motion at the elbow consists of rotation of the ulna about the humerus during flexion-extension, and rotation of the radius about the ulna during supination-pronation. The geometric congruity of the articulating surfaces, together with the compressive force exerted by the muscles and ligaments spanning the joint, confine the joint motion to almost pure rotation. The humeroulnar joint is constrained by the saddle-shaped geometry of the trochlea. This forms a perfect hinge joint, which can be described by a single rotational axis.[9,14] The radius, confined by the annular ligament and the articulation between the concave radial head and spheric humeral capitulum, rotates about the ulna. Here forearm supination-pronation is achieved by the motion of the distal end of the radius about the distal end of the ulna. Forearm motion can also be described by a single axis of rotation.[14] Because flexion-extension and forearm supination-pronation each occur about a single, indepen-

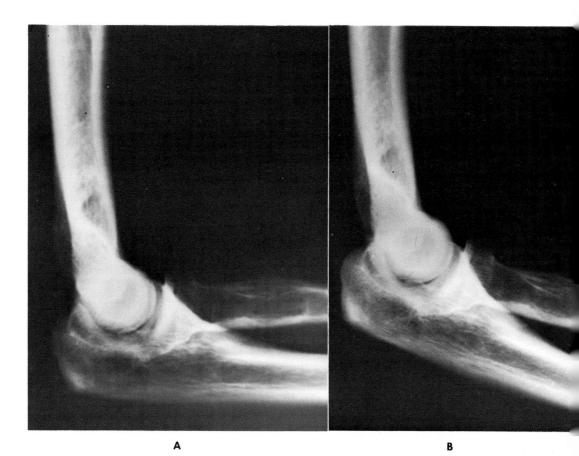

A   B

Fig. 14-14. Lateral roentgenogram of the elbow at 75 and 60 degrees of flexion.

dent rotational axis, the kinematics of the joint motion can best be analyzed by use of instant centers of rotation.

The technique of instant centers of rotation assumes the humerus and forearm to represent two rigid bodies linked together at the elbow joint. For flexion-extension one can determine the motion of the ulna relative to the humerus by utilizing successive roentgenographic projections at two different flexion positions. Care should be taken to obtain lateral roentgenograms with the humeral capitulum and trochlea aligned and superimposed to form two concentric circles (Fig. 14-14). Successive roentgenograms can then be taken after small flexion angle changes and the humerus superimposed from two successive films to provide a description of the motion of two points on the ulna (Fig. 14-15). The intersection of the perpendicular bisectors of the line connecting the motion of each point defines the instant center of rotation. This is continued for each successive position of rotation, providing a locus of points defining the instant center for the entire range of flexion-extension (Fig. 14-16).[13] Similar studies have been conducted for the knee joint[2,4] and for the ankle.[11]

Each position of the instant center defines the instantaneous axis of rotation

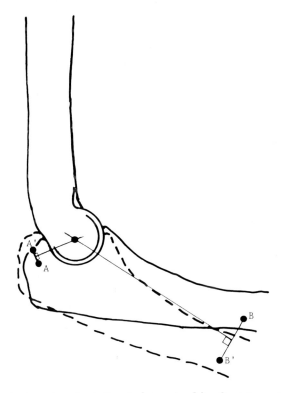

Fig. 14-15. The instant center of rotation is determined by the intersection of the perpendicular bisectors of the line connecting the motion of points *A* and *A'* and *B* to *B'*, shown during extension from 75 to 60 degrees of flexion.

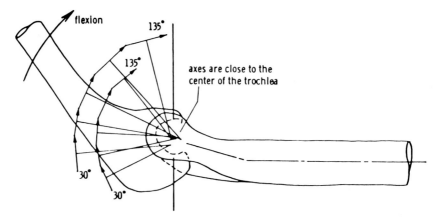

Fig. 14-16. Geometric construction for the determination of the locus of instant centers of rotation for the normal range of motion. (From Walker, P.S.: Human joints and their artificial replacements, Springfield, Ill., 1977, Charles C Thomas, Publisher.)

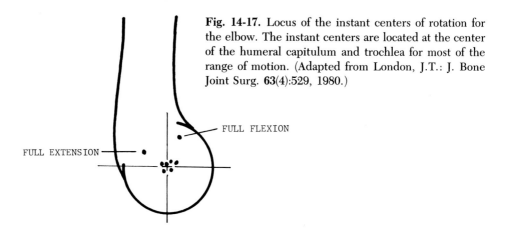

Fig. 14-17. Locus of the instant centers of rotation for the elbow. The instant centers are located at the center of the humeral capitulum and trochlea for most of the range of motion. (Adapted from London, J.T.: J. Bone Joint Surg. **63**(4):529, 1980.)

about which the elbow moves for a particular increment of joint rotation (Fig. 14-17). Except at the extremes of motion the locus of instant centers lies at the approximate center of the concentric circles formed by the lateral projections of the humeral capitulum and trochlea. This locus of instant centers indicates a smooth sliding motion at the articular surface. Only at full extension and full flexion are the instant centers displaced from the center of the concentric circles, indicating impingement of the ulna on the humerus at the extremes of motion. Thus during most of the range of normal flexion-extension the articulating surfaces glide smoothly over one another with a single axis of rotation.

When viewed from the frontal plane, this rotational axis is found to be medially or internally rotated 4 to 8 degrees with respect to the longitudinal axis of the humerus (Fig. 14-18).[7] Morrey and Chao[9] stated that the carrying angle varied from approximately 11 degrees of valgus in full extension to 6 degrees of varus in full flexion when viewed from the anterior direction (Fig. 14-19). However, with

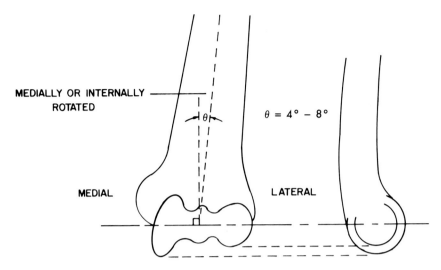

Fig. 14-18. Position of the axis of rotation for flexion-extension. The axis is rotated medially or internally with respect to the long axis of the humerus.

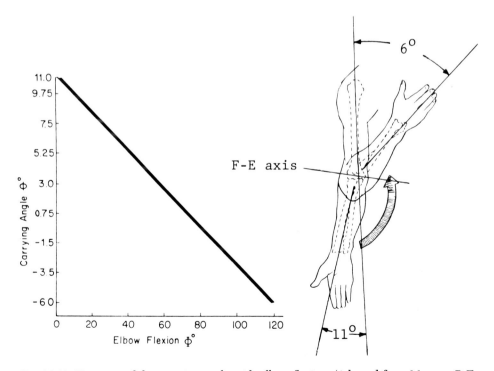

Fig. 14-19. Variation of the carrying angle with elbow flexion. (Adapted from Morrey, B.F., and Chao, E.Y.S.: J. Bone Joint Surg. **58A:**501, 1976.)

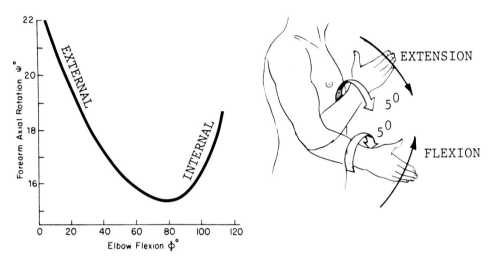

Fig. 14-20. Forearm axial rotation with elbow flexion. (Adapted from Morrey, B.F., and Chao, E.Y.S.: J. Bone Joint Surg. **58A:**501, 1976.)

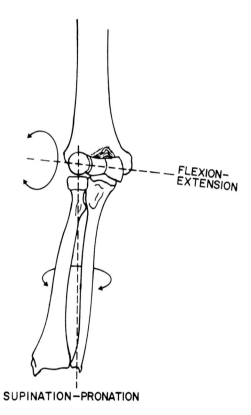

SUPINATION–PRONATION

Fig. 14-21. The axis of rotation for supination-pronation is directed along a line connecting the distal end of the ulna and the center of the humeral capitulum.

respect to this internally rotated axis the carrying angle is probably constant throughout the normal flexion-extension range.

During the normal range of elbow flexion and extension the forearm internally and externally rotates approximately 5 degrees about the neutral position (Fig. 14-20).[9] Forearm axial rotation is most likely attributable to supination-pronation of the radius about the ulna[7,14] and not to any incongruities in the humeral articular surfaces or ligament constraints.[9] Youm and others,[14] using instant centers of rotation, found the longitudinal axis of forearm rotation for pronation-supination to be directed along a line connecting the distal end of the ulna and the center of the humeral capitulum (Fig. 14-21). With respect to the neutral position the forearm pronated an average of 70 degrees while forearm supination averaged 45 degrees. No ulna movement was detected during pronation-supination, nor any axial rotation or mediolateral movement during flexion-extension.

It would appear therefore that the humeroulnar joint is a "perfect" hinge with respect to the internally rotated flexion-extension axis described. Forearm supination-pronation is also a purely rotational motion described by a single longitudinally directed axis. These two motions are independent and uniaxial, and so the elbow joint is restricted to two degrees of freedom.

SUMMARY

The biomechanical analysis presented here is an endeavor to illustrate some of the aspects of the forces generated about the elbow joint during normal physiologic function and to define the kinematic motion of the elbow joint during flexion-extension and supination-pronation.

From the static analysis of the muscle and joint reaction forces we can conclude with the following:

1. Muscle and joint reaction forces can be several times body weight during normal activity
2. Joint forces are greatest in extension; thus the flexed elbow can tolerate a higher load than the extended elbow can.
3. Joint forces are greatest in pronation because of the decreased moment arm of the biceps muscle.
4. Twisting moments about the humeral axis are probably high, being a significant factor when the prosthetic design is considered.
5. A distal transfer of the biceps muscle attachment decreases the joint reaction forces; however, near full extension this mechanical advantage may be reversed.
6. Joint positional changes may cause this reversal to occur at greater flexion angles.

From the kinematic analysis of elbow motion we can conclude with the following:

1. Flexion-extension occurs about a single axis through the centers of the humeral trochlea and capitulum. This axis is internally rotated 4 to 8 degrees with respect to the long axis of the humerus.

2. Sliding occurs at the joint surfaces until the extremes of full flexion and extension are reached, at which point bony impingement occurs.
3. The humeroulnar joint is a perfect hinge, with little or no extraneous relative motion during pronation-supination or flexion-extension.
4. The carrying angle (ulna relative to the humerus in the coronal plane) varies from approximately 11 degrees of valgus in full extension to 6 degrees of varus in full flexion.
5. The carrying angle is relatively constant with respect to the flexion-extension axis.
6. The forearm axially rotates (supination-pronation) about a single axis during elbow flexion-extension.

REFERENCES

1. Amis, A.A., Dowson, D., Wright, V., and Miller, J.H.: The derivation of elbow joint forces and their relation to prosthesis design, J. Med. Eng. Tech. **3:**229, 1979.
2. Arnoczky, S.P., Torzilli, P.A., and Marshall, J.L.: Biomechanical evaluation of anterior cruciate ligament repair in the dog: an analysis of the instant center of motion, J. Am. Animal Hosp. Assoc. **13:**553-558,1977.
3. Arvikar, R., and Seireg, A.: Evaluation of upper extremity joint forces during exercise, 1978 Advances in Bioengineering, American Society of Mechanical Engineers, Winter Annual Meeting, San Francisco, Calif., 1978, pp. 71 to 73.
4. Frankel, V.H., Burstein, A.H., and Brooks, D.B.: Biomechanics of internal derangement of the knee: pathomechanics as determined by analysis of the instant centers of motion, J. Bone Joint Surg. **53A:**945-963, 1971.
5. Hui, F.C., An, K.N., and Chao, E.Y.: Three-dimensional force analysis of the elbow under isometric functions, 1977 Biomechanics Symposium, New York City, American Society of Mechanical Engineers—Applied Mechanics Division **23:**94-98, 1977.
6. Hui, F.C. Chao, E.Y.S., and An, K.N.: Muscle and joint forces at the elbow during isometric lifting, Twenty-fourth meeting of the Orthopaedic Research Society, Dallas, Texas, 1978, pp. 167.
7. London, J.T.: Kinematics of the elbow, J. Bone Joint Surg. **63**(4):529, 1981.
8. Morrey, B.F., and Bryan, R.S.: Total joint arthroplasty: the elbow, Mayo Clin. Proc. **54:**507, 1979.
9. Morrey, B.F., and Chao, E.Y.S.: Passive motion of the elbow joint, J. Bone Joint Surg. **58A:**501, 1976.
10. Nicol, A.C., Berme, N., and Paul, J.P.: A biomechanical analysis of elbow joint function. In Joint replacement in the upper limb, London, 1977, Mechanical Engineering Publications, Ltd.
11. Sammarco, G.J., Burstein, A.H., and Frankel, V.H.: Biomechanics of the ankle: a kinematic study, Orthop. Clin. North Am. **4:**75-96, 1973.
12. Schwab, G.H., Bennett, J.B., Woods, G.W., and Tullos, H.S.: Biomechanics of elbow instability: the role of the medial collateral ligament, Clin. Orthop. Rel. Res. **146:**42, 1980.
13. Walker, P.S.: Human joints and their artificial replacements, Springfield, Ill., 1977, Charles C. Thomas, Publisher.
14. Youm, Y., Dryer, R.F., Thambrajah, K., Flatt, A.E., and Sprague, B.L.: Biomechanical analysis of forearm pronation-supination and elbow flexion-extension, J. Biomechanics **12:**245, 1979.

PART FOUR

The hand and wrist

15. Anatomy of the metacarpophalangeal joint in rheumatoid arthritis: etiology of ulnar drift

Lee Ramsay Straub, M.D.

In the group of diseases that we classify as rheumatoid arthritis the villain is diseased synovium. Just as each of these diseases has subtle variations, so too are there differences in the synovium. Some have acute and expansile synovitis causing rapid joint enlargement; others have chronic dry synovitis, similar to a pannus overlying articular cartilage. In some there is exuberant joint enlargement with little other articular change. It is here that early synovectomy may be an effective procedure. On the other hand, the "dry" type tends to stiffen joints and may lead to ankylosis.

ULNAR DRIFT

Abnormal synovium is the common denominator of all deformities in the rheumatoid hand. There has been much written about the cause of ulnar drift. Many authors have proposed a single cause of this deformity. Smith and his colleagues[5,6] at the University of Michigan did careful mechanical and mathematical studies of the forces applied by the long flexor tendons to the volar plate of a diseased joint. This accounted for forward displacement of the base of the phalanx on the meta-carpal head and for ulnar drift attitude of the index, long, and ring fingers; it did not, however, account for ulnar drift in the little finger. Shapiro[4] and his group, working in Heinola, Finland, related the ulnar deviation of the phalanges to radial collapse of the carpus and indicated that the collapse may be the causative factor of ulnar drift.

To come to any conclusion as to the cause of this rather consistent deformity in the rheumatoid patient, one must first observe with minuteness the normal anatomy around the metacarpophalangeal joint. This can only be done in fresh anatomic specimens because the tissues in preserved cadavers are usually hardened, a condition precluding minute observation.

SOME FEATURES OF NORMAL ANATOMY AT THE METACARPOPHALANGEAL JOINT

A proximal phalanx is stabilized on the metacarpal head by a number of fibrous structures. The metacarpal head is monocondylar opposing the phalanx in extension. In flexion, however, the shape of the metacarpal heads forms two condyles that provide strong stability when the metacarpophalangeal joints are flexed to 90 degrees and the collateral ligaments are intact. The volar plate (or volar ligament) is particularly important. It is a very strong and clearly demarcated structure. It is firmly attached to the volar base of the proximal phalanx. Proximally, it is thinned and has loose attachment. With flexion and extension it slides like a window blind. A number of other structures attach and contribute fibers to this volar plate as it lies in front or volar to the metacarpal head. The transverse fibers of the dorsal hood and the joint capsule surround the metacarpal head and make attachment to each side of the volar plate. The radial and ulnar collateral ligaments make similiar attachment to the plate margins. The very strong transverse and cruciate fibers of the A1 and A2 pulleys of the flexor tendon sheath make rigid attachment to the volar plate from its palmar surface. Finally, and most importantly, the transverse intervolar plate ligament blends its fibers with that of each volar plate as it crosses

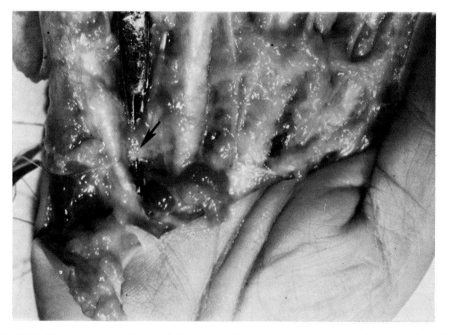

Fig. 15-1. Hemostat passed beneath the intervolar plate ligament, *arrow*, between the volar plates of the fourth and fifth metacarpophalangeal joints.

deep in the palm (Figs. 15-1 and 15-2). This ligament is very strong and thick between the little finger and the ring finger and between the ring finger and the long finger. It is usually thinner between the long finger and the index finger. The tendon of the powerful abductor digiti minimi muscle makes firm attachment to the volar plate of the little finger and, through it, exerts a strong ulnar force to the other volar plates through the transverse ligament (Fig. 15-3). This ligament is an important stabilizer of the ulnar half of the hand in power grip.

As each of the tendons of the interosseous muscles pass by their respective metacarpal heads, they lie directly on the dorsum of the intervolar plate ligament at its juncture to that volar plate. At this point these tendons give firm attachment to the capsule and the side of the volar plate before passing distally into the lateral band of the finger. It is here that the interosseous muscles exert their greatest force for metacarpophalangeal flexion.

Study of the collateral ligaments show that they have partial synovial coverage in their sulci on the metacarpal head. This coverage is nearly complete around the radial collateral ligament and much less around the ulnar collateral ligament. This may suggest that compression and enzymatic penetration by a diseased synovium causes earlier destruction of the radial collateral ligament than of the ulnar. This is borne out almost universally in dissection of the diseased joints at surgery.

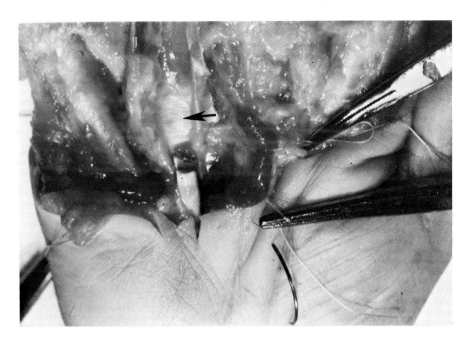

Fig. 15-2. With the long flexor tendons divided and reflected, the volar plate is visualized, *arrow*. Ulnar retraction of the neurovascular bundle exposes the confluence of the ulnar intervolar plate ligament into the volar plate of the fourth metacarpophalangeal joint.

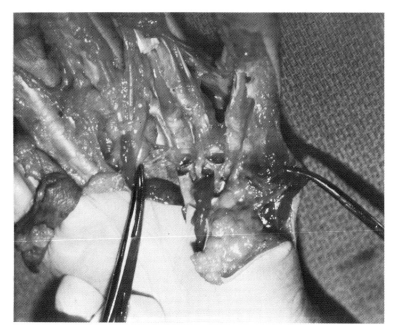

Fig. 15-3. Tension on abductor digiti minimi causes ulnar traction, *A*, on volar plates, *B*, through the intervolar plate ligaments. If joints are unstable, ulnar drift ensues. (Ring finger tendons resected.)

THE STRESS POINT

Early in the rheumatoid process, through a massive infiltration of inflammatory and plasma cells into the synovium, joint enlargement and tension may occur. Toxic enzymes produced by cell breakdown may destroy ligaments, cartilage, and even bone. Distension of the joint capsule produces an eventual shift in the volar plate position. The joint capsule is weakened in a number of areas, but mostly on the dorsal and radial side of the joint. The radial collateral ligament is attenuated by its surrounding synovial membrane, which is both compressive and destructive. The dorsal support of the joint capsule and hood to the radial side of the volar plate are gradually weakened. It is this juncture of the dorsal fibers of hood, capsule, and collateral ligament with the volar plate to which I refer as the stress point. With dorsal support gone, the volar and ulnar forces take over to produce ulnar drift, flexion, and eventual forward dislocation of the proximal phalanx.

The basic process is as follows. The attachment of the volar plate to the volar base of the proximal phalanx remains strong. With the joint expansion and ligamentous weakening caused by the inflammatory process and with the pain and muscle spasm related to it, an ulnar and flexor drag of the proximal phalanx begins. Primary involvement is to the third, fourth, and fifth metacarpophalangeal joints.

The process at the index metacarpophalangeal joint is slightly different (see below). The abductor digiti minimi and the associated hypothenar muscles working through the intervolar plate ligaments exert a strong ulnar force to the volar plates. This drags the proximal phalanx into ulnar drift. The ulnar interosseous muscles also enhance this motion. At the same time the flexor force of the flexores digitorum profundus and superficialis is applied to the volar plate through the flexor sheath attachments. With weakening of the dorsal hood especially on its radial side a forward shift of the base of the phalanx begins. Since the hood is most weakened on its dorsal radial aspect, ulnar deviation becomes part of this movement. Early in this process before actual ulnar angulation of the phalanges develops, shift of the long extensor tendons starts to deviate toward the ulnar valleys. This may begin as a "snapping" phenomenon especially over the fourth and fifth metacarpal heads. Eventually all the four extensor tendons shift into their respective ulnar "valleys." In extreme deformities these tendons may be found dislocated forward on the ulnar side of the metacarpal head, there becoming a flexor and ulnar deviating force rather than an extensor.

ULNAR DRIFT AT INDEX FINGER

Synovial expansion and tissue change has the same deleterious effect on the structures of the second metacarpophalangeal joint as it does elsewhere. Flatt and his associates[1] have demonstrated that in the normal hand the index finger rests in slight ulnar angulation to its metacarpal. The first dorsal interosseous, a powerful muscle, would naturally be expected, through its attachment to the base of the proximal phalanx, to prevent any ulnar angulation at that metacarpophalangeal joint. Further, this intervolar plate ligament was almost wanting in most of our dissections.

In observing the course of the ulnar drift deformity over a period I would suggest that the index finger is usually the slowest to develop a severe ulnar drift deformity. The fact that the deformity occurs at all has led to a great deal of conjecture and controversy. Some years ago Flatt[1] had suggested the possibility of denervation of the first dorsal interosseous muscle by synovial pressure on its nerve supply. This theory has not been supported by muscle biopsy at the time of corrective surgery.

Eiler and Markee[2] indicated that the insertion of the first dorsal interosseous was entirely to bone. Our dissection and our findings at clinical surgery would indicate that in passing the metacarpophalangeal joint level the fibers of the insertion of the first dorsal go to bone only after first becoming intimately related with fibers of the dorsal hood and capsule of the radial aspect of the joint (Fig. 15-4). When weakening and distention of the joint occurs and when the phalanx starts to shift slightly forward on the metacarpal head, the interosseous insertion tends to drop forward and loses its strong abductor force. At operation the abductor tendon is found to lie forward of its normal position. With this, pronation of the index finger has occurred. With simultaneous destruction of the radial collateral ligament

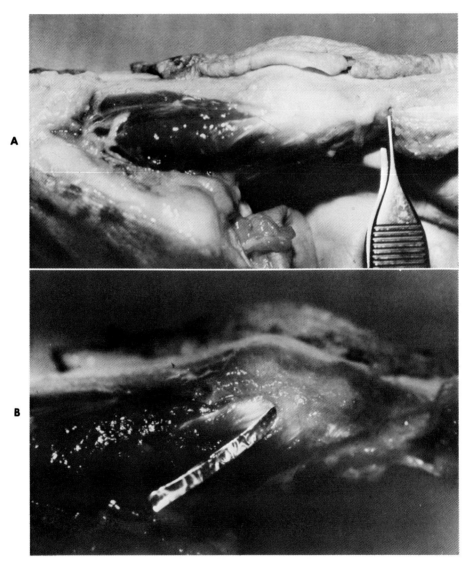

Fig. 15-4. Tendon of first dorsal interosseous muscle passing beneath arc of transverse fibers of the dorsal "hood," to insert into the joint capsule and thence to the base of the proximal phalanx of the index finger.

and the attenuation of the radial dorsal hood, the flexor force of the long flexor tendons passing through the pulleys to the volar plate produces an ulnar pull and eventual forward dislocation of the base of the phalanx on the second metacarpal head.

It must be recalled that preceding and concomitant with these deformities synovitis in all these joints has reduced the height of the articular cartilage and, with simultaneous articular erosion, synovitis has greatly reduced the inherent stability of the joints.

If all the previously mentioned factors are analyzed and are as we believe true, ulnar drift is a result of a complicated interaction of the effects of synovitis on all the articular and periarticular structures. Although there is the theory that the Z-wrist collapse may have a relaxing affect on the long tendons passing the metacarpophalangeal joint, I do not believe that it is related to the cause of the ulnar drift deformity; rather it is a concomitant event resulting from synovitis locally at the wrist.

Correction of the ulnar drift deformity requires a careful understanding of the anatomy of this disease. In the early stage of the disease before serious deformity of the metacarpal head, synovectomy (reconstruction of the radial hood and capsule) is accompanied by intrinsic transfer. "Intrinsic transfer" refers to transfer of the ulnar interosseous muscle of each of the fingers to the radial hood or intrinsic tendon of its ulnar neighboring finger. At the little finger the abductor digiti minimi is divided and a section of its muscle belly removed.

In the severely dislocated metacarpophalangeal joint where implants are to be placed, the ulnar intrinsic muscle is transferred or at least resected.

METACARPOHALANGEAL JOINT OF THE THUMB

Normally the forces exerting flexion at the base of the proximal phalanx of the thumb are far greater than those forces of extension. The adductor attaching to the medial sesamoid and those of the abductor pollicis brevis attaching to the lateral sesamoid transmit a great flexor force to the volar plate, which is firmly attached to the base of the proximal phalanx. Furthermore, the flexor pulley attaches in the same area so that the flexor pollicis brevis also exerts a forward force at this point.

Synovial expansion in the metacarpophalangeal joint of the thumb first expands and weakens the capsule and the transverse fibers of its dorsal hood. The extensor pollicis brevis tendon, which intermingles with the fibers of the hood, soon looses its attachment to the base of the proximal phalanx. As the collateral ligaments are weakened by their local synovitis, the flexor forces overpower the extensor forces. Flexion of the joint occurs along with forward displacement of the phalanx on the metacarpal head and eventual dislocation. There may or may not be lateral instability of the joint depending on the status of the collateral ligaments. The attachments of the short muscles slide forward with the dislocation. Should there be good preservation of articular cartilage as may occur in the early dislocation, reconstruction of the soft tissues with imbrication of the dorsal extensor hood may be sufficient. Should there be any articular surface change, arthrodesis is recommended. In the normal hand this joint often has very limited motion, indicating that fusion is well tolerated.

EVALUATION

Rheumatoid arthritis is a relentless disease. It is rare indeed to hear of a "burnt-out" case. Synovitis with its destruction of bone, ligament, and tendon behaves as a multicentric cancer. There may be long periods of remission, but sudden "flares" may occur at any time. For the seriously involved patient to whom I refer in this chapter, drugs have done but little good. They may temporarily relieve pain and temporarily slow disease activity, but they have done nothing to eliminate the disease. In our efforts at corrective surgery we are often frustrated as the disease continues its slow inexorable progress. Short-term postoperative evaluations of 1 to 3 years may seem most promising. Follow-up determinations of 10 years and longer are almost invariably disappointing. This has been well demonstrated in most rheumatoid joints even where prosthesis of one type or another have been employed. What we need obviously are procedures that will last the lifetime of the patient. As was the case with poliomyelitis, what we really need is a successful vaccination.

REFERENCES

1. Ellison, M.R., Flatt, A.E., and Kelly, K.J.: Ulnar drift of the fingers in rheumatoid disease: treatment by crossed intrinsic tendon transfer, J. Bone Joint Surg. **53A**(6):1061, Sept. 1971.
2. Eyler, D.L., and Markee, J.E.: The anatomy and function of the intrinsic musculature of the fingers, J. Bone Joint Surg. **36A**(1):1-9, 18-20, Jan. 1954.
3. Shapiro, J.S.: Ulnar drift: report of a related finding, Acta Orthop. Scand. **39**:346, 1968.
4. Shapiro, J.S.: A new factor in the etiology of ulnar drift, Clin. Orthop. **68**:32, 1970.
5. Smith, E.M., Juvinall, R.C., Bender, L.F., and Pearson, R.: Role of the finger flexors in rheumatoid deformities of the metacarpal phalangeal joints, Arthritis Rheum. **7**(5):467, 1964.
6. Smith, E.M., Juvinall, R.C., Bender, L.F., and Pearson, R.: Flexor forces and rheumatoid metacarpophalangeal deformity: clinical implications, J.A.M.A. **198**(2):130, Oct. 10, 1966.

16. History, design and development of Steffee metacarpophalangeal prosthesis

Arthur Steffee

Two decades ago, finger joint replacement was in its infancy. From 1956 to 1959, Colonel E.W. Brannon[1] performed the first surgery on military patients with traumatic arthritis. His prosthesis was a stainless-steel hinge. Although the initial reports were encouraging, after a few years bone resorption and migration of the prosthesis became a serious problem. Adrian Flatt[2] modified that prosthesis by designing a steel hinge with two steel pins on either side for anchoring the prosthesis into the intramedullary canal. His prosthesis was used in rheumatoid hands, and the reports in 1961 were encouraging. However, all stresses, whether lateral, anterior, posterior, or rotational, were dissipated through the stems in the bone, causing migration into the bone, and loosening occurred. Eventually, the hinge-and-pin design developed mechanical problems.

These problems suggested a need for a new design, one that would have a "soft" socket to allow the external forces to be absorbed by the socket itself, rather than in the stems anchoring the socket to the bone. The new design simply snapped together, eliminating the use of hinge pins and the rigid interconnection between the proximal and distal components. The stems were designed to fit snugly into the intramedullary canal, along with bone grafts intended to grow across the perforation in the stem, anchoring it firmly, much like the stem of the Austin-Moore hip prosthesis.

The original models, made of Teflon sockets molded on chrome-cobalt alloy stems, had many technical problems in the manufacturing process. These were solved by George Laure of Laure Prosthetics (Kalamazoo, Michigan). The socket design did allow for almost complete reproduction of normal range of motion and lateral deviation in extension, but with increased flexion, loss of all lateral deviation, hyperextension of 15 to 20 degrees, and flexion to 100 degrees.

In 1965, a series of prostheses were implanted into the middle finger on each hand of eight chimpanzees at the Delta Primate Center in Covington, Louisiana (Fig. 16-1, A). The prostheses survived 1 year of implantation. All eventually became infected by *Serratia marcescens*, a nonpathogenic bacteria. Despite the in-

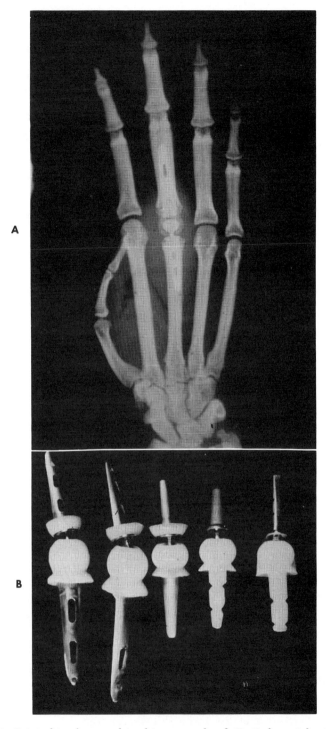

Fig. 16-1. A, Original implant used in chimpanzee hand. **B,** *Left to right,* Original implant for use with bone grafts, chrome-cobalt stems, and Teflon socket; first human implant of chrome-cobalt high-density polyethylene plastic; 1970 model, first used with polymethylmethacrylate cement; dropped center of rotation and all-plastic proximal component; latest model.

fection, mechanically the prostheses functioned well and withstood the various forces applied to it. At that time, Sir John Charnley was noting foreign-body reactions in his patients with Teflon acetabulum components, but he was encouraged by high-density polyethylene. At his suggestion, the sockets were changed from Teflon to RCH-1000, which is still used today.

In 1968, the first prosthesis was implanted into a hand severely destroyed by rheumatoid arthritis (Fig. 16-1, *B*). In 1971, because of the success with bone cement in other areas of total joint replacement, stem modifications were made to utilize cement rather than bone grafts. After implantation of several prostheses, the problem of extensor lag became apparent. Flatt, of the University of Iowa, and the Department of Hand Surgery of the Mayo Clinic suggested a basic design alternation to lower the center of rotation. This gave the extensor tendon a better moment arm for extending the finger (Fig. 16-2).

Flatt and Fisher, in 1969, determined that the center of rotation of the metacarpophalangeal joint was very close to the center of the "ball" of the metacarpal head. Subsequent studies (supported by funds from the DePuy Manufacturing Company, Warsaw, Indiana) using Shonander x-ray technique of various metacarpophalangeal prostheses have shown that the center of rotation of the Steffee prosthesis very nearly approximates that of a normal joint.[3]

The initial goal was to design a prosthesis that reproduced the motion of the normal joint—one that was simple to insert; one that would be well tolerated and could function for the life of the patient. The reproduction of the motion of the normal joint was not difficult to obtain. With many years of experience, it has now become apparent that insertion is not easy. Although each component, including

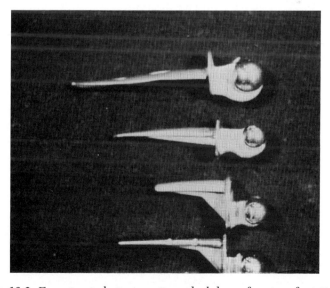

Fig. 16-2. From top to bottom, note gradual drop of center of rotation.

cement, is well tolerated, there is a tendency for a relatively large number of prostheses to loosen. Three main factors causing loosening seem to be:

1. Poor bone stock in the rheumatoid hand
2. Technical errors in reaming
3. Excessive angular and torque forces at the bone-cement interface

One cannot look at a destroyed rheumatoid hand, replace four metacarpophalangeal joints, and expect the hand to function well. Should the wrist be destroyed and in fixed radial deviation, the wrist must either be fused or be replaced before the metacarpophalangeal joints are corrected. Without correction of the radial deviation, recurrent ulnar drift at the metacarpophalangeal level is certain to occur. Tendon transfers at the wrist (bridle procedure) should be done in conjunction with metacarpophalangeal joint replacement if radial deviation is not fixed. Distal to the metacarpophalangeal joint, swan-neck or boutonnière deformities must also be repaired, whether then or at a later time.

Perhaps the most important concept to understand at the metacarpophalangeal level is that of Zancolli's force nucleus[4] (Fig. 16-3). It is the point on the volar aspect where the volar plate, transverse metacarpal ligament, transverse fiber of the extensor hood, collateral ligaments, and fibro-osseous flexor canal coalesce. When the joint is destroyed by rheumatoid arthritis, not only does the extensor mechanism slide down over the ulnar side below the center of rotation, but the force nucleus, also migrating volarly and ulnarly, gives the flexors a much greater mechanical advantage as well. Therefore it is not sufficient to replace the joint without exercising great care in reconstructing the soft tissue around it on both the flexor and extensor surfaces. Because this is so important, a small "wing" has been placed on both sides of the plastic socket to enable the surgeon to maintain the flexor compartment immediately under the prosthesis and to restoring a more normal flexor moment arm (Fig. 16-4). If this is not done, extensor lag and flexion attitude of finger with recurrent ulnar drift will probably be the result.

Through the years, some prostheses have failed because of migration of either the proximal or the distal component, or of cement and all, through the volar aspect of the bone (Fig. 16-5). In most cases, this can be traced to excessive and vigorous reaming with high-speed burrs. Because of the anatomic configuration of the intramedullary canal, it is easy for one to inadvertently "ream out" the volar cortex of the bone, thereby losing all support for the prosthetic stem and cement (Fig. 16-6). In most cases of rheumatoid arthritis, reaming with anything other than a curette is contraindicated.

Breakage of the prosthesis has not been a significant problem. Breakage, when it has occurred, has been only at the juncture of the plastic socket and stem. There have been bench tests that show adequate strength when angular and linear forces are applied to the plastic proximal component. One metacarpophalangeal joint, placed in a flexing apparatus in an air environment and flexed through 90 degrees of motion with 35 pounds of compressive forces for 30 million cycles, has shown no measurable wear.

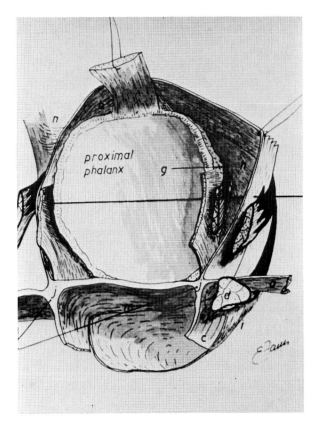

Fig. 16-3. Force nucleus of metacarpophalangeal joint. (From Zancolli, E.: Structural and dynamic bases of hand surgery, Philadelphia, 1968, J.B. Lippincott Co.)

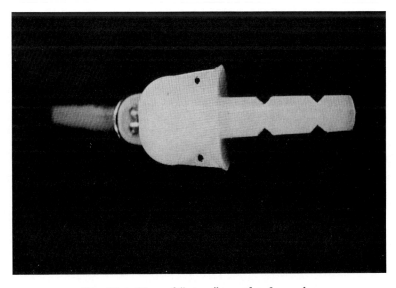

Fig. 16-4. View of "wings" on side of capsule.

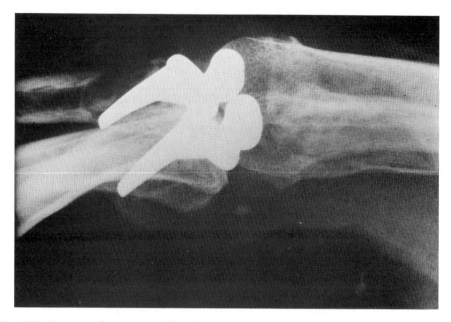

Fig. 16-5. Excessive loosening of distal component and migration of cement through volar aspect of bone.

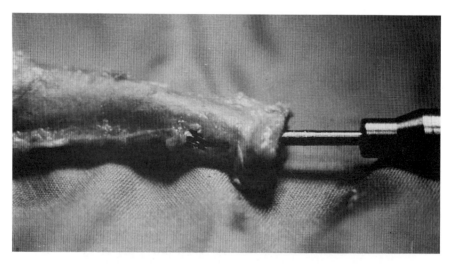

Fig. 16-6. Reamer through volar aspect of bone.

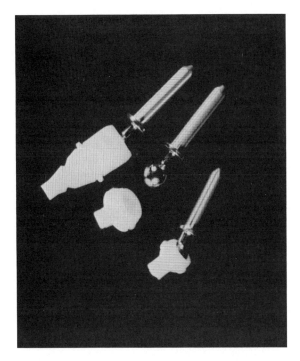

Fig. 16-7. Ball-and-socket joint for carpometacarpal joint replacement of thumb.

The concept of hard joint, as opposed to Silastic spacers, has been carried to the proximal interphalangeal and carpometacarpal joints of the thumb. The proximal interphalangeal joint differs from the metacarpophalangeal only in that motion is allowed in flexion and extension. The carpometacarpal joint, resembling a small total hip, allows complete rotary motion (Fig. 16-7). The plastic socket is designed to be cemented into the trapezium with the metal distal component implanted into the metacarpal. This prosthesis, designed in 1974, has been implanted since 1975 with excellent results. Allowing almost immediate function, it restores stability at the base of the thumb. Loosening has not been a problem because most forces are compressive, not angular or torque. Many surgeons have speculated that reaming the trapezium to accept the plastic socket will cause avascular necrosis. This has not yet occurred in over 100 cases. As with metacarpophalangeal joints, reaming must be done with great care.

Experimental and clinical experience with hard joints now spans 15 years. The largest series of metacarpophalangeal joints of this design has been studied by the Department of Hand Surgery of the Mayo Clinic. They have been involved since 1972, and their results are reported in another paper. The basic design of the metacarpophalangeal prosthesis seems to be adequate; the method of fixation does not. Loosening has been a problem with all total joint replacements, such as those for hips, knees, and shoulder. Those in the hand are no exception.

In May 1981, at the postgraduate course "Upper Extremity Joint Replacement" in Denver, Colorado, all Steffee finger joints were "removed from the market" with the exception of the carpometacarpal joint. It has become apparent that with the use of the "hard joints" cemented into the hand, one can obtain excellent early results, but after 2 to 3 years, the failure rate becomes unacceptably high.

I do not believe this to be attributable to the design of the prosthesis as much as to the means of fixation. Subsidence, as seen in the hip joint, is a very real problem at the metacarpophalangeal and proximal interphalangeal joint levels. Frequently, the entire mass of prosthesis and cement will migrate down the intramedullary canal. This most likely is caused by the difference in the modulus of elasticity between the hard cement and the soft osteoporotic rheumatoid bone. Angular forces and torque also play a major role in this loosening, since it occurs also in "normal" bone of degenerative and traumatic arthritis but not so rapidly.

Considerable effort is being expended today to find a means of anchoring a prosthesis to bone. Bone will not grow into methyl methacrylate cement. It does grow into porous materials, such as cintered metals and some plastics, for example, polysulfone. The basic problem with rheumatoid bone is its deterioration, its thin cortex, and its virtual absence of a cancellous structure. It is difficult to imagine that rheumatoid bone would have the ability to grow and penetrate into any type of biomaterial.

There is no experimental model available that duplicates the poor quality rheumatoid bone. Therefore new prostheses and means of fixing them to bone must be tried experimentally in the patient. Advancement in hand surgery, as in all other disciplines, requires that innovation not be stifled. New designs must be encouraged and new materials tried, until the design of the day needs no further improvement.

REFERENCES

1. Brannon, E.W., and Klein, G.: Experiences with a finger-joint prosthesis, J. Bone Joint Surg. **41A:**87-101, 1959.
2. Flatt, A.E.: The prosthetic replacement of rheumatoid finger joints, Rheumatism **16:**90-97, 1960.
3. Gillespie, T.E., Flatt, A.E., Youm, Y., and Sprague, B.L.: Biochemical evaluation of metacarpophalangeal joint prosthesis designs, J. Hand Surg. 4(6):508, 1979.
4. Zancolli, E.: Structural and dynamic bases of hand surgery, ed. 2, Philadelphia, 1979, J.B. Lippincott Co.

17. Metacarpophalangeal arthroplasty with Steffee prostheses

Ronald L. Linscheid, M.D.
Robert D. Beckenbaugh, M.D.
James H. Dobyns, M.D.
William P. Cooney III, M.D.

A dissatisfaction with the results achieved using various methods of arthroplasty in rheumatoid arthritis led us to consider the usage of a metalloplastic device for metacarpophalangeal arthroplasty.[1] In 1973 the decision to proceed on this course was made with considerable deliberation and only after an in-depth study of results of some 150 hands in which resectional arthroplasty and interposition arthroplasty had been performed. It was also preceded by careful review of the then existing biomechanical studies[2,6] and a close monitoring of total joint arthroplasty performed in other anatomic areas at our institution.

The Steffee device, which consisted of a metal stem for the proximal phalanx and a molded polyethylene snap-fitting metacarpal head with a metallic stem proximally (Mark I), was felt to be suitable (Fig. 17-1). During the early development period, positioning the device for correct extension moment arm length did not prevent metacarpophalangeal flexion deformities and recurrent swan-neck deformities from developing.[3-5]

A redesign with an offset distal and proximal stem and shortened overall length was obtained by conversion of the proximal component to a single polyethylene piece (Mark II). This became available in 1975.[5] It also had a shorter distal stem for easier one-piece insertion. It was believed that the lowered center or rotation provided by this design would overcome the problems previously seen.

In September 1977, the distal stem was lengthened (Mark III) after it was noted that occasional loosening and a palmar tilt of the distal stem were being seen.[5]

This study encompasses a review of the new Steffee devices, which were designated Mark II and Mark III. There were 141 patients in whom 585 Mark II joints were inserted and 42 patients in whom 143 MARK III joints were inserted. The age (in years) ranged from 22 to 83 and the mean was 56. Most patients had rheumatoid arthritis with only five joints with traumatic arthritis and two joints with

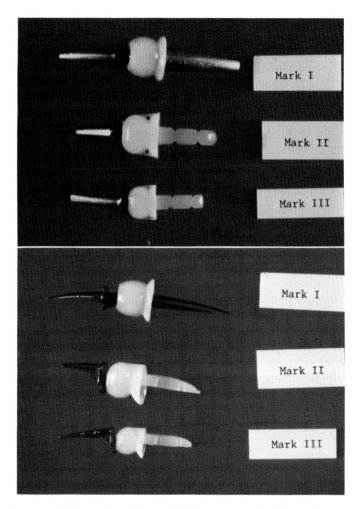

Fig. 17-1. Metacarpophalangeal prostheses (Steffee design). Mark I was the initial design by Arthur Steffee, M.D. Mark II shows shortening of the distal component. The shortened hub area required less bone resection. The polyethylene proximal component has dorsally offset stems to lower the center of rotation as does the distal stem. The short distal stem was to ease insertion. The Mark III has the lengthened distal stem for improved fixation and stability and lateral flanges on the proximal component for securing the volar plate in reduced position.

degenerative arthritis replaced (Fig. 17-2). All patients were shown the device and given an explanation of the procedure before surgery.

Standard operative technique for total joint replacement included filtered surgical air, hoods and masks, double gloving, and preoperative and postoperative prophylactic antibiotics.

The metacarpophalangeal joint was usually exposed by incision of the radial sagittal band on the radial aspect of the extensor tendon with a separate incision through the capsule, usually in the site of synovial destruction. The metacarpal head and neck resection length was generally dictated by the degree of subluxation and shortening present at the individual joints. Although it was sometimes possible

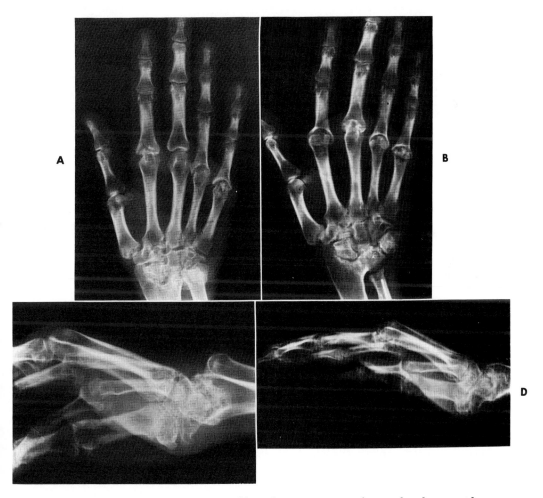

Fig. 17-2. Business manager, 36 years old, with progressive multiarticular rheumatoid arthritis. **A** and **B,** Initial appearance of roentgenogram. **C** and **D,** Thirty-three months later there is metacarpophalangeal subluxation, ulnar drift, and decreasing functional capability.

Continued.

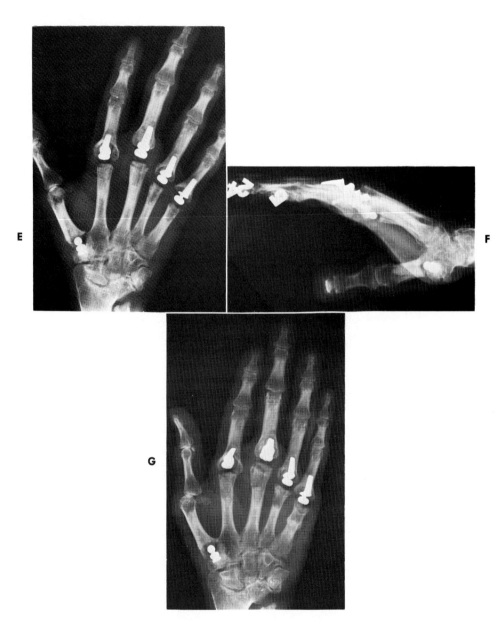

Fig. 17-2, cont'd. **E** and **F**, Three months after metacarpophalangeal arthroplasties. Improved strength, mobility, and function with excellent pain relief. **G** and **H**, At 1 year, rotation and loosening of distal components of index and long finger with some increased extensor lag. **I** and **J**, Three months after revision with Mark III stems she has no pain and has satisfactory motion. **K** and **L**, No further evidence of loosening.

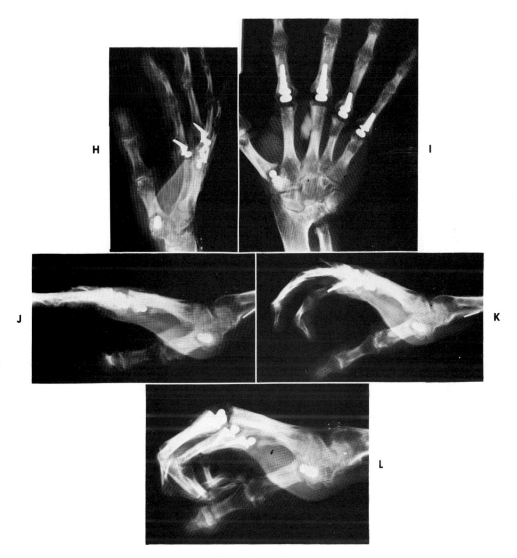

Fig. 17-2, cont'd. For legend see opposite page.

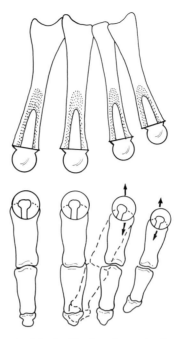

Fig. 17-3. Rotational alignment of both distal and proximal components is critical to the prevention of overlap of the fingers during flexion. The transverse articular bar of the distal component must be parallel to the flexion axis of the phalanges. This is best estimated by insertion with the finger passively flexed. The stem is placed adjacent and parallel to the dorsal cortical surface. The proximal components are more difficult to align because of the curvature of the distal metacarpal arch. This is often accentuated in the rheumatoid hand because of the laxity of the metacarpocarpal joints of the fourth and fifth rays. If the slot is rotated when the device is assembled, finger overlap will occur.

to insert the device in one piece, shortly after beginning the study we elected to cement in the distal component and the proximal component separately to achieve more careful control of alignment and placement (Fig. 17-3). We were particularly anxious to prevent any toggling from occurring during insertion, which would change the position of the center of rotation. After prosthesis insertion and assembly, capsulorrhaphy to tighten the radial collateral ligament was followed by centralization of the extensor tendons.

Additional soft tissue and joint procedures included release of the ulnar wing tendons, release of the ulnar phalangeal interosseous tendons, proximal interphalangeal arthrotomy, arthrodeses of the distal interphalangeal joints, proximal interphalangeal joints, and thumb joints, and occasionally replacement of the wrist or proximal interphalangeal joints.

In postoperative management the dressings were changed at the second or fourth day. Isoprene dynamic and resting splints were fabricated within the first week. The slings about the proximal phalanges of the dynamic splints were fitted to hold the fingers in extension and slight radial deviation. Alternating flexion slings were added at 2 weeks if needed. The static splint is used to hold the fingers in a relaxed functional position for rest. Supervised exercises during the first three weeks concentrate on restoring finger motion and control.

Patients were asked to return at 6 weeks for assessment and reinstruction and at 3 months for an x-ray examination and reassessment. All patients were asked to return at 1 year for a recheck examination and a number of patients have been followed at 2, 3, and 5 years.

The average follow-up was 30 months. Standard forms for preoperative and postoperative evaluation were filled out for each visit. The preoperative range of active motion averaged −48 to 95 degrees and postoperative −20 to 64 degrees. Ulnar deviation was seen in a large number of the patients with a preoperative range of 31 degrees. Postoperatively, ulnar deviation averaged 19 degrees (normal 8 to 10 degrees) and recurred to some extent in a substantial percentage of patients. Grasp strength preoperatively averaged 2.2 kg and postoperatively at 1 year 2.6 kg. Pinch strength averaged 1.2 kg preoperatively and 1.8 kg postoperatively.

Patients were asked to rate their results. At 1 year these were much better 47%, better 50%, no change 0%, and worse 3%. At 2 years these were much better 56%, better 36%, no change 5%, and worse 3%. The motion achieved at the metacarpophalangeal joint seldom improved significantly after 3 months, and only rarely did proximal interphalangeal joint motion significantly improve after this time. Further deterioration of other hand joints continued in many patients.

Extension lag remained the most common problem associated with this arthroplasty. It was follwed by recurrence to varying degrees of swan-neck deformity and ulnar drift. Motion at the metacarpophalangeal joint was usually best at the index and long fingers where extension lag was more common. Flexion of the little and ring fingers was more likely to be limited, and this limitation may explain some of the inability to achieve significant improvement of power grip.

In the Mark II prosthesis loosening of the distal stem within the proximal phalanx occurred in 19.3% and of the proximal stem in the metacarpal in 2%. This was accompanied by flexion of the device and occasional penetration of the palmar cortex. In one patient this resulted in a rupture of the flexor profundus to the index finger, and in others this seemed to merely accentuate the extensor lag (Fig. 17-4). There was, however, little discomfort associated with this problem.

The longer stemmed Mark II has shown a sharply diminished tendency toward loosening of the prosthesis, 1% at the distal stem and 2% at the proximal stem. Fracture or failure of the metacarpal head occurred in 0.1%, and infection in 0.3% of the patients. Revision was performed in 7.6% by recementing or replacement.

DISCUSSION

Accurate rebalancing of the three-joint finger system deteriorated by the rheumatoid process is quite difficult, in large part because of the complexity of the anatomy at the metacarpophalangeal joint (Fig. 17-5 and 17-6). The pathologic al-

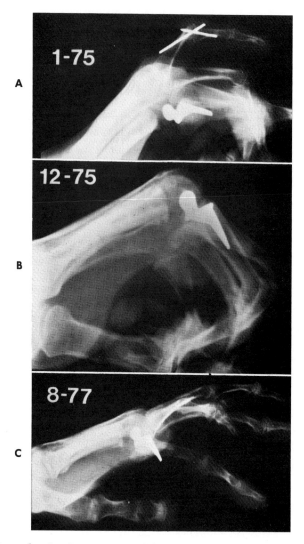

Fig. 17-4. A, Immediately after insertion of the Steffee type of prosthesis in the index finger. **B,** At 11 months there is loosening of distal stem of device, and, **C,** at 2½ years the distal stem has eroded through volar cortex. This is associated with loss of extension. The problem can be prevented, at least in part, when one leaves some cortical bone at the base of the proximal phalanx to retain methacrylate cement plug by ensuring adequate filling of the intramedullary cavity with cement and by using longer stem on distal portion of prosthesis. (From Linscheid, R.L., and Dobyns, J.H.: Mayo Clin. Proc. **54:**516-526, Aug. 1979; by permission.)

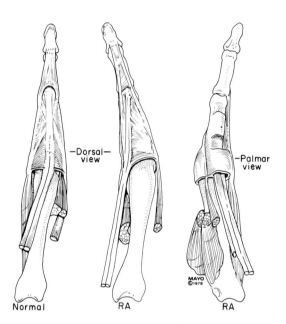

Fig. 17-5. On normal index or long finger, extensor tendon is well centralized over dorsum of joint, and intrinsic muscles are balanced to either side. With progressive deformity, extensor tendon slips into intermetacarpal groove, where it no longer has significant ability to extend metacarpophalangeal joint but increases tendency toward ulnar deviation. Palmar view shows progressive subluxation of volar plate complex to ulnar side of finger as well. This is not appreciated as readily as is ulnar subluxation of extensor tendon unless one palpates tendon on palmar aspect of hand and notes its relationship to overlying metacarpophalangeal joint. *RA*, Rhematoid arthritis. (From Linscheid, R.L., and Dobyns, J.H.: Mayo Clin. Proc. **54:**516-526, Aug. 1979; by permission.)

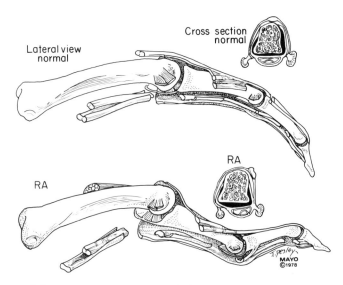

Fig. 17-6. Sagittal drawing, *top,* shows normal alignment of metacarpals and phalanges obtained through ligamentous constraints about joints. Tendons are closely applied about joint. Sagittal drawing, *bottom,* indicates progressive deformity associated with rheumatoid arthritis, *RA,* in which there is volar subluxation at metacarpophalangeal joint and lengthening of capsular ligaments through attenuation by synovitis. There is secondary loss of cartilage height by erosion and frequently secondary change in bony architecture, producing flattening of metacarpal head and settling and erosion of dorsal lip of proximal phalanx. This results in proximal migration and volar subluxation of proximal phalanx, often associated with synovitis in flexor tendon sheath and volar distraction of flexor tendons. This provides much larger flexion moment arm at metacarpophalangeal joint. Ulnar drift of finger is attributable to ulnar bowstringing of flexor tendons and ulnar pull on intermetacarpal ligament by hypothenar musculature. On cross section, volar plate is displaced volarly and ulnarly on stretched collateral ligaments and radial sagittal band of extensor apparatus. This tends to be associated with progressive myofascial contracture of ulnar interosseous muscles and displacement of attachment of radial interosseous muscles. (From Linscheid, R.L., and Dobyns, J.H.: Mayo Clin. Proc. **54:**516-526, Aug. 1979; by permission.)

terations include elongation and attenuation of the collateral ligaments, palmar displacement and ulnar translation of the flexor tendon complex, and also contraction of the ulnar aspect of the extensor mechanism and concomitant attenuation of the radial aspect with ulnar displacement of the extensor tendon. Destruction of the articular surfaces leads to progressive shortening of the osseous elements and variable myofibrosis of the intrinsic musculature, particularly on the ulnar aspect.

Secondary changes at the proximal interphalangeal joint, in both the soft tissues and the joint architecture may dispose toward limited improvement in proximal interphalangeal flexion and to maintenance of the swan-neck deformity.

Perhaps the largest single factor in attempting to determine the outcome of the

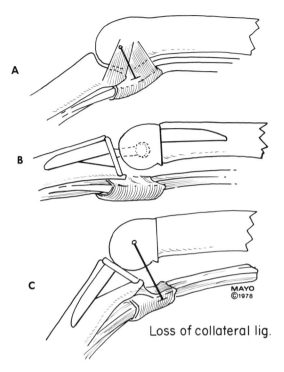

Fig. 17-7. A, Normal moment arm for flexor tendons as they cross metacarpophalangeal joint is determined by attachment of collateral and accessory collateral ligaments to volar plate. **B,** When metacarpal head is removed, fixation of collateral ligaments is loosened or lost, and volar plate and flexor tendon sheath may subluxate volarly, greatly increase moment arm of flexor tendons, and tend to induce flexion contracture at joint, **C.** (From Linscheid, R.L., and Dobyns, J.H.: Mayo Clin. Proc. **54:**516-526, Aug. 1979; by permission.)

procedure is the position of the flexor tendon mechanism. Resection of the metacarpal head releases the already attenuated origins of the collateral ligaments so that the flexor mechanism is further loosened (Fig. 17-7). Diminished gliding of the tendons within the tendon sheath because of tenosynovitis short circuits the flexor tendons and encourages metacarpophalangeal flexion. Metacarpophalangeal extension is often inhibited by the preoperative stretching of the extensor apparatus and the concurrent contracture of the flexor apparatus and intrinsics. The shortening of the metacarpal aggravates the persisting extensor lag. Diminished laminar excursions within the extensor apparatus caused by the contracted state and postoperative adhesions inhibit independent proximal interphalangeal flexion and encourage maintenance of the swan-neck deformity. The ability to more accurately control the subluxation tendency of the flexor mechanism might allow for distinct improvement in results of all arthroplasties.

Changes in bone remodeling as a result of stress in the intramedullary cavities is a persisting concern after prosthetic replacement, especially in the younger individuals who will use the joints with greater stress over a longer time. Although it appears that longer stems and better cement packing have a definite salutary effect on the stability of the cemented devices, pressure distribution against the endosteal bone may vary greatly. The disruption of the ligamentous tension force with metacarpal head resection may also interfere with the maintenance of normal cortical thickness by change in the feedback mechanism to normal osteogenesis.

Although the results and complications reported in this series of patients are cause for concern, there are a number of patients in whom the results appear to have results appear to have resulted in performance equal or superior to that obtained with other mehtods of arthroplasty. In general, we have been disappointed with the resultant grip and pinch strengths. The more secure fixation within bone should supply more than the modest increase in strength that has been apparent.

In general, cemented metacarpophalangeal arthroplasty appears to be a technique that should be reserved for older patients because of the danger of loosening. One should approach it in a methodical manner to ensure correct placement, alignment, and secure fixation through forceful cement packing. Loose cement and debris must be removed and careful soft-tissue reconstruction with supervised postoperative therapy are necessary. Pain relief has been good, and a more functional arc of motion and improved alignment of the fingers usually results. Wear characteristics and strength of the components has been good. Strength of grip and pinch has been improved but still is disappointing. Soft-tissue balance problems are not solved by insertion of prostheses.

REFERENCES

1. Beckenbaugh, R.D., Dobyns, J.H., Linscheid, R.L., and Bryan, R.S.: Review and analysis of silicone-rubber metacarpophalangeal implants, J. Bone Joint Surg. **58A**(4):483-487, June 1976.
2. Flatt, A.E.: The pathomechanics of ulnar drift: a biomechanical and clinical study. Final report, Social and Rehabilitation Services Grant No. RD226M, 1971.
3. Linscheid, R.L.: Preliminary results with Steffee arthroplasty in rheumatoid arthritis (Abstract), Clin. Orthop. Rel. Res. **119**:273, 1976.
4. Linscheid, R.L., and Dobyns, J.H.: Total joint arthroplasty—the hand, Mayo Clin. Proc. **54**:516-526, 1979.
5. Steffee, A.D., Beckenbaugh, R.D., Linscheid, R.L., and Dobyns, J.H.: The development, technique and early clinical results of a total joint replacement for the metacarpophalangeal joints of the fingers, Orthopaedics **4**:175, Feb. 1981.
6. Zancolli, E.: Structural and dynamic bases of hand surgery, Philadelphia, 1968, J.B. Lippincott Co.

18. Total metacarpophalangeal joint arthroplasty with limited metacarpal head resection

Robert J. Schultz, M.D.

Rheumatoid arthritis is a deforming disease that produces changes at the metacarpophalangeal joint, resulting in narrowing of the span of the palm. As a result of this decrease in palm span, the rheumatoid patient frequently becomes two-handed in activities of daily living for which people with normal hands are one-handed (Fig. 18-1).

In an attempt to improve function, surgical treatment may be indicated, the goals of which are to permit the patient to have fine pinch, a grasp with strength and stability, and the ability to hold large objects. Therefore, in addition to gaining as much flexion as possible, the rheumatoid patient must also obtain metacarpophalangeal joint extension to widen the palm in order to place the hand around large objects.

The primary deformities in rheumatoid arthritis at the metacarpophalangeal joint are volar dislocation and ulnar drift (Fig. 18-2). These deformities are produced by a variety of causes, for example[3-6,9]:

1. On the extensor surface of the hand, displacement of the extensor tendons into the valleys between the metacarpal heads
2. On the flexor surface of the hand, intrinsic contractures and the force of the natural volar and ulnar vectors of the flexor tendons acting on unstable metacarpophalangeal joints caused by failure of the collateral ligaments or destruction of the joint architecture
3. At the wrist, carpal subluxation with radial deviation of the wrist and compensatory ulnar deviation of the digits

One should understand that these forces are constantly acting and must be neutralized in the treatment plan.

SURGICAL CONSIDERATIONS

Surgery in the form of resection arthroplasty or prosthetic replacement is indicated when the rheumatoid process has irreparably destroyed the articular sur-

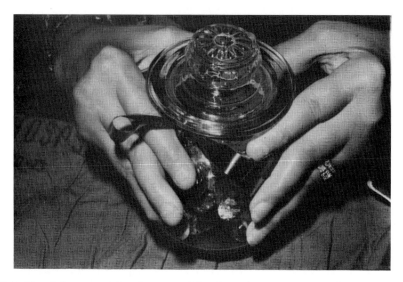

Fig. 18-1. The deformity of the rheumatoid hand results in a narrow palm span, requiring the patient to use two hands for an otherwise one-handed activity.

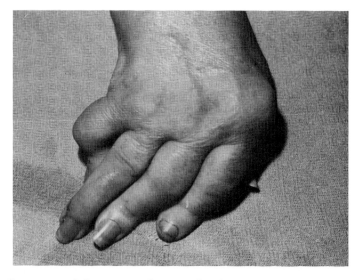

Fig. 18-2. The primary deformities in rheumatoid arthritis at the metacarpophalangeal joint are volar dislocation and ulnar drift.

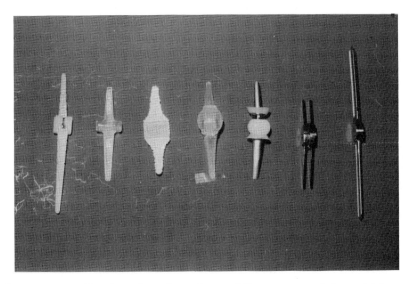

Fig. 18-3. A variety of implants have been designed for metacarpophalangeal joint replacement. These range from extremely rigid to flexible implants.

faces, or where joint instability has occurred, resulting in dislocation or subluxation of the metacarpophalangeal joint beyond the possibility of soft-tissue correction. In resection arthroplasty, the metacarpal head is resected and the soft tissues are reconstructed to produce stability. Joint replacement arthroplasty includes the implantation of a prosthesis or spacer after preparation of the joint. These procedures in most instances require complete metacarpal head resection.[2,10] A variety of implants, ranging from flexible to rigid, have been designed (Fig. 18-3).

EXPERIMENTAL EVALUATION OF METACARPOPHALANGEAL JOINT

Prosthetic replacement requires an understanding of the joint involved; thus a study of the metacarpophalangeal joint was undertaken and evaluated biomechanically and anatomically. To accomplish this, we developed a goniometer that permitted direct-measurement recordings of the metacarpophalangeal joint in the three-dimensional planes. Based on the recorded data, a computer-simulated model of the joint was developed. This model established a method of predicting the orientation of the proximal phalanx in relation to the metacarpal for any given instantaneous point in the axis of motion of the metacarpophalangeal joint. In addition, it demonstrated the effect of the collateral ligaments and their contribution to joint motion and stability.[8]

The recorded data, in conjunction with the computer model, demonstrated several points:

1. For a given hand, the angle of lateral deviation (abduction and adduction) remained the same as the finger passes from 0 degrees to approximately 70 degrees of flexion.

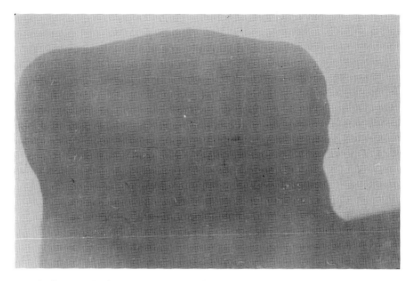

Fig. 18-4. Shadowgraph demonstrating the bicondylar contour of the metacarpal head at approximately 70 degrees of flexion.

2. After 70 degrees, a sharp decrease in lateral deviation occurred.
3. During metacarpophalangeal joint flexion and extension there is an instantaneous change in the axis of rotation, with the motion being one of combined rolling and sliding.

The surface characteristics of the metacarpal head was further studied with a shadow profilometer. These studies demonstrated that from 0 to 70 degrees of flexion, the metacarpal head is essentially spheric in shape. At 70 degrees, however, the contour of the metacarpal head changes if one assumes a bicondylar shape similar to the head of the proximal phalanx (Fig. 18-4).

The collateral ligaments were also evaluated by the computer model as well as by anatomic dissection. Contrary to the commonly accepted view that the collateral ligaments are slack in extension, permitting a large range of lateral deviation, and tight in flexion, restricting this motion, the collateral ligaments were found to be taut at all times, supporting the joint in extension, flexion, and intermediate positions.

The stabilizing effects of the collateral ligaments were evaluated by placement of dissected specimens of the metacarpophalangeal joint under stress in various planes. Restraint to volar subluxation readily occurred, since this displacement was in the direction of the collateral ligament fibers and would require a stretch of the fibers. Longitudinal distraction and dorsal subluxation of the extended joint was possible though the collateral ligaments were taut, since these motions were not in the direction of, and therefore not restricted by, the collateral ligament fibers. In

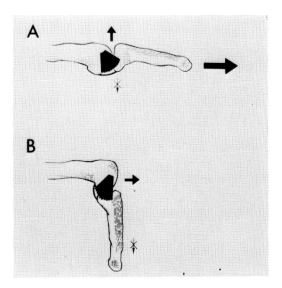

Fig. 18-5. When stress is placed on the metacarpophalangeal joint, volar subluxation is restricted, since this displacement is in the direction of the collateral ligament fibers. Distraction and dorsal displacement are possible, since these movements are not in the direction of the fibers.

flexion, longitudinal distraction and volar subluxation are restricted, since these motions are in the direction of the collateral ligament fibers (Fig. 18-5).

This concept that the collateral ligament is taut in all ranges is further supported by our knowledge of the living hand. If the collateral ligaments are slack in extension, the constant volar vector of the flexor tendon forces of the living hand would produce volar subluxation of the metacarpophalangeal joint in extension or intermediate flexion positions, until the point is reached where the ligaments would be assumed tight. This subluxation we know does not occur unless the collateral ligaments or the joint surfaces are damaged. Thus, how can the differences in lateral deviation during abduction and adduction, with the finger in extension or flexion, be explained? The explanation rests with the principle that the linear displacement of a point rotating about an axis is the product of the angle of displacement and the perpendicular distance from the point to the axis.

Multiple goniometric measurements with the spatial goniometer demonstrated that from 0 to 70 degrees of metacarpophalangeal joint flexion the angle of displacement (lateral deviation of the phalanx on the metacarpal) for a given hand is constant. The phalanx in abduction-adduction rotates about a vertical axis (Fig. 18-6). As the metacarpophalangeal joint flexes, the distance from the tip of the finger to the vertical axis decreases. In extension, the tip of the finger is 90 degrees to the vertical axis and is at its greatest distance from the vertical axis. Therefore the linear lateral displacement is at a maximum. As the finger flexes, the fingertip approaches the vertical axis and causes the shortening of the distance from the

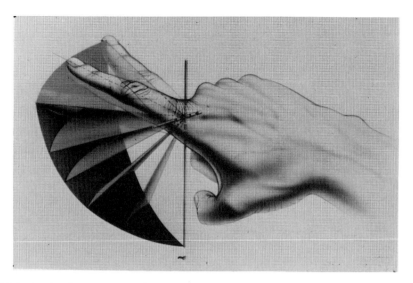

Fig. 18-6. As the finger rotates about its vertical axis, the linear lateral displacement for a given angular displacement decreases as the tip of the finger approaches the vertical axis.

point to the axis, producing a decrease in the linear lateral displacement. After 70 degrees of flexion, as previously noted, the configuration of the metacarpal head changes, becoming bicondylar in shape producing a block to angular displacement.

PROSTHETIC DESIGN

In view of these studies, we believed that a prosthesis should be constructed of low-friction materials, provide motion, and have no static forces to overcome. The prosthesis should provide stability in pinch and grasp, as well as against the forces that will be continually acting in the rheumatoid hand to produce recurrent deformity. To provide further stability, the collateral ligaments should be retained if possible. Articulation of the prosthesis during surgery should be accomplished easily. The prosthesis should have a minimum of moving parts and have an instantaneous change in the axis of motion.

To accomplish this, a two-component prosthesis was developed, composed of a metacarpal component of molded ultrahigh molecular weight polyethylene and a phalangeal component of stainless steel (Fig. 18-7). The head of the metacarpal component is designed such that the phalangeal component has a snap-fitting articulation and runs in a tract, producing an instantaneous change in the axis of motion. The medullary stem of the prosthesis comes in interchangeable sizes, with the articulating surfaces being identical. The snap-fitting articulation eliminates the need for fixation screws or bars.

A further design characteristic of the prosthesis permits insertion of the implant with a limited resection of the metacarpal head (Fig. 18-8). Limited metacarpal

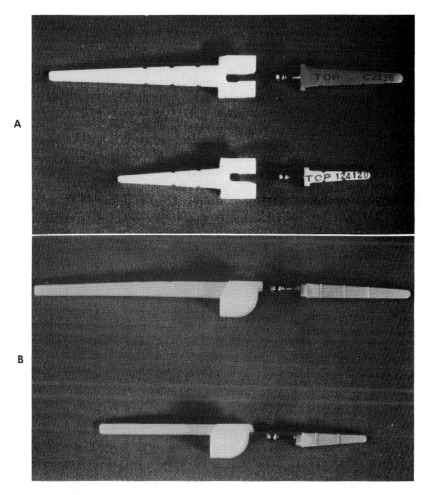

Fig. 18-7. Two-component metacarpophalangeal joint prosthesis demonstrating the metacarpal and phalangeal components. Note that the articulating surfaces are identical, permitting interchangeability of the sizes. **A,** Top view. **B,** Side view.

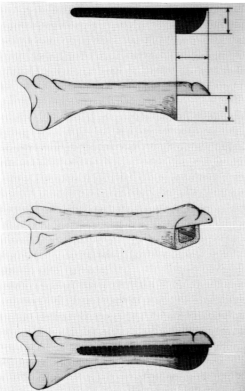

Fig. 18-8. Limited metacarpal head resection seats the prosthesis beneath the ledge of the metacarpal head. This permits the axis of rotation of the prosthesis to better coincide with the axis of rotation of the joint, prevents the extensor tendons from contacting the prosthesis, and permits retention of the collateral ligaments.

Fig. 18-9. Anatomic specimen demonstrating how limited head resection permits retention of the collateral ligaments. The area of resection is outlined.

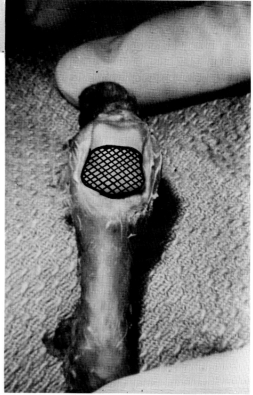

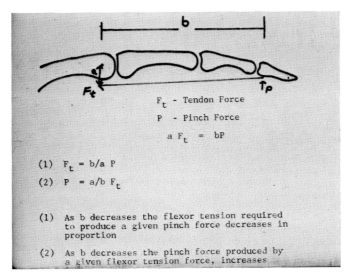

F_t - Tendon Force

P - Pinch Force

a F_t = bP

(1) $F_t = b/a\ P$

(2) $P = a/b\ F_t$

(1) As b decreases the flexor tension required to produce a given pinch force decreases in proportion

(2) As b decreases the pinch force produced by a given flexor tension force, increases

Fig. 18-10. Resection distal to the axis of rotation of the prosthesis gives an increased pinch force for the same unit tendon force.

head resection provides several advantages: (1) there is more accurate seating of the prosthesis with the axis of rotation of the prosthesis more closely coinciding to the axis of rotation of the natural metacarpophalangeal joint, (2) the ledge of the metacarpal head provides a fulcrum for the extensor tendons, (3) limited resection permits retention of the collateral ligaments since the collateral ligaments arise from the superior margin of the metacarpal head (Fig. 18-9), and (4) less bone is resected leaving more available if a salvage procedure is necessary.

At times, there is a flexion contracture that cannot be overcome by soft-tissue releases alone, requiring bone resection. In these cases, bone resection is performed at the base of the proximal phalanx and not at the metacarpal neck. Resection in this location results in a shorter lever distal to the axis of rotation of the prosthesis, with the effect of an increased pinch force for the same unit tendon force, thus increasing the mechanical advantage of the flexor and extensor tendons (Fig. 18-10).

To establish a fixed fulcrum, an anchoring mechanism for the implant is needed. At the present time, polymethylmethacrylate provides immediate fixation for the prosthesis. Without the use of cement or another form of fixation, pistoning of the prosthesis will occur during flexion and extension of the digit.

In view of the narrow cortical wall of the tubular bones of the hand and concern about the effects of the heat generated during cement curing, the thermal effects of polymerization of methyl methacrylate in small long bones was studied both physically and histologically in living and nonliving tissue.[7] These studies demonstrated that small volumes of methyl methacrylate produce a small rise in temperature, a shorter duration of temperature rise, and in vivo no damage to the cells as a result of heat generation during curing. Thus, when small long bones were exposed to slight temperature increases as a result of cement curing, the maximum temperature rise was found to be within the tolerance level for living bone cells. Since smaller cement volumes also cool more rapidly, it further reduced the deleterious temperature affects. The histologic in vivo animal studies showed no recognizable thermal effects on cells and only demonstrated changes consistent with surgically induced ischemia and vascularization.

REPLACEMENT OF METACARPOPHALANGEAL JOINT
Indications

Primarily, prosthetic replacement of the metacarpophalangeal joint is indicated for hands incapacitated by rheumatoid arthritis. These hands have painful, stiff, or contracted metacarpophalangeal joints in which the rheumatoid process has irreparably destroyed the articular surfaces, or produced joint instability resulting in subluxation or dislocation advanced beyond the possibility of soft-tissue correction. Traumatic destruction of the joint surfaces may also be reconstruected by joint replacement.

Contraindications

Contraindications to joint replacement are poor-quality and nonviable tissue or obvious skin defects in the operative area, bone or joint infections, an intramedullary canal size or bone stock insufficient to receive the medullary stem, and absent or unrepaired tendons that cannot be reconstructed before or after joint replacement.

Surgical procedures

A standard hand-operating table is used. Although the surgeon may elect to sit at the axillary side, it is preferable to sit at the end of the table so as to view the hand in its long axis. One or more joints can be replaced at a single operation.

After the sterile preparation, the hand and forearm are draped to allow for free movement of the extremity. With the metacarpophalangeal joints flexed, an incision is made distal to the metacarpal heads at the level of the metacarpophalangeal joint (Fig. 8-11). Skin flaps are developed and procedures on the intrinsic tendons can be readily performed, if necessary, through this incision[1,2,5] (Fig. 8-12). Care should be taken to preserve the intermetacarpal vessels.

Each digit is done in similar fashion. The joint is exposed through the customary incisions on either the radial or ulnar side of the extensor tendon. A synovectomy of the readily accessible synovium is performed. The collateral ligaments should be left intact.

Preparation of metacarpal heads. To perform the limited head resection, the inferior half of the metacarpal head is removed with a sharp rongeur entering into the cancellous bone. No attempt is made to shape the metacarpal head at this time.

The medullary canal is entered longitudinally and prepared with a finger-ream-

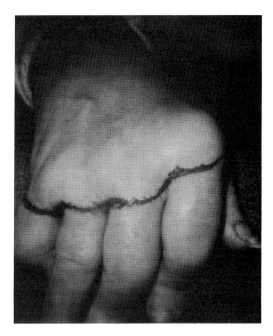

Fig. 18-11. The incision is made distal to the metacarpal heads at the level of the metacarpophalangeal joints.

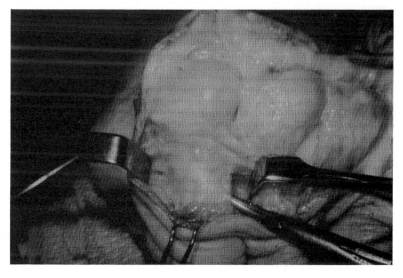

Fig. 18-12. With the skin flaps developed, the extensor mechanism is readily demonstrated. Procedures on the intrinsic tendon can be easily performed through this incision.

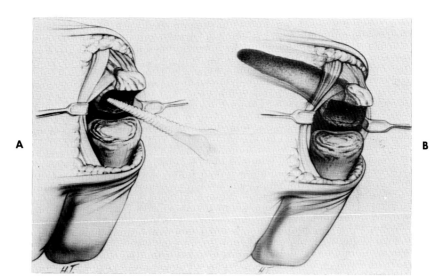

Fig. 18-13. A, The inferior half of the metacarpal is resected and the medullary canal prepared before final shaping of the metacarpal head. **B,** The lateral inferior cortices are cut back equal to the length of the head of the prosthesis.

ing burr or a metacarpal reamer (Fig. 18-13). Once the medullary canal is fully outlined, the inferior and lateral cortices of the metacarpal head are well visualized and can be fashioned into their proper contour. The cortices are cut back equal to the length of the head of the prosthesis, which is usually to a point just distal to the flair of the metacarpal head-neck junction, with the superior ledge of metacarpal head being retained.

Sufficient resection of the superior ledge is assessed by use of the metacarpal reamer inserted into the medullary canal. If the resection is complete, the reamer will be parallel to the medullary canal and superiorly will contact the ledge of bone. This will ensure that the stem and head of the prosthesis will be inserted parallel to the medullary canal. The medullary canal should be widened larger than the stem of the metacarpal implant to accommodate the methyl methacrylate. A trial metacarpal component is inserted to test the length and proper seating beneath the metacarpal ledge. The head of the prosthesis, when in place, should be parallel to the superior ledge of the metacarpal in the transverse plane and the shaft longitudinally (Fig. 18-14).

If a block to implantation is encountered, one must check the following areas (Fig. 18-15):

1. The medullary canal should be sufficiently widened.
2. The proper length of prosthesis has been chosen.
3. Sufficient and smooth resection of the lateral and inferior cortices of the

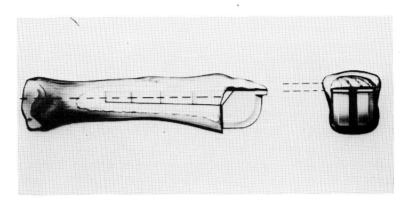

Fig. 18-14. The trial metacarpal component should be inserted to test length and proper seating. A properly seated prosthesis should be parallel to the superior ledge of the metacarpal in the transverse plane and the shaft longitudinally.

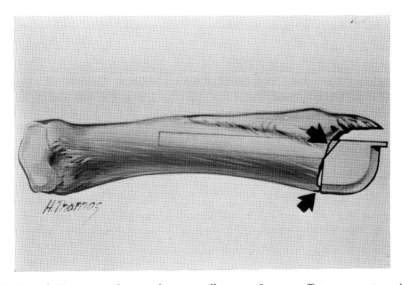

Fig. 18-15. Inability to seat the prosthesis usually arises from insufficient resection of either the inferior aspect of the metacarpal or the corners between the lateral surface and the ledge of metacarpal head.

metacarpal has been accomplished (especially the inferior cortex and the corners between the lateral cortex and the ledge of metacarpal head). This feature is most commonly responsible for inability to seat the prosthesis.

A trial prosthesis is inserted into each metacarpal and the proper size determined.

With the inferior aspect of the metacarpal head removed, the increased visibility permits completion of the synovectomy. The collateral ligaments and the base of the proximal phalanx are also better visualized.

Preparation of proximal phalanges. The base of the phalanges are perforated and the opening enlarged, so that the entire articular surface is removed. This large opening will facilitate the insertion of the polymethylmethacrylate into the medullary canal. The medullary canal is widely reamed, irrigated, and cleansed of all excess fragments of bone. All peripheral exostoses should be excised.

A trial phalangeal component is inserted for a test and should be loose and sink well into the phalanx. The additional space is to accommodate the cement (Fig. 18-16).

Implantation of prosthesis. Before insertion of the prosthesis, a trial reduction of the proximal phalanx on the metacarpal is performed. The collateral ligaments should be left intact if possible. Soft-tissue releases are performed, initially of the volar plate, and then the collateral ligaments, if a flexion deformity cannot be overcome. If, after the soft-tissue releases are performed, a contracture still exists, further relaxation can be obtained by bone resection of the proximal aspect of the proximal phalanx.

It is advisable to insert the prosthesis sequentially from index toward small or vice versa.

The medullary canals are irrigated and suctioned dry. The polymethylmethacrylate is prepared and inserted, under pressure, into each of the prepared medullary canals utilizing a tapered syringe. It is necessary to insert the cement under pressure to get good filling, starting deep in the canal and withdrawing the syringe as the cement is being inserted.

Phalangeal insertion. The phalangeal components are inserted first, and care must be taken to obtain the proper alignment. The prosthesis should be placed straight in the medullary canal with its superior surface parallel to the dorsal surface of the phalanx (Fig. 18-17). This can be accomplished with little difficulty if care is taken. The tip of the stem is inserted into the cement, and changes in position are made at this time. Once there is satisfaction with the alignment, complete insertion of the prosthesis is completed and all excess cement is removed.

Metacarpal insertion. Fixation of the metacarpal component is also accomplished by use of polymethylmethacrylate, which is inserted under pressure into each of the prepared medullary canals. The cement should be inserted just short of the inferior and lateral cortices and not to the level of the metacarpal ledge. This will prevent the cement from oozing into the channel in the prosthetic head when the prosthesis is inserted.

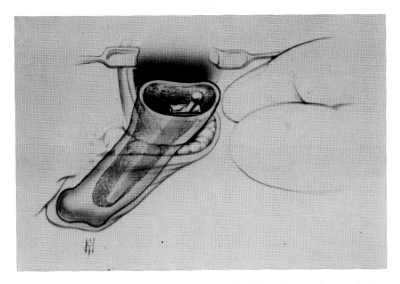

Fig. 18-16. The trial phalangeal component should fall well into the medullary canal to provide room for the polymethylmethacrylate.

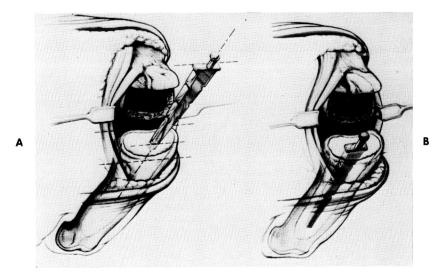

A   B

Fig. 18-17. The phalangeal component is aligned, **A,** so that the prosthesis will be straight in the medullary canal and parallel to the dorsal surface of the phalanx, **B.**

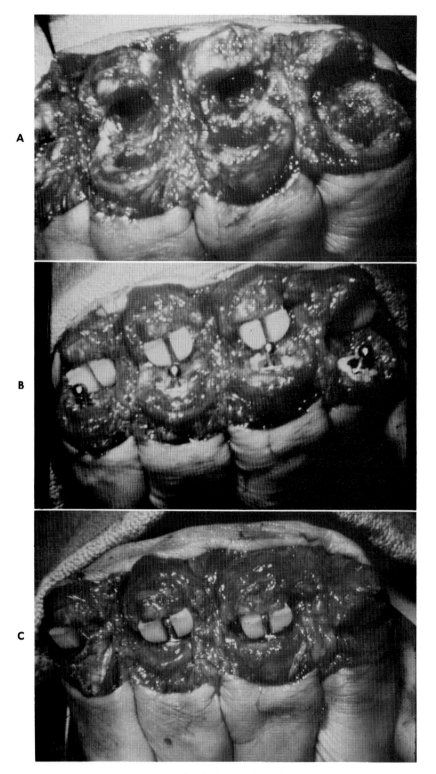

Fig. 18-18. A, Intraoperative view. The ledges and medullary canals have been prepared. **B,** The metacarpal and phalangeal components are inserted. **C,** Articulation of the two-component prosthesis.

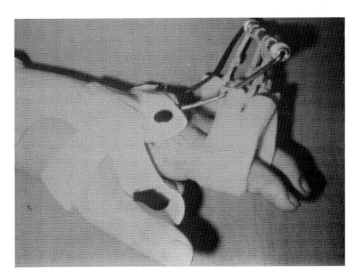

Fig. 18-19. On the fourth or fifth postoperative day, the patient is fitted with a dorsal orthosis and extension outrigger.

The metacarpal components should be properly aligned, and any changes in position should be done before the final seating. The metacarpal components should be held in under pressure, and all excess cement must be removed from the articular surfaces and the tract.

Articulation of prosthesis. The prosthesis is articulated by a snap-fit of the ball and neck of the phalangeal component through the space provided in the superior part of the head of the metacarpal component (Fig. 18-18). Once it is articulated, one should make a test flexion and extension to see that there is free glide of the prosthesis.

Closure. The wound is closed by recentralization of the extensor tendons. A closed-system suction drain should be placed beneath the proximal skin flap and the skin closed. A pressure dressing is applied, with the fingers maintained in moderate flexion at the metacarpophalangeal joints.

Postoperative management

Motion is begun on the fourth or fifth postoperative day. The patient is placed in a dorsal splint with a finger-extension outrigger, which is removed two to three times a day for active and gentle passive motion (Fig. 18-19). The passive motion is performed by gentle movement of the finger in flexion and extension, followed by gentle pressure on the dorsum of the proximal phalanx until 60 to 70 degrees of flexion is achieved. The patient, at this time, should attempt to maintain this position with active finger flexion. The splint is worn constantly for 4 to 6 weeks and at night for another 4 to 6 weeks. After this, all splinting is removed and patients are encouraged to use their hands as naturally as possible.

SUMMARY

Prosthetic replacement of the metacarpophalangeal joint provides patients with improved hand function and relief of pain in joints deformed or destroyed beyond the ability of soft-tissue repair. The anatomy, function, and biomechanics of the metacarpophalangeal joint must be carefully assessed when one is considering the design characteristics of a prosthesis for metacarpophalangeal joint replacement. Limited head resection can offer the advantages of accurate seating of the prosthesis, a fulcrum to assist metacarpophalangeal joint extension, retention of the collateral ligaments to assist in stability, and less bone resection so that other procedures can be performed if necessary.

REFERENCES

1. Ellison, M.R., Flatt, A.E., and Kelly, K.S.: Ulnar drift of the fingers in rheumatoid disease treatment by crossed intrinsic transfer, J. Bone Joint Surg. **53A:**1064-1082, 1979.
2. Flatt, A.E.: The care of the rheumatoid hand, ed. 3, St. Louis, 1974, The C.V. Mosby Co.
3. Flatt, A.E.: Some pathomechanics of ulnar drift, Plast. Reconstr. Surg. **37:**285-303, 1966.
4. Hakstian, R.W., and Tubiana, R.: Ulnar deviation of the fingers: the role of the collateral ligaments, J. Bone Joint Surg. **49A:**299-316, 1967.
5. Hastings, D.E., and Evans, J.A.: Rheumatoid wrist deformities and their relation to ulnar drift, J. Bone Joint Surg. **57:**930-935, 1975.
6. Pahle, J.A.: The influence of wrist position finger deviation in the rheumatoid hand, J. Bone Joint Surg. **51B:**664-676, 1969.
7. Schultz, R.J., and Storace, A.: A new viewpoint on metacarpophalangeal joint motion and the role of the collateral ligaments, J. Hand Surg. **3:**291, 1978.
8. Schultz, R.J., Rangaswamy, L., and Storace, A.: The thermal effects of polymerization of acrylic cement in small long bones (a physical and histological analysis), Orthop. Trans. **1:**Feb. 1977.
9. Smith, R.J., and Kaplan, E.B.: Rheumatoid deformities at the metacarpophalangeal joints of the fingers: a correlative study of anatomy and pathology, J. Bone Joint Surg. **49A:**31-47, 1967.
10. Swanson, A.B.: Flexible implant resection arthroplasty in the hand and extremities, St. Louis, 1973, The C.V. Mosby Co.

19. Joint replacement in the rheumatoid metacarpophalangeal joint

Alfred B. Swanson, M.D.
Genevieve de Groot Swanson, M.D.

The quest for improvement of methods to achieve the ideal goals for joint re construction has stimulated the pursuit for new materials, concepts, and methods. The industrial development of synthetic materials that can be used in the human body has given the researcher tools for human engineering and has opened up great possibilities for functional joint restoration. To bring the subject of implant arthroplasty into perspective, we have attempted to classify the implant materials available, the types of implants available, their fixation, and the basic methods of implant arthroplasty.

BASIC CONCEPTS OF ARTHROPLASTY METHODS
Classification of implant materials

Implant materials that can be used in reconstructive surgery of the extremities can be classified according to their physical characteristics: (1) rigid—metals, (2) semirigid—high-density polymers, and (3) flexible—elastic polymers (elastomers). There are different applications for each type of implant material. The rigid and semirigid materials have been most commonly used for total joint replacement type of prostheses. The flexible materials (silicone elastomers) have been used as an adjunct to resection arthroplasty. These two methods of arthroplasty differ significantly as discussed further.

Classification of arthroplasty implants

The possible combination of various types of implants materials and basic designs could be infinite. However, some basic arthroplasty implant concept and design can be classified as follows: (1) interposition arthroplasty, (2) condylar replacement implant, (3) ball and socket implant, (4) interlocking hinge with or without transfixion pin, and (5) flexible hinge (Fig. 19-1).

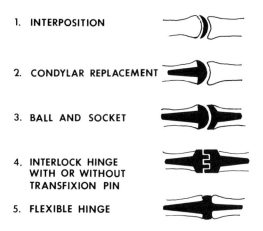

1. INTERPOSITION

2. CONDYLAR REPLACEMENT

3. BALL AND SOCKET

4. INTERLOCK HINGE
   WITH OR WITHOUT
   TRANSFIXION PIN

5. FLEXIBLE HINGE

Fig. 19-1. Classification of arthroplasty implants.

Classification of implant fixation

Stabilizing the implant in the desired position for function is an important consideration for both total joint replacement procedures and flexible implant arthroplasty. This may be obtained in many ways: (1) fasteners—pins, screws, bolts, nails, sutures, and so on; (2) mechanical interlocking—with a stem, collar, sleeve-like cap, or grooving on the implant; (3) cementing—physical bonding at the interface between the material and host with cement such as methyl methacrylate; (4) direct chemical bonding—organic fixation of synthetic material with host tissues being possible with some of the new ceramic materials, but the interface remains and the permanence of this bond is unlikely; (5) ingrowth of tissue into the implant, composed of fibers of loosely woven textiles or metallic fiber materials (The properties of such material must be seriously considered when such material is used inside a synovial cavity, which rejects these relatively inert materials if they have rough surfaces and therefore an increased surface area. The time of immobilization necessary for tissue ingrowth results in joint stiffness and delays rehabilitation.); (6) encapsulation around a smooth surface silicone implant with the use of capsuloligamentous reconstruction (It should be noted that all implants become encapsulated.)

Classification of arthroplasty methods for metacarpophalangeal joint

It appears that three different concepts of arthroplasty have emerged: resection arthroplasty, fixed-axis articulated joint replacement, and flexible-implant resection arthroplasty. These methods differ significantly in their concepts, designs, applications, material characteristics, and postoperative management.[36]

Surgical resection of bone in a stiffened contracted joint can improve motion by shortening skeletal structures, relatively lengthening soft parts, providing new gliding surfaces, and allowing nature to develop a new joint space with a supportive fibrous joint capsule. Regular joint resection arthroplasty works well in the hand if the joint space and alignment can be maintained. However, this method frequently requires excessive postoperative fixation with pins and external support. The fixation, if overused, will compromise the expected range of motion. In a considerable number of cases the joint space gradually narrows and stiffness and subluxation may result. Bone absorption and remodeling at the amputated bone end is a frequent occurrence, resulting in further shortening and joint instability. Good results do occur occasionally, however, and are related to the development of a supportive fibrous joint capsule organized during the period of guarded range of motion. The unpredictable results that have followed simple resection arthroplasty methods in finger-joint reconstruction have been a challenge for continued research.

Fixed-axis articulated joint replacement is a method in which the function of a joint is completely substituted by that of a mechanical model. This approach has certain attractive possibilities from the engineering standpoint and has found success in the weight-bearing knee and hip joints. A problem remains, however, with the total dependency on insubstantial synthetic materials at the boundary between it and the human tissues. As a result, any implanted device is only as successful as its biomechanical and biologic tolerance by human host tissues. The method used to replace small joints of the extremities with mechanical hinges or partial implants, has met with mixed success and limited acceptance; in many cases the bone has not tolerated the hard material. Bone absorption and material breakdown have negated many of the early good results obtained. Articulated implants made of rigid materials that are designed to replace the small joints of the hand have proved technically difficult for the operator and biomechanically unforgiving. If it were possible to reproduce anatomically the human joint with synthetic materials and if these could be permanently fixed in position as to simulate the required motions, this could be ideal. However, the use of this method has shown that it is extremely difficult to cement implants into small bones without either injuring the bone or failing to get an adequate permanent fixation. The problem with polyethylene materials is that they have a tendency to permanently deform because of cold flow of the plastic material.

In our earlier observations of the simple resection arthroplasty technique, it appeared to us that if we could in some way provide internal support to guide the healing process, the ideal joint substitute could perhaps be found. From this, Alfred Swanson originated in 1962 a research project to design and develop *flexible (silicone) implants* to be used as an adjunct to resection arthroplasty. This is an easier and safer alternative to help nature build a joint system through the resection arthroplasty concept. The method provides an excellent functional restoration though not an anatomic one. By minimizing the demands of the synthetic materials and simulating the biomechanics of the human joint system, it is much more likely that the improved resection arthroplasty will be long lived and free of disastrous complications.

FLEXIBLE (SILICONE) IMPLANT ARTHROPLASTY

Since 1962, the senior author has led a full-time research project to develop flexible implants for reconstructive surgery of the extremities. The experience gained with silicone elastomer implants for end-bearing stumps both in dogs and in humans and for overgrowth problems in the long bones of the juvenile amputees has prompted us to study the possibilities of applying silicone elastomer as an interpositional material to enhance the resection arthroplasty concept.[28,36] The concept of flexible implant arthroplasty has been responsibly developed into a reality because we proceeded in a reasonable orderly course in our department. This included a study of proper anatomic configuration, mechanical and engineering principles and design, physical characteristics of the material, biologic reaction of the tissues to the material, and the effect of loads applied on joint activity through the implant on bone. Serial evaluation of the joints by clinical, radiographic, and laboratory studies demonstrated the tolerance of the implants by soft tissues, bone, and cartilage. The retrieval study has included the early and long-term study of our cases and those operated in a special field clinic structure.[33,35,36]

Basic concepts

One of the most important functions of a flexible implant is to maintain proper joint alignment and spacing while early motion is started, with the implant acting as a dynamic spacer. The finger-joint silicone rubber intramedullary stemmed implant is a flexible hinge that acts as an internal mold around which a new capsuloligamentous system develops (Fig. 19-2). Early motion is essential in promoting the development of a new, functionally adapted fibrous capsule.[17] The intramedullary stems of the implant help maintain alignment and prevent joint displacement. In the postoperative course, the implant continues to support the important functionally adapted fibrous capsule and maintains the integrity of the new joint space. This important phenomenon has been named the "encapsulation process."[30] The flexible-implant resection arthroplasty concept could be simply expressed in the following:

$$\text{Bone resection} + \text{Implant} + \text{Encapsulation} = \text{New joint}$$

Proper orientation of the capsule is extremely important in the early stages of healing. The immediate postoperative positioning and control of joint movement during the 6- to 8-week rehabilitation period are as important as the surgery itself, and these are achieved by dynamic bracing and physiotherapy. The useful adaptability of the capsuloligamentous stabilization should further be emphasized. When increased mobility is desired such as in the finger joint arthroplasty, early motion is started. When greater stability than mobility is desired, as in the carpal bones, radiocarpal joint, or first metacarpophalangeal joint[43] reconstructions, the postoperative immobilization is carried out longer. The concepts of fixation of any implant must take into consideration the same requirements as the design of the implant itself, that is, anatomic, engineering, material, and physiologic considerations and

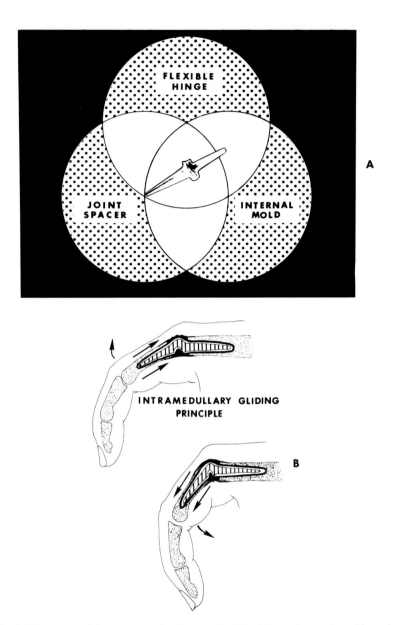

Fig. 19-2. A, Function of finger joint implant as flexible hinge, internal mold, and joint spacer can be represented in Venn diagram. Insertion of implant assists nature in development of more predictable and reproducible resection arthroplasty, which has been proved pain free, stable, mobile, and salvageable. **B,** Intramedullary gliding principle. The implant becomes completely surrounded by the new capsuloligamentous system. The distribution of forces around the implant are spread over a broader surface causing less stress at the interface with bone and less stress on the implant.

the patient's needs. Fixation of a device must be functionally and permanently stable. If the fixation points are receiving loads beyond their tolerance, a localized rigid fixation will gradually break down. Rigid fixation must be distributed over a wide area; otherwise loosening and wobbling of the device will eventually occur. Because the flexible implant becomes so well stabilized by the capsuloligamentous system and the surrounding bone, it is believed that no other permanent fixation of the implant is required; in fact, it is contraindicated. However, temporary fixation of certain implants, such as those for carpal bones (trapezium, scaphoid, lunate) can be beneficial in certain cases. Our early experiences with permanent fixation of flexible implants with cross pins, cement, or Dacron cover on the intramedullary stems of the implants and some nonabsorbable suture fixations have led to early breakage of the implants. In fact, lateral stability decreased in time because of bone absorption at the fixation site. Most of these implants have been removed, and it has been found that Dacron in a synovium-lined cavity can cause severe inflammatory reaction, which in turn enlarges the joint capsule and results in instability. An implant should cause no inflammatory reaction if it is to be long tolerated.

Stability of a reconstructed joint cannot be dependent on any implant if it is to be tolerated on a long-term basis. Long-standing host-implant reciprocal tolerance requires achievement of joint stability from the extrinsic capsular ligamentous and musculotendinous systems. The flexible-implant concept respects this biologic requirement. The smooth flexible implant is completely included in the encapsulation process. The slight amount of movement of the stems increases the life of the implant because forces that develop around the implant on motion are not concentrated in any particular area but rather spread over a broader section, and because the flexible hinge implants can find the best position with respect to the axis of rotation of the joint. This distribution of forces on the implant is also reflected at its interface with the bone or cartilage. The bone is less likely to react at the juncture with the implant if the forces are within the strain tolerance of the bone. Furthermore, the intramedullary stem of the implant has a supportive action on the cut end of the amputated bone; it prevents the excessive resorption and remodeling phenomena that frequently occur after amputation as noted in a 15-year study of the finger joint arthroplasty (Fig. 19-3). The low-modulus implant is softer than bone and has force-dampening characteristics that further protect the bone or cartilage and soft tissues. It is therefore preferable to avoid interface problems by distribution of the forces of stabilization of the implant over a broad area with a low-modulus material.

Salvageability of an arthroplasty procedure must be one of the important considerations; this implies preservation of bone and soft tissues so that a secondary procedure can be performed. This requirement was of particular importance in the flexible-implant arthroplasty method. The capsuloligamentous structures around any flexible implant can be reconstructed to improve the stability, alignment, and durability of the arthroplasty, and revision procedures to further reinforce, release, or realign the capsule and ligaments when necessary are easily performed. Because

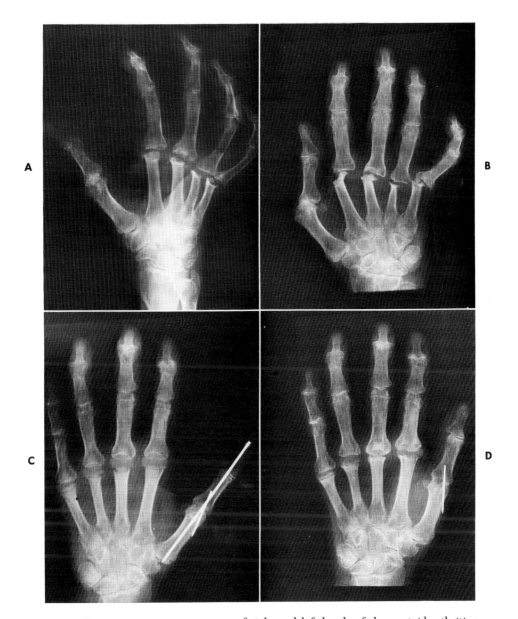

Fig. 19-3. Comparative roentgenograms of right and left hands of rheumatoid arthritic patient soon after surgery and 5 years later. A simple resection arthroplasty was carried out on right hand. **A,** Roentgenogram of hand taken 6 months after resection arthroplasty of metacarpophalangeal joints of index, middle, ring, and little fingers. **B,** Roentgenogram showing simple resection arthroplasty 5 years later. Note pronounced remodeling of amputated metacarpal ends. **C,** Early postoperative roentgenogram showing flexible implant arthroplasty of four metacarpophalangeal joints and fusion of thumb metacarpophalangeal joint. **D,** Roentgenogram 5 years after flexible implant resection arthroplasty. Note maintenance of squared-off appearance of bone ends and controlled bone remodeling around implant stems. Note fracture of implant of long finger; patient presented no clinical changes. Contour of bone ends has been maintained as compared to progressive penciling seen in opposite hand because implant continues to maintain joint space and integrity of capsular structure and bone.

the implants are not firmly attached to bone, replacement of an implant for either infection, fracture, or subluxation is a relatively simple procedure. Furthermore, if a fracture of an implant develops or removal become necessary, a functioning resection arthroplasty remains. In case of fracture, the implant continues to function by maintaining the joint space and the integrity of the capsular space. In case of implant removal, the implant has fulfilled much of its mission as a spacer to support the development of the capsule-ligament system. The bone-stock removal is minimal, and bone absorption practically never occurs, and so an arthrodesis procedure with a bone graft can easily be accomplished.

Implant material, testing, and durability

Medical-grade silicone elastomer was selected as the ideal material for flexible implants because of its long history of excellent biocompatibility and biodurability both in laboratory animals and in 25 years of clinical use as an implant material. However, it had not been previously evaluated from the view-point of orthopaedic applications. We have been concerned about implant material and testing of implant devices since the beginning of our research project in 1962. Hundreds of implants have been tested mechanically in our laboratory. Host-tissue response has been studied in laboratory animals including a long-term study of the end-bearing amputation cushion in dogs; the 10-year study of two of these animals showed at autopsy the excellent inertness of the materials with no peripheral spread to lymph nodes or any of the organs. Similar results were observed in the postmortem study of a 68-year-old rheumatoid patient who had bilateral metacarpophalangeal arthroplasties 15 years ago. An in vivo retrieval study has shown no correlation between lipid levels in the implants or the patient's serum and either the incidence of breakage or duration of the implantation.[20,45] The capsular reaction around the implant was very mild.

A field clinic study involving 293 participating clinics throughout the world was originated in 1965 to enlarge the clinical experience with flexible implant arthroplasty methods.[1-16,18,19,21-26,47-50] Later, in 1974, a computer study was initiated for storage and retrieval of clinical data. The results of these studies are presented later.

The retrieval study has included the early and long-term evaluation of our cases and those operated on in the participating field clinics. Serial evaluation of the joints by clinical, radiographic, and laboratory studies was carried out. The tolerance of the implants by soft tissues, bone, and cartilage has been studied. These comprehensive studies have shown that the medical-grade silicone elastomer that we have been using is well suited and tolerated for human implantation. Further studies were done to evaluate the biologic characteristics of the high-performance silicone elastomer.

A study of implant fractures, which were relatively rare in our cases, was undertaken. We believe that fractures of the silicone materials are the result of propagating tears in the elastomer. These tears are most often produced by pinching and cutting of the implant by sharp bone edges across a tight subluxating joint or a joint that has become loosened by recurrent synovitis.

In an effort to improve the durability of the implants, the manufacturer instituted an intense research effort to increase the tear-resistance characteristics of the silicone elastomer and, at the same time, maintain its other physical characteristics and medical grading. A higher performance material that was developed has approximately 400% greater tear-propagation resistance than the previous material did. A 6-year clinical and laboratory study has shown this material to be a true scientific breakthrough and further enhances the flexible implant resection arthroplasty method.

FLEXIBLE IMPLANT ARTHROPLASTY OF METACARPOPHALANGEAL JOINT
General considerations

If arthroplasty is to be considered, the patient must be cooperative and in good general condition. The skin and neurovascular status must be adequate, and the elements necessary to produce a functional musculotendinous system must be available along with adequate bone stock to receive and support the implant. Adequate facilities must also be available for the operative and postoperative therapy.

Reconstructive procedures of weight-bearing joints of the lower extremity that will require walking with crutches, should precede upper extremity reconstruction. Excessive manual labor and awkward hand weight bearing, as seen in some crutch walkers, should be avoided after surgery. If crutch walking cannot be avoided, special platform crutches should be used. Multiple reconstructive procedures must be appropriately staged.[27,29] Tendon repair and synovectomy of tendon sheaths should be done 6 to 8 weeks before joint reconstruction in the rheumatoid hand. However, if the extensor tendons are ruptured and the metacarpophalangeal joints are dislocated, arthroplasty of the metacarpophalangeal joints is done before the finger joints. In swan-neck deformity, arthroplasties of the metacarpophalangeal and proximal interphalangeal joints are done at the same stage. However, in boutonnière deformity, it is preferable to reconstruct the proximal interphalangeal joint before the metacarpophalangeal joint.

Metacarpophalangeal joint implant arthroplasty

The finger-joint distributing-load flexible hinge is a one-piece intramedullary stemmed implant made of high-performance silicone elastomer and is available in 11 sizes (00 through 9). This implant has been tested for up to 600 million flexion repetitions to 90 degrees without evidence of material failure (Fig. 19-4).

Indications. The following are painful rheumatoid or posttraumatic disabilities: (1) fixed or stiff metacarpophalangeal joints; (2) radiologic evidence of joint destruction or subluxation; (3) ulnar drift, not correctable by surgery of soft tissues alone; (4) contracted intrinsic and extrinsic musculature and ligament system; and (5) associated stiff interphalangeal joints.[31,32,34,37-40,42,44,46]

Surgical technique. A long transverse skin incision is made on the dorsum of the hand over the necks of the metacarpals. The dissection is carried down through subcutaneous tissue to expose the extensor tendons. The dorsal veins, which lie between the metacarpal heads, are carefully released by blunt longitudinal dissection and are retracted laterally. The extensor hood is exposed to the base of the proximal phalanx. Its radial portion is usually stretched out and the extensor tendon dislocated ulnarward. A longitudinal incision is made in the extensor hood fibers parallel to the extensor tendon on its ulnar aspect (Fig. 19-5, A). In the little

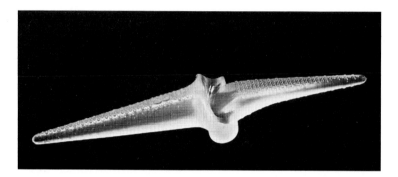

Fig. 19-4. Design features of our distributing-load flexible-hinge finger-joint implant. The distal stem is shown on the right and the proximal stem on the left. A compromise between flexibility and stiffness is achieved by proper distribution of the material at the midsection. The area of the distal stem into the midsection is thickened volarly and is accommodated on flexion by a depression in the proximal middle area of the volar aspect of the midsection. This design decreased flex load and increased the flex life of the implant while maintaining its strength and stability. These implants have been tested for more than 600 million flexion repetitions without evidence of fatigue failure.

Fig. 19-5. A, Extensor hood is incised on ulnar side, parallel to extensor tendon. The ulnar intrinsics of the index and middle fingers are preserved whenever possible; however, if severely tight, they are sectioned at the myotendinous junction. In closure the extensor hood is reefed to relocate the extensor tendon slightly to the radial side of the center of the joint. **B,** The metacarpal heads are removed, with part of the flair of the metaphysis being left. A synovectomy of the joint is performed. It is essential to completely reduce the joint by resection of bone and release of all soft-tissue contractures. On passive extension of the joint, there should be no impingement of the midsection of the implant by the bone edges. **C,** Measures to correct pronation deformity of the index and middle fingers. Proper rectangular and axial reaming of the intramedullary canal is necessary to stabilize the implant stems and maintain slight supination. The axis of the rectangle is placed high on the dorsal ulnar side of the base of the proximal phalanx and low on its radial palmar side. A distally based flap made of collateral ligament and related structures is released from neck of metacarpal and sutured to its dorsoradial aspect through small drill holes. The preserved radial capsule can be included in this repair. This reconstruction further helps maintain supination of these digits.

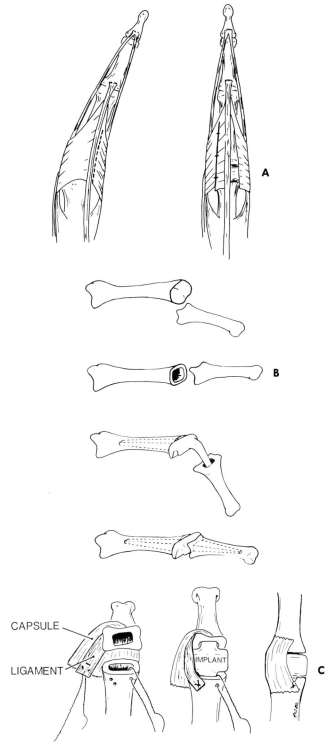

Fig. 19-5. For legend see opposite page.

finger, the approach is made between the extensor communis and proprius tendons. The hood fibers and capsule are carefully dissected from the underlying synovium and retracted to the radial side. The joint is exposed and the head of the metacarpal identified.

The neck of the metacarpal is exposed subperiosteally and transected with an air drill, motor saw, or bone-cutting forceps, leaving part of the metaphyseal flare. Care should be taken to avoid splintering the bone. The head of the metacarpal is grasped, and the collateral ligaments and capsule attachments are incised and preserved. The head of the metacarpal along with the hypertrophied synovial material is thereby removed en masse (Fig. 19-5, *B*). Further involved synovia of the joint cavity and surrounding tissues is removed. A pituitary rongeur has been found to be useful for this purpose.

A comprehensive soft-tissue release procedure must be done at this stage so that the base of the proximal phalanx can be displaced dorsally above the metacarpal. This may require incision of the palmar plate and collateral ligament attachments from the proximal phalanx. This release should be symmetric and complete. The ulnar intrinsic tendon is identified, pulled up into the wound with a blunt hook, and sectioned at the myotendinous junction if tight. However, it is important to know that the ulnar intrinsic of the index and middle fingers (first and second volar interosseous) normally apply a supinatory force to these digits; therefore to avoid the tendency for postoperative pronation deformity, these must be preserved whenever possible.

In some patients who have demonstrated evidence of a flexor synovitis, the flexor sheath can be incised longitudinally in its dorsal aspect. The long flexor tendons can be identified and pulled up gently into the wound with a blunt hook. The degree of involvement of the flexor tendons can be evaluated. In some cases a partial synovectomy and tendon sheath release or injection of corticosteroids is done through this incision.

The tendon of the abductor digiti minimi is exposed on the ulnar aspect of the fifth metacarpophalangeal joint, pulled into the wound with a blunt hook, and sectioned. Care should be taken to avoid the ulnar digital nerve in the dissection. It is believed that this tendon eventually reattaches but in a lengthened position. The tendon of the flexor digiti minimi is preserved because of its importance to obtain flexion at the metacarpophalangeal joint of the little finger.

Bony resection of the base of the proximal phalanx is not usually performed except for marginal osteophytes, which might interfere with the implant. Occasionally in patients with osteoporosis and long-standing dislocation, deformities of the base of the proximal phalanx will be severe. In these cases a shaping of the base of the phalanx may be necessary. The intramedullary canal of the metacarpal is prepared in a rectangular fashion with a curette, broach, and an air drill with a smooth leader point burr to prevent inadvertent perforation through the cortex. The occasional constriction in the intramedullary canal of the proximal third of the metacarpal can easily be enlarged with the burr. The canal of the ring metacarpal is frequently small and requires careful preparation. Care should be taken to avoid too much reaming of the canal, especially in patients with thin bones. Test implants are used to select the proper size. The implant stems should fit well down into the canal so that the transverse midsection of the implant abuts against the bone end. The largest implant possible should be used. Implants of sizes 4 through 9 are generally used. A rectangular hole is then made in the joint surface of the proximal phalanx with an osteotome, knife, broach, or air drill. The intramedullary canal is reamed in the same fashion as the metacarpal to receive the distal stem of the implant selected for the metacarpal. Any sharp points or rough surfaces on the bone ends should be completely smoothened.

In the index and middle fingers, the intramedullary canal is reamed so that the rectangle is positioned high on the ulnodorsal side of the base of the proximal phalanx and low on its radiopalmar side (Fig. 19-5, *C*). This proper rectangular and axial configuration of the intramedullary canal is necessary to stabilize the implant stems and help maintian slight supination of the digit. Attention to this detail of the technique again will help prevent the occurrence of postoperative pronation deformity. Contrarily, in the little finger, a position of slight pronation is desired and the intramedullary rectangle is positioned high on the dorsoradial side and low on the ulnopalmar side.

The wound is thoroughly irrigated with saline to remove all debris. Blunt instruments should be used with a "no-touch technique" when one is inserting silicone finger-joint implants. First the implant is firmly inserted into the intramedullary canal of the metacarpal, and then by slight traction on the finger, the joint is distracted and the implant is flexed so that the distal stem can easily be inserted into the proximal phalanx. With the joint in extension, there should be no impingement of the implant. If there is, soft-tissue release or bone resection has not been adequate.

The radial portion of the sagittal fibers of each extensor hood is reefed in an overlapping fashion so that the extensor tendon is brought slightly to the radial side of the center of the joint. Three to five 4-0 Dacron sutures with a buried-knot technique are used. In the index and middle fingers it is most important not to overcorrect the position of the extensor tendon too far radially; this would result in a deforming force in favor of pronation. In certain cases of severe or long-standing flexion deformity, the extensor tendons may become stretched and an extensor tendon lag may persist if not corrected. In these cases, the extensor tendon should be reefed not only transversely as described, but also longitudinally. Exceptionally one can accomplish an extensor tendon tenodesis by suturing it to the dorsal base of the proximal phalanx through small drill holes. Perfect balance of the extensor mechanism is essential.

Rheumatoid patients often present an inadequate first dorsal interosseous muscle or have a tendency for pronation deformity of the index finger and occasionally of the middle finger; a reconstruction of the radial collateral ligament is then indicated. A distally based flap made of the collateral ligament and related structures is prepared when it is released from the neck of the metacarpal and sutured to the dorsoradial aspect of the neck of the metacarpal through small drill holes using 3-0 Dacron sutures. The radial capsule that has been preserved, may also be included in this repair. Occasionally the radial collateral ligament is not incised; however, if loose, it is reefed with a suture passed through drill holes in the neck of the meta-carpal similarly as above. The sutures are placed before the implant is inserted and are tied as the finger is held in supination and abduction. Note that the first dorsal interosseous muscle fibers that attach to the ligament become dorsally relocated with this repair. When the radial collateral ligament is inadequate, a palmar plate flap may be used to reconstruct this ligament. This procedure has seemed to be important in correction of pronation deformities and provides some improved lateral stability for pinch. It seems to decrease flexion of the index metacarpophalangeal joint by 10 to 20 degrees when the capsule is tightened, but this loss is outweighed by increased stability and a better correction of the pronation deformity. Meticulous evaluation and correction of the balance of the capsuloligamentous and musculotendinous structures will be rewarded by improved results.

The skin incision is closed with interrupted 5-0 nylon sutures: two small drains made from strips of silicone elastomer sheeting are inserted into the wound under the skin. A nonadherent dressing such as rayon is applied over the wound along with a nitrofurazone (Furacin) or alternate gauze overlay. A voluminous hand-conforming dressing is applied, with avoidance of pressure on the radial side of the index. A narrow plaster splint is included on the palmar aspect.

Postoperative care and bracing. Immediate and continous elevation of the hand and the forearm during the postoperative course is very important. The wound is usually checked on the second day and the drains removed. Swelling is generally minimal, and so use of the dynamic brace can begin on the third to fifth postoperative day. A light dressing is applied to the hand and forearm, and the dynamic brace is fitted and adjusted enabling the patient to start finger movements in a protected area. Because of space limitation, refer to previous publications for the important details of the postoperative care,[36,41] and to Chapter 20 of this book.

Results

The presentation of results is limited to those obtained with high-performance silicone elastomer implants in a group of patients operated on in the Grand Rapids Clinic and participating field clinics and whose results were evaluated by the computer retrieval method. In the first group there were 160 patients with 511 metacarpophalangeal flexible-implant resection arthroplasties followed for an average of 29 months after surgery. Of this same group, a smaller group of 37 patients with 100 metacarpophalangeal reconstruction with an average of 4 years of follow-up was isolated. Data were reported on specially designed preoperative postoperative evaluation forms. The program was written in a PL-1 language for the IBM 370 computer.

In this review data pertinent to implant fractures, clinical abnormalities, bone response, and range of motion are reported.

Table 19-1. Fracture incidence in 511 high-performance metacarpophalangeal implant arthroplasties with an average of 29 months of follow-up.

Index	5/132
Middle	5/139
Ring	1/120
Little	1/120
Total	12/511 (2.35%)

Implant fractures. Fractures of the high-performance finger-joint implant were reported in 12 of the 511 (2.35%) metacarpophalangeal joints reconstructed; these were distributed over the index, middle, ring, and little fingers as shown in Table 19-1. In the 4-year follow-up group of 100 reconstructed joints, only one fracture was reported. On the other hand it is interesting to note the findings of a 1976 study released by the Grand Rapids Clinic. A long-term series of 868 metacarpophalangeal joints reconstructed with the original silicone elastomer showed an overall fracture rate of 7.6%; on the other hand, the fracture rate in 638 metacarpophalangeal joints reconstructed with the high-performance silicone implant dropped to 1.6%. Surgeons in the home clinic and also in the field clinics observed that fractures occurred in a small group of patients who use their hands roughly or in those who have extremely thin bones. One of our patients broke all four earlier elastomer implants in both hands and subsequently fractured two of the replacement implants for a total of 10 fractured implants in a single patient. It has also been noted that, in reconstructed joints prone to develop fractured implants, this will usually occur in the first 2 years. Patients with stable and functional joints at the end of 2 years can reasonably expect to maintain good durability of the reconstructed joints.

It is our feeling that fractures of silicone implants result from propagating tears in the elastomer. Although this has been greatly decreased by the introduction of the high-performance material, the causative mechanism remains the same. The tears are most often initiated by pinching or cutting of the implant by sharp bone edges across a tight subluxating joint or a joint that has become loosened through recurrent synovitis. In a joint that presents a tendency for subluxation, the implant midsection becomes impinged by the bone ends. The implant alone cannot stabilize the joint, and if the joint is deformed, it will receive unusual high stress that can result in tears and eventually fracture of the implant. The tendency for subluxation can be attributable to inadequate surgical correction of the deformity or to increased progression of the synovial disease; this can also be seen when the more proximal joints fall victim to the destructive process resulting in collapse of the longitudinal arch with secondary tendon imbalances distally as seen in the swan-neck deformity. Consequently all efforts should be made to obtain an adequate joint space with smooth bone edges, to properly release the contractures, to provide a well-balanced musculotendinous and capsuloligamentous support around the reconstructed joint, and to handle the implant with an atraumatic technique. At-

Table 19-2. Alignment in 511 high-performance metacarpophalangeal joint implant arthroplasties with an average of 29 months of follow-up.

Residual subluxation	2
Recurrent subluxation	10
Residual ulnar deviation	21
Recurrent ulnar deviation	16
Radial overcorrection	16

Table 19-3. Alignment in 100 high-performance metacarpophalangeal joint implant arthroplasties with an average of 47 months of follow-up.

Residual ulnar deviation	3
Recurrent ulnar deviation	1
Radial overcorrection	1
Perforated bone cortex	1

tention to the postoperative dressing and rehabilitation are equally important. Patients with severe rheumatoid disease and thin sharp bones in tight joints are prone to develop implant fractures. For this reason, a project to develop a smooth bone liner (grommet) of a synthetic material is currently in progress, and early clinical trials appear promising. It has been noted, however, that the implant that is not perfectly intact continued to perform as a spacer and also supported the intramedullary canal of the cut bone end to preserve its squared-off shape.

Correction of deformities. Clinical deformities noted in 511 operated metacarpophalangeal joints are reported in Table 19-2. Note that this group presented 23 (5%) residual deformities and 42 (8%) recurrent deformities. The ulnar drift remained corrected to less than 10 degrees of ulnar deviation in 92.8% of the joints. The subluxation of the metacarpophalangeal joint remained corrected in 97.6% of the digits. Radial overcorrection was present in 3.1% of the joints. In the group of 37 patients with 100 metacarpophalangeal joint arthroplasties, residual ulnar deviation was reported in 3%, recurrent ulnar deviation in 1%, and radial overcorrection in 1%. There was one report of surgical perforation through the bone cortex (Table 19-3).

Note that the role of the implant in preventing these deformities is minimal. The importance of proper surgical technique and postoperative care cannot be sufficiently stressed. These deformities are usually attributable to inadequate soft-tissue release, inadequate reefing of the extensor mechanism, and improper postoperative bracing. The cases of recurrent subluxation are attributable to inadequate soft-tissue release or bone removal. Radial overcorrection is often associated with a pronation deformity, especially in the index and middle fingers.

Bone response. Bone response was evaluated by review of roentgenograms done at an average of 29 months for 379 reconstructed metacarpophalangeal joints

Table 19-4. Bone response in 379 high-performance metacarpophalangeal joint implant arthroplasties with an average of 29 months of follow-up.

	Resorption	Production
Around stems	4	39
Proximal bone end	8	27
Distal bone end	12	3

Table 19-5. Bone response in 48 high-performance metacarpophalangeal joint implant arthroplasties with an average of 49 months of follow-up.

	Resorption	Production
Around stems	0	14
Proximal bone end	0	13
Distal bone end	4	0
None	54	43

shown in Table 19-4. The roentgenographic findings in a group of 32 patients with 58 metacarpophalangeal reconstructions are shown at an average of 49 months post-operatively in Table 19-5.

Minimal bone production around the intramedullary stems is expected in most cases and is further evidence of the encapsulation process. Moderate bone production was shown in a total of 39 cases. This is also desirable because it is evidence of the tolerance of the bone interface to the soft flexible hinged implant. This response further contributes to the strength and stability of the reconstruction without interfering with joint function. In some cases bone production is somewhat increased, in others it is not evident, and in a few cases there is minimal bone resorption. This finding contrasts considerably with joint replacement implants having rigid stems or cases in which the stem fixation has failed with either cement or tissue ingrowth methods. Considerable bone resorption has been reported in the majority of these types of implants that have been followed for 2 years or more. As rigid implant stems become progressively looser, the joint becomes unstable and the function of this implant is lost; further destruction ensues with activity of the patient. Resorption of bone is also noted in a resection arthroplasty done without any implant and is caused by excessive bone remodeling in the absence of normal forces transmitted to the bone in joint function. This is seen as shortening, narrowing, and spiking of the bones. This does not occur when the flexible implant is used because it supports the bone, both in the intramedullary canal and at the bone ends to continue to maintain the bone shape.

Range of motion. The average range of motion in a group of 327 metacarpophalangeal joints was from a 31-degree lack of extension to 84 degrees of flexion preoperatively; after an average of 29 months after implant arthroplasty, there was an average of a 3-degree lack of extension to 65 degrees of flexion. Note that the arc of motion, though increased by 9 degrees, has been most importantly been relo-

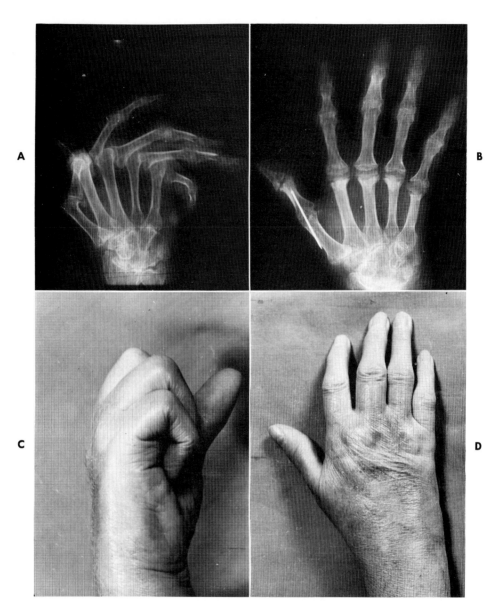

Fig. 19-6. A 52-year-old woman with severe rheumatoid arthritis of 20 years' duration. **A,** Preoperative roentgenogram shows typical subluxation and deviation at the metacarpophalangeal joints and boutonnière deformity of the thumb. **B,** An 8-year postoperative roentgenogram showing excellent correction of deformities and tolerance of deformities and tolerance of the metacarpophalangeal implants. Note the fusions of the metacarpophalangeal joint of the thumb. **C** and **D,** She maintains an excellent functional and cosmetic result and is free of pain.

cated in a functional zone for activities of daily living. This corrected area of movement along with excellent stability and relief of pain provided the patients with a very rewarding functional improvement (Fig. 19-6).

Although there was an average improvement in the strength of grip and pinch, we believe that this measurement is not a consistent index for evaluation of the metacarpophalangeal joint because of the progressive nature of the disease and multiple involvement of other joints in the same extremity.

Surgical complications. In these series there were no reports of infection or of implant subluxation. However, one should note that when implant dislocation occurs it is always the result of a technical error and occurs immediately. It can be caused by incomplete correction of deformities, too small a size implant, improper manipulation of the hand, failure to insert the implant in the intramedullary canal, or improper application of the operative dressing.

Infections can usually be controlled by measures of wound drainage and antibiotic therapy both systemic and in a closed irrigation system. If there are signs of bone infection on roentgenograms, the implant should be removed. If indicated, the implant can be easily reinserted when all signs of infection have cleared. However, this is often not necessary if the capsular formation has occurred because the joint can continue to function adequately as a simple resection arthroplasty.

SUMMARY

The basic concepts and principles of flexible implant resection arthroplasty have been discussed. The surgical indications and techniques for flexible implant arthroplasty of the metacarpophalangeal joint have been detailed. A computer analysis of the results of metacarpophalangeal joint arthroplasty obtained in a special field clinic study have been analyzed.

Flexible implants have been used in more than 600,000 patients in most countries in the world. The results of metacarpophalangeal implant arthroplasty have shown that this method can provide a painfree, durable, mobile, stable, and salvageable arthroplasty. This method has received an overwhelming acceptance as the method of choice throughout the world.

REFERENCES

1. Allieu, Y., Dimeglio, A., and Pech, J.: Les arthroplasties des metacarpophalangiennes avec implants de Swanson dans la main rhumatismale, Ann. Chir. **28**:873-882, 1974.
2. Bocca, M., and Salvi, V.: Le endoprotesi in Silastic di Swanson nelle lesioni articolari di natura degenerative e traumatica, Riv. Chir. Mano **9**:243-254, 1971.
3. Bolten, H.: Arthroplasty of the metacarpophalangeal joints: the hand, J. Br. Soc. Surg. Hand **3**:131-134, 1971.
4. Bouwer, S.: Silicone implants in the hand, Acta Orthop. Belg. **38**:27-32, 1972.
5. Braun, R.M., and Chandler, J.: Quantitative results following implant arthroplasty of the proximal finger joints in the arthritic hand, Clin. Orthop. **83**:135-143, 1972.
6. Comtet, J.J., Monatte, J.P., and Machenaud, A.: Utilisation des implants de Swanson au niveau des articulations interphalangiennes proximales dans les sequelles de traumatisme, voie d'abord—resultats—indications, Ann. Chir. **29**:471-474, 1975.

7. Cugola, L., and Vecchini, L.: Impiego di endoprotesi di Swanson un caso di pseudoartrosi trapezio-metacarpale, Riv. Chir. Mano **9**:149-150, 1971.

8. Curtis, R.M.: Joints of the hand. In Flynn, J.E., editor: Hand surgery, ed. 2, Baltimore, The Williams & Wilkins Co.

9. de Salamanca, R.E.: Artritis rheumatoide (prótesis de Swanson), Madrid, 1971, Editorial Oteo, pp. 299-308.

10. Girzadas, D.V.: Limitations of the use of metallic prosthesis in the rheumatoid hand, Clin. Orthop. **67**:169-171, 1969.

11. Gschwend, V.N., and Zimmermann, J.: Analyse von 200 MCP Arthroplastiken, Hand Chir. **1**(6):7-14, 1973.

12. Haimovici, V.N.: Die Fingergelenk-Endoprothese bei der Dupuytrenschen Krankheit und bei angeborenen Missbildungen der Hand, Med. Orthop. Technik **95**:87-89, 1975.

13. Inglis, A.E., Ranawat, C.S., and Straub, L.R.: Silastic prosthetic implants in the metacarpophalangeal joint of the hand, Rev. Hosp. Special Surg. N.Y. **1**:80-87, 1971.

14. Iseline, F.: Les prothèses articulaires des doigts, Vie Med. **34**:4657-4666, 1970.

15. Jakubowski, V.S.: Silikonendoprothesen der Fingergelenke, Orthop. Traumatol. **3**(18):148-151, 1971.

16. MacFarland, G.B., Jr.: Early experiences with the silicone rubber prosthesis (Swanson) in reconstructive surgery of the rheumatoid hand, South. Med. J. **65**:113-117, 1972.

17. Madden, J.W., and Peacock, E.E., Jr.: Studies on the biology of collagen during wound healing: dynamic metabolism of scar collagen and remodeling of dermal wounds, Ann. Surg. **174**:511-520, 1971.

18. Mannerfelt, L., and Andersson, K.: Silastic arthroplasty of the metacarpophalangeal joints in rheumatoid arthritis (long-term results), J. Bone Joint Surg. **57A**:484-489, 1975.

19. Matev, I.B.: Silicon implantatum a kéz helyreállító sebészeteben, Traumatologia **14**:222-223, 1971.

20. Meester, W.D., and Swanson, A.B.: In vivo testing of silicone rubber joint implants for lipid absorption, J. Biomed. Mater. Res. **6**:193-199, 1972.

21. Michon, J., Delgoutte, J.P., and Jandeaux, M.: Les implants en Silastic de Swanson en traumatologie de la main, Ann. Chir. Plast. **19**:13-21, 1974.

22. Millender, L.H., Nalebuff, E.A., Hawkins, R.B., and Ennis, A.: Infection after silicone prosthetic arthroplasty in the hand, J. Bone Joint Surg. **57A**:825-829, 1975.

23. Millesi, H.: Wiederherstellung der Fingergelenkfunktion durch Silikon-gummi-interponate nach Swanson, Chir. Plast. Allem. **1**:157-165, 1972.

24. Rhodes, K., Jeffs, J.V., and Scott, J.T.: Experience with Silastic prostheses in rheumatoid hands, Ann. Rheum. Dis. **31**:103-108, 1972.

25. Salvi, V.: Principi del trattamento chirugico nelle artropatie croniche della mano, Rheumatisma **22**:208-222, 1970.

26. Swanson, A.B.: The need for early treatment of the rheumatoid hand, J. Mich. Med. Soc. **60**:348-351, 1961.

27. Swanson, A.B.: A flexible implant for replacement of arthritic or destroyed joints in the hand, N.Y. Univ. Inter-Clin. Inform. Bull. **6**:16-19, 1966.

28. Swanson, A.B.: Improving end-bearing characteristics of lower-extremity amputation stumps, N.Y. Univ. Inter-Clin. Inform. Bull. **5**:1-7, 1966.

29. Swanson, A.B.: Silicone rubber implants for replacement of arthritic or destroyed joints in the hand, Surg. Clin. North Am. **48**:1113-1127, 1968.

30. Swanson, A.B.: Finger joint replacement by silicone rubber implants and the concept of implant fixation by encapsulation, Ann. Rheum. Dis. (supp.) **28**:47-55, 1969.

31. Swanson, A.B.: Silicone rubber implants for replacement of arthritic or destroyed joints in the hand. In Tubiana, R., editor: The rheumatoid hand, Group d'Etude de la Main monograph no. 3, Paris, 1969, L'Expansion Scientifique Française, pp. 176-189.

32. Swanson, A.B.: Arthroplasty in traumatic arthritic joints in the hand, Orthop. Clin. North Am. **1**:285-298, 1970.

33. Swanson, A.B.: The results of silicone rubber implant arthroplasty in the digits, J. Bone Joint Surg. **53A**:807, 1971.

34. Swanson, A.B.: Surgery of established rheumatoid deformities in the hand. In Cruess, R.L., and

Mitchell, N., editors: Surgery of rheumatoid arthritis, Philadelphia, 1971, J.B. Lippincott Co., pp. 177-198.

35. Swanson, A.B.: Flexible implant arthroplasty of arthritic finger joints: rationale, technique and results of treatment, J. Bone Joint Surg. **54A:**435-455, 1972.
36. Swanson, A.B.: Flexible implant resection arthroplasty in the hand and extremities. St. Louis, 1973, The C.V. Mosby Co.
37. Swanson, A.B.: Flexible implant arthroplasty in the hand, Clin. Plast. Surg. **3:**141-157, 1976.
38. Swanson, A.B.: Reconstructive surgery in the arthritic hand and foot, Ciba Clin. Symp. **31**(6), 1979.
39. Swanson, A.B., and de Groot, G.: Flexible implant resection arthroplasty in the upper extremity in hand surgery. In Flynn, J.E., editor: Hand surgery, ed. 2, Baltimore, 1975, The Williams & Wilkins Co.
40. Swanson, A.B., and de Groot Swanson, G.: Disabling osteoarthritis in the hand and its treatment, Symposium on Osteoarthritis, St. Louis, 1976, The C.V. Mosby Co.
41. Swanson, A.B., de Groot Swanson, G., and Leonard, J.: Postoperative rehabilitation program in flexible implant arthroplasty of the digits. In Hunter, J.M., Schneider, L.H., Mackin, E.J., and Bell, J.A., editors: Rehabilitation of the hand, St. Louis, 1978, The C.V. Mosby Co.
42. Swanson, A.B., and de Groot Swanson, G.: Flexible implant resection arthroplasty; a method for reconstruction of small joints in the extremities, The American Academy of Orthopaedic Surgeons Instructional Course Lectures, **27:**27-60, St. Louis, 1978, The C.V. Mosby Co.
43. Swanson, A.B., and Herndon, J.H.: Flexible (silicone) implant arthroplasty of the metacarpophalangeal joint of the thumb, J. Bone Joint Surg. **59A**(3):362-368, April 1977.
44. Swanson, A.B., and Matev, I.B.: The proximal interphalangeal joint in arthritic disabilities and experiences in the use of silicone rubber implant arthroplasty in the upper extremity, J. Bone Joint Surg. **52A:**1265, 1970.
45. Swanson, A.B., Meester, W.D., de Groot Swanson, G., Rangaswamy, L., and Schut, G.E.D.: Durability of silicone implants: an in vivo study, Orthop. Clin. North Am. **4:**1097-1112, 1973.
46. Swanson, A.B., and Yamauchi, Y.: Silicone rubber implants for replacement of arthritic or destroyed joints (Abstract), J. Bone Joint Surg. **50A:**1272, 1968.
47. Tubiana, R., Achach, P., and Rousso, M.: Les arthroplasties par implants en silicone au niveau de la main, Chirurgie **96:**1000-1004, 1970.
48. Vainio, K., and Pulkki, T.: Surgical treatment of arthritis mutilans, Ann. Chir. Gynaecol. Fenn. **48:**361-368, 1959.
49. Weigert, M., and Gronert, H.J.: Silicon-Kautschuk in der Handchirurgie, Arch. Orthop. Unfall-Chir. **73:**189-200, 1972.
50. Wessinghage, D.: Der Fingergelenkersatz als funktions-bessernde Massnahme, Phys. Med. Rehabil. **7**(14):209-211, 1973.

20. Postoperative rehabilitation program for flexible implant arthroplasty of the fingers

Alfred B. Swanson, M.D.
Genevieve de Groot Swanson, M.D.
Judy Leonard, O.T.R.

The postoperative care and rehabilitation program are critical for the quality of the result of finger joint arthroplasty. In the flexible implant arthroplasty method, the implant acts as a dynamic spacer that separates the bone ends while maintaining alignment of the joint, and as an internal mold to support the development of the new joint capsule, and as a flexible hinge (see Chapter 22). As with simple resection arthroplasty, if motion is restricted during the healing phase, there will be poor mobility of the joint. Therefore the host tissue or collagen reaction must be used advantageously; the fact that the collagen capsule can be reinforced at surgery and trained postoperatively is used prospectively in the formation of the new joint.[1-5]

Variations of the arthritic involvement presented by many patients demand great mastery of the factors involved. In patients who have a "complex hand" with involvement of both the metacarpophalangeal and proximal interphalangeal joints, the metacarpophalangeal joint should have priority in the surgical reconstructive and rehabilitation program. Any tendon imbalance or bone and joint malalignment must be corrected; otherwise it will affect the long-term result of joint replacement. Precise anatomic dissection, adequate soft-tissue release, respect for gliding surfaces, prevention of edema, and early guided movement in functional planes are essential for good results in arthroplasty procedures. From the early stages of treatment, every measure should be taken to decrease, if not prevent, unnecessary residual stiffness in the hand, wrist, elbow, and shoulder joints. Knowledge and strict application of certain basic principles of hand care are therefore essential and include proper operative dressing, immobilization in a functional position, postoperative elevation, early motion, and exercises.

The postoperative dressing should give support to the arches of the hand, control alignment, and provide adequate compression without constriction; it is fashioned with Dacron batting applied longitudinally; it includes a small palmar plaster splint to maintain the wrist in a neutral position. Pressure on the radial side of the hand should be avoided; proper alignment of the digits can be supported by application of Webril strips to the ulnar side of the digits. Proper elevation of the hand and extremity will enhance venous return and reduce edema. The use of a special arm sling that can be attached to an intravenous infusion stand has been very helpful. Slings should not routinely be worn when the patient is in the upright position because they may prevent use of the extremity. Early active motion is important to maintain muscle length, reduce edema, prevent ligament contracture, prevent adhesions of tendons and other gliding surfaces, and maintain hand architecture. Passive motion is avoided in the very early postoperative phase. Motion should be encouraged not only distally but also at the level of the wrist, elbow, and shoulder joints so that sympathetic dystrophy is avoided. The patient should be frequently examined for any loss of mobility of the elbow and shoulder; even a few degrees of loss of abduction and external rotation may signal an impending shoulder-hand syndrome. Circumduction exercises of the shoulder, active movements of the digits, especially with the hand elevated, if done early and continued throughout the treatment program, will avoid many of the disastrous effects seen in improperly treated patients. Specific exercises for the reconstructed part must follow an organized and supervised regimen.[6]

The greatest challenge in postoperative rehabilitation of finger joint arthroplasty is to maintain a proper balance between good healing of the surrounding scar tissue and at the same time apply proper amounts of tension across the scar to obtain the desired range of motion. Controlled motion during this period will train the new capsule to have sufficient looseness for flexion and extension and sufficient tightness in the mediolateral plane for rotation and angular stability. An adjustable dynamic brace is necessary to guide the motion of the joint in desired planes and to prevent recurrent deformity during the early postoperative course. Scar formation will vary accourding to the joint involved, the type of surgery performed, and the differences in collagen reaction in each patient. The associated tendon deficiencies also vary. It is therefore the responsibility of the operating surgeon to control the process by providing a well-organized and preplanned rehabilitation program for his patients. The patients receive specific instructions and are regularly followed in the early postoperative period. They are instructed to sit comfortably to stabilize the proximal joints, including the shoulder, elbow, and wrist to concentrate the movement at the reconstructed joints. Once the sutures are removed, the patients can precede their exercises with an oil or lotion massage. The follow-up should be meticulous and include objective measurements of the patient's progress. This is as important to the final result as the surgical procedure. To fail to understand these basic facts is to miss the opportunity of the pleasure of a complete success.

DYNAMIC BRACE
Function

We have designed a brace to facilitate early postoperative motion in our cases of finger joint implant resection arthroplasty. Its use has greatly improved the anatomic and functional results. The brace prevents undue stretching of associated reconstructed tendons and ligaments and also assists the digital extensors and flexors, which are frequently weak because of long-standing deformity, an accompanying tenosynovitis, and fibrosis. The dynamic brace has three major functions: (1) to provide complete and adjustable correction of residual deformity, (2) to control motion in the desired plane and range, and (3) to assist flexor and extensor power.

Construction

The basic brace for finger joint arthroplasty consists of a dorsal splint that provides a stable base for outriggers and supports the wrist. The brace is available in three basic sizes.* Three transverse straps attached to the dorsal splint are made of malleable metal to be easily adjusted to the shape and size of the forearm; adjustable Velcro straps are attached to these transverse straps to hold the brace in position; two Velcro straps are placed around the forearm and one across the palm, with the last having a palmar pad to help maintain the arches of the hand and prevent rotation of the brace. A transverse bar to which finger slings are attached is fitted onto a dorsal arm. The position of the transverse bar can be adjusted in all three planes. The finger slings are made of soft plastic with multiple perforations and are connected to the transverse bar with rubber bands. Small radially placed outriggers may be added for correction of pronation deformity often present in the index and middle fingers of rheumatoid hands. A longer bar can be used for thumb abduction. All these outriggers are attached with thumb screws. A flexion cuff is used to help correct flexor weakness. This sheepskin cuff is attached to the dorsal splint, passes around the digits, and draws them into flexion by the pull of a Velcro strap attached through a loop on the proximal portion of the brace. With this cuff, the finger joints can be passively brought into flexion for prescribed periods of time during the day. A figure-of-eight elbow strap is used to prevent distal migration of the brace when the cuff is used.

METACARPOPHALANGEAL JOINT POSTOPERATIVE PROGRAM
Goals and special considerations

The results of an organized postoperative program for these patients are so much better than those of any other method that all attempts should be made by the surgeon to provide this type of care for his patient.

The ideal motion to be obtained after implant resection arthroplasty at the metacarpophalangeal joints would provide adequate flexion of the ulnar digits, allowing the surface of their pulps to touch the palm at the distal palmar crease for adequate grasp of smaller objects. Full flexion of the index and middle fingers is less critical for grasping because these digits are mainly used for pinch activities. A degree of speading of the fingers into abduction, especially of the index finger, is important. Full extension at these joints is also important for the performance of normal hand activities and for maintenance of the balance of the distal joints.

---

*Parke, Davis & Co., Pope Division, Box 368, Greenwood, South Carolina 29646.

Chronic flexion deformity of the metacarpophalangeal joints can further aggravate hyperextension tendencies at the proximal interphalangeal joints. Pronation deformity of the index finger and occasionally the middle finger can be a problem in the rheumatoid hand and can, to some degree, be corrected in the postoperative program.

Brace fitting and postoperative treatment

The voluminous conforming operative hand dressing is left on until the postoperative swelling has decreased, usually in 3 to 5 days. The dynamic brace is applied over a lightly padded dressing after removal of the postoperative dressing. If the brace is not available, guided early motion may still be obtained by application of a light-weight, short arm cast fitted with outriggers and similar rubber band slings.

The dorsal wrist splint, with a $^1\!/_4$-inch felt pad placed between the forearm and the brace, should be applied loosely enough so that it is not constrictive and yet tightly enough so that it does not rotate on the forearm and hand. If there is a tendency toward continued swelling, the limb may be elevated with the wrist supported in extension against an intravenous infusion stand. Active exercises in the elevated position may then be carried out.

The rubber band slings are placed on the proximal phalanges to guide the alignment of the digits into the desired position. The pull of the slings should be adjusted in a slight radial deviation to prevent recurrent ulnar drift. The tension of the rubber bands should be tight enough to support the digits and yet loose enough to allow 70 degrees of active flexion; this is especially true of the little finger, which may have weak flexion power (Fig. 20-1). The brace may require adjustment once or twice a day in the early postoperative course.

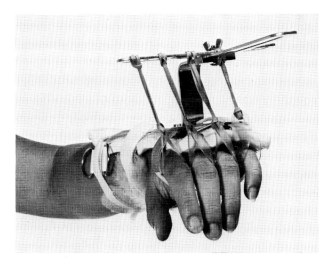

Fig. 20-1. The finger slings of the dynamic brace are placed on the proximal phalanges to assist metacarpophalangeal joint extension and guide the alignment of the digits. The slings are adjusted to pull from the radial side to prevent ulnar deviation. Padding underneath the brace with a light-weight dressing or a dorsal strip of felt may be necessary.

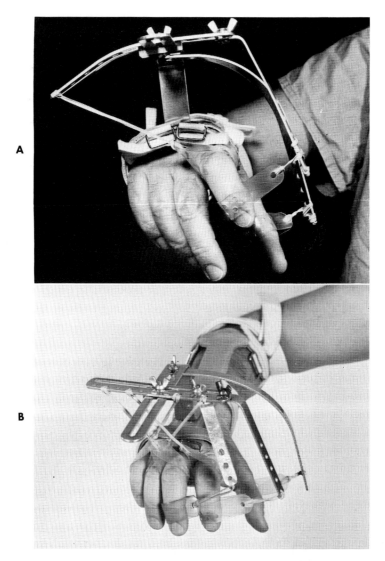

Fig. 20-2. A, Method of using the combined pull of two slings on one digit to form a couple producing a supination torque force without interfering with flexion and extension movements. This technique can be used to assist in correction of pronation deformity, which is often seen in the index and middle fingers in rheumatoid hands. **B,** Dynamic brace with all outriggers attached for correcting ulnar drift and rotation deformity of the index and middle fingers and for controlling abduction of the thumb. (From Swanson, A.B., Swanson, G. de Groot, and Leonard, J.: In Hunter, J.M., et al.: Rehabilitation of the hand, St. Louis, 1978, The C.V. Mosby Co.)

The thumb outrigger is usually applied in all cases because of the patient's tendency to bring the thumb over the fingers on flexion. This should be avoided because the lateral pressure of the thumb on the index finger could result in recurrent ulnar drift deformity. If there is a tendency toward medial rotation (pronation) in the index or middle fingers, additional outrigger bars are applied to provide a rotation force at the metacarpophalangeal joint according to the concept of a force couple; a force couple is defined as two equal and opposite forces that act along parallel lines and is obtained by application of the loops to the digit that shows a tendency for pronation (Fig. 20-2). A rubber band sling is fitted from an additional outrigger to the distal phalanx of the digit showing a pronation tendency. This combined pull of two slings provides a torque force in the direction of supination on the digit without interfering with flexion and extension movements.

The extension portion of the brace is worn continuously day and night for the first 3 weeks alternating with specific flexion measures. The flexion exercises in the brace with the extension slings in position are carried out, starting at 3 days postoperatively, both actively and passively (with no more than 2 pounds of force) on an hourly basis (Fig. 20-3). The ideal goal of 0 degrees of extension to 70 degrees of flexion is constantly stressed. The patient is seen at least three times by the physician or the therapist during the first week, and the brace is carefully readjusted as necessary. Only exceptionally, if there is considerable flexor weakness of the little finger with adequate extensor stability, can the extension sling be removed from this digit during the exercise periods.

During the second and third weeks, the extension portion of the brace is also worn continuously day and night. If there is severe flexor weakness and good extension, the extensor sling can be removed 1 to 2 hours a day to achieve greater active flexion of the metacarpophalangeal joints. If the patient appears not to be obtaining 70 degrees of flexion, several measures can be taken. Should most of the motion be occurring at the proximal interphalangeal joints, these joints may be immobilized with small dorsal taped-on padded aluminum splints to help localize the flexion force at the metacarpophalangeal joints. The rubber bands may be lengthened to decrease the extension force applied. Occasionally, temporary Kirschner wire fixation of the proximal interphalangeal joints can also be used for the same functional purpose.

At 3 weeks any residual lack of flexion should be energetically treated. The flexion cuff may be worn 1 to 2 hours twice a day to flex the metacarpophalangeal joints passively. When this cuff is used, the figure-of-eight elbow strap should be applied to prevent distal migration of the brace (Fig. 20-4, A). The patient may use the flexion cuff to obtain further flexion during the active flexion exercises. Other useful devices to improve flexion in the presence of adequate extension include the use of traction devices. Finger slings on the proximal phalanges can be attached volarly to the loop of a special Velcro wrist strap or to the wrist strap of the dynamic brace (Fig. 20-4, B). If the distal and proximal interphalangeal joints are stable, dressmaker hooks can be glued to the fingernails with a cyanoacrylate

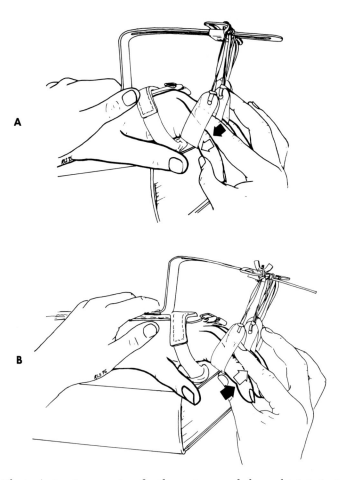

Fig. 20-3. Flexion/extension exercises for the metacarpophalangeal joint. **A,** Active and passive flexion exercises are carried out in the brace starting at 3 days postoperatively. No more than 2 pounds of force should be applied to assist passive flexion. The arm is positioned over a book to help stabilize the proximal joints so that movement of the digits is allowed. Proper adjustment of the tension of the rubber bands is essential to allow full range of motion. The extension portion of the brace is worn continuously for the first 3 weeks. **B,** Active and passive extension exercises are carried out in the brace. (**A** and **B** from Swanson, A.B., Swanson, G. de Groot, and Leonard, J.: In Hunter, J.M., et al.: Rehabilitation of the hand, St. Louis, 1978, The C.V. Mosby Co.)

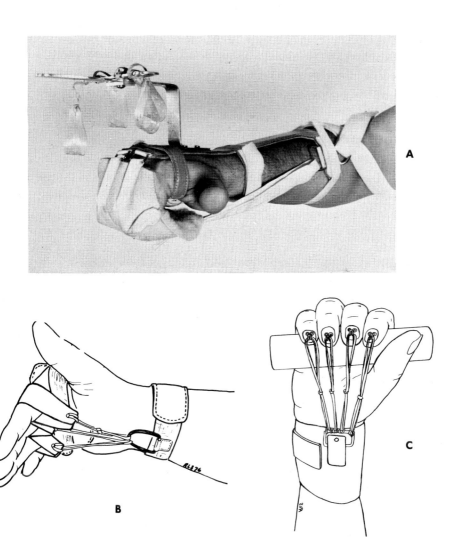

Fig. 20-4. Passive flexion devices that can be used starting at 3 weeks postoperatively. **A,** Flexion cuff is in place to passively assist flexion of the joints. The Velcro strap pulls to the radial side and may be used by the patient to gradually increase the stretching effort. Figure-of-eight elbow strap should be used to prevent distal migration of the brace. **B,** Finger slings placed on the proximal phalanges are attached to the loop of a special Velcro wrist strap or to the strap of the dynamic brace to provide flexion traction. **C,** An extremely efficient method of obtaining passive flexion of the metacarpophalangeal joints after arthroplasty provided that the interphalangeal joints are stable. (**A** and **B** from Swanson, A.B., Swanson, G. de Groot, and Leonard, J.: In Hunter, J.M., et al.: Rehabilitation of the hand, St. Louis, 1978, The C.V. Mosby Co.)

adhesive. Individual rubber bands are then attached from the loop of the special wrist strap to the nail hooks (Fig. 20-4, C). Initially this is done over a 1¼-inch wooden dowel to encourage flexion. As the flexion increases, the size of the dowel is progressively reduced to obtain even further flexion. A finger crutch can also be substituted for the dowel. Eventually this traction device is used without any grasping device. A small Band-Aid is applied over the hooks so that one can avoid snagging them between exercise periods. The just-described traction methods give better control of the alignment and the desired amount of flexion pull for each individual finger. These traction methods are especially useful and can be started during the early postoperative course in certain cases presenting severe preoperative stiffness or flexor weakness, with an adequate extensor mechanism. In these difficult cases a functional compromise can be reached after a few degrees of extension have been given up.

The extension portion of the brace is usually worn at night only, starting on the fourth postoperative week for another 3 weeks. In certain few cases, where there is a persistent extensor lag or a tendency for flexion contracture or deviation of the digits, continued part-time support by the use of the brace must be prescribed for several more weeks or even months. The patient should follow a continued exercise and stretching program for 3 months postoperatively to maintain the movement obtained in the early phase. After this time the final range of motion will have been established.

PROXIMAL INTERPHALANGEAL JOINT PROGRAM

The type of postoperative care for the proximal interphalangeal joint depends upon several factors. There are three basic situations: (1) reconstruction of a stiff proximal interphalangeal joint, (2) reconstruction of a swan-neck deformity, and (3) reconstruction of a boutonnière deformity.

When the implant arthroplasty has been performed without a tendon reconstruction for a *stiff proximal interphalangeal joint,* active movements of flexion and extension should be started within 3 to 5 days after surgery. The ideal range of motion after this surgery is 0 degrees of extension to 70 degrees of flexion. Small, taped-on padded aluminum splints to hold the digit in extension are worn mainly as night splints and may be used for several weeks postoperatively, depending on the degree of extensor lag present (Fig. 20-5). There almost always are a few degrees of extensor lag in this type of surgery. The same splint may also be applied slightly to the ulnar or radial side of the dorsum of the digit to correct any associated angular deformity. Active flexion and extension exercises can be performed with a variety of exercise devices such as described further in this chapter. If necessary, the distal interphalangeal joint may be temporarily pinned with a Kirschner wire to concentrate the action of the flexor profundus at the proximal interphalangeal joint. These pins can be removed after approximately 3 weeks.

If the implant resection arthroplasty of the proximal interphalangeal joint has been done for a *swan-neck deformity* in association with a tendon reconstruction

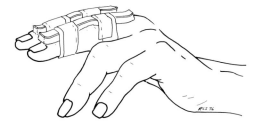

Fig 20-5. Tapped-on padded aluminum splint to hold the digits in extension is worn as night splint or continuously depending on the degree of extensor lag present. The splint may also be applied slightly to the ulnar or radial side of the digit to correct associated angulation deformities.

procedure, a padded taped-on aluminum splint is usually placed on the digit after the postoperative edema has subsided. The joint is immobilized in 10 to 20 degrees of flexion, and the splint is left on for 10 days until the exercises are begun. It is important to obtain at least 10 degrees of flexion contracture of these joints in order to prevent recurrent hyperextension tendencies. Unless the central slip has been released, there may be an imbalance of the joint in favor of extension. During the healing phase the digit should be held in the flexed position with the aluminum splints at least on a part-time basis. The distal interphalangeal joint must not remain in severe flexion and may be temporarily pinned in a neutral position. This will localize the flexion forces at the proximal interphalangeal joint and help the recovery of movement. The metacarpophalangeal joint should be supported in extension with the rubber band slings of the brace or with the reverse lumbrical bar. After the second week, gentle passive flexion exercises of the proximal interphalangeal joint can be started if it appears necessary.

If the implant resection arthroplasty procedure has been done to correct a *boutonnière deformity*, it is important to maintain the extension of the proximal interphalangeal joint and to allow flexion of the distal interphalangeal joint. The distal interphalangeal joint, if in severe hyperextension, should be released by sectioning of the central tendon over the middle phalanx or by relative lengthening of the lateral tendons. The reconstruction of the extensor mechanism should be protected for approximately 10 days with an extension splint applied after the postoperative swelling has decreased. The aluminum splint, in this situation, should immobilize only the proximal interphalangeal joint in extension for 3 to 6 weeks, depending on the degree of extension lag present. The distal joint should be allowed to flex freely. Active flexion and extension exercises are usually started from 10 to 14 days after surgery in alternation with the use of the extension splint, which should be worn at night to hold the proximal interphalangeal joint in extension until the position of the joint is stable, a result that may require 10 weeks. A Kirschner wire passed into the flexor sheath through the fingertip can be used as a temporary internal splint for immobilization of either the distal interphalangeal or proximal

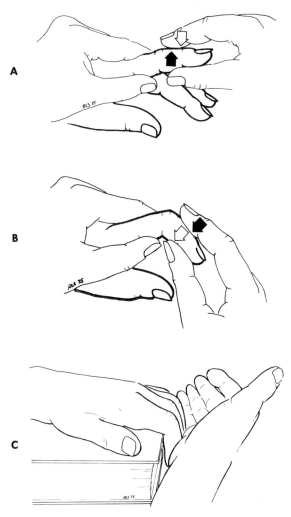

Fig. 20-6. Flexion and extension exercises for the proximal interphalangeal joint. **A,** Active and passive extension exercises are carried out while the proximal phalanx is stabilized. **B** and **C,** Passive flexion exercises can be carried out with the opposite hand while the proximal phalanx is stabilized either over the edge of a book, by an assistant, or with a dowel. **D,** The reverse lumbrical bar can be used to support the proximal phalanges and eliminate motion of the metacarpophalangeal joints during flexion exercises. Note the palmar pad used to maintain the transverse arches of the hand and to assist in preventing rotation of the brace. **E,** Flexion of the proximal interphalangeal joints over a reverse lumbrical bar. The flexion cuff can be applied to gently force flexion if it appears to be necessary. **F,** We designed a "finger crutch" to help support the proximal phalanx in extension during flexion exercises. (**A** to **F** from Swanson, A.B., Swanson, G. de Groot, and Leonard, J.: In Hunter, J.M., et al.: Rehabilitation of the hand, St. Louis, 1978, The C.V. Mosby Co.)

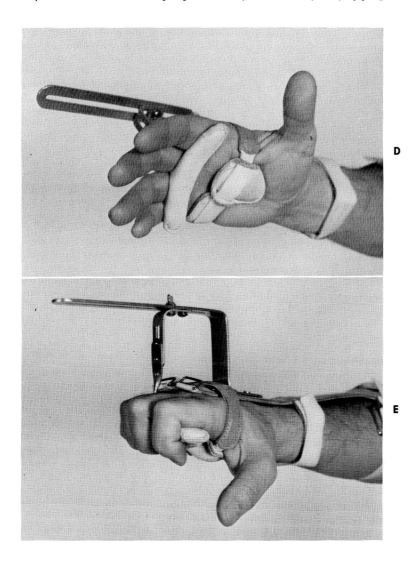

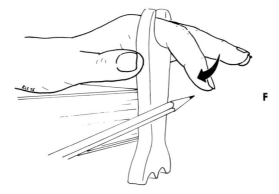

Fig. 20-6, cont'd. For legend see opposite page.

interphalangeal joints. A 0.035-inch wire is very carefully passed through the fingertip from distal to proximal; the wire should end up touching the palmar aspect of the proximal end of the proximal phalanx and is left in place for several days or until the postoperative swelling has decreased sufficiently so that splints with circumferential bandaging can be used.

The exercises for the proximal interphalangeal joint can be carried out actively and passively, with care always being taken to support the metacarpophalangeal joint in extension. This can be done with the opposite hand, over the edge of a book, or with a variety of orthotic devices (Fig. 20-6). Extension of the metacarpophalangeal joints can be supported with the reverse lumbrical bar attached to the dynamic brace or to a special wrist splint. Passive flexion can then be obtained with the flexor cuff or with rubber band traction to fingernail hooks. A dowel can also be used to support the metacarpophalangeal joints. We have developed a small "finger crutch," which we have used in a similar fashion to the Bunnell wood block to support the proximal phalanx during exercises; this is made of ¼-inch plywood or hard rubber material. Passive stretching of flexion contractures of the proximal interphalangeal joint can be carried out when hyperextension of the metacarpophalangeal joint is blocked with the standard lumbrical bar and extension force is applied to the middle phalanx with the extension rubber band slings of the dynamic brace (Fig. 20-7).

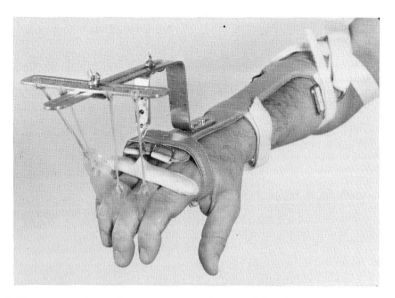

Fig. 20-7. Passive stretching of a joint requires the use of the three-point principle of pressure application. The brace can be adjusted to stretch the proximal interphalangeal joints in extension with the lumbrical bar in normal position for cases of flexion deformities. This adaptation of the brace should not be used after metacarpophalangeal joint arthroplasty because it may produce a palmarward subluxation of the base of the proximal phalanx. (From Swanson, A.B., Swanson, G. de Groot, and Leonard, J.: In Hunter, J.M., et al.: Rehabilitation of the hand, St. Louis, 1978, The C.V. Mosby Co.)

OTHER MODALITIES OF POSTOPERATIVE TREATMENT

Physical and occupational therapy modalities should be considered in most patient. If a therapist is not available, most patients can be managed by the surgeon. Some simple heat applications may be of benefit in the postoperative course after complete wound healing. We occasionally will use paraffin or contrast baths for their heating and analgesic benefits. The following method for these baths is described:

Paraffin bath for hands

Materials: 4 cartons of paraffin and one 10-ounce bottle of baby oil.
Directions:
1. Put these materials in a large can or double boiler. Heat slowly to melting point, approximately 100 to 110 degrees.
2. Dip hand in quickly in 2 inches beyond the wrist, keeping hand over can; repeat 12 times or until $1/4$ inch of wax remains on hand.
3. Wrap the paraffin-covered hand for 15 minutes with a plastic or waxed paper and a large bath towel. Exercise fingers with wax on.
4. Remove paraffin by stripping it off, holding the hand over the can.
5. Massage and exercise warm fingers. Elevate the arm if the hand is swollen. Wear gloves to maintain the heat, especially if going out of doors in cold weather.

This bath may be repeated two or three times a day. There should be no open wounds or unusual swelling of tissue or skin reaction.

Contrast baths for hands

1. Sit at the side of a sink that has a mixing faucet to regulate hot and cold water.
2. Run the faucet at moderate speed, mixing hot and cold water to a temperature of approximately 105° F.
3. The hands should be placed under the water. Active flexion and extension movements of the finers with the hands together in a "wringing of the hands" movement should be done.
4. The hot water should be used for 4 minutes; switch to cold water for 1 minute, hot water for 4 minutes, cold water for 1 minute, and hot water for 4 minutes.
5. The hands are then dried and a small amount of hand lotion can be rubbed into the skin.

Active exercises

The patient may increase the range of motion and strength of the reconstructed joints by exercise over a variety of devices such as the Bunnel block or modifications thereof, cylinders of progressive sizes, or a variety of commercially available hand exercisers. These devices should maintain the architecture of the hand and should not force the digits into deformed positions. To be efficient, they must

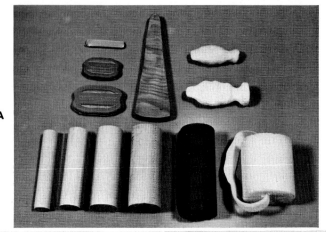

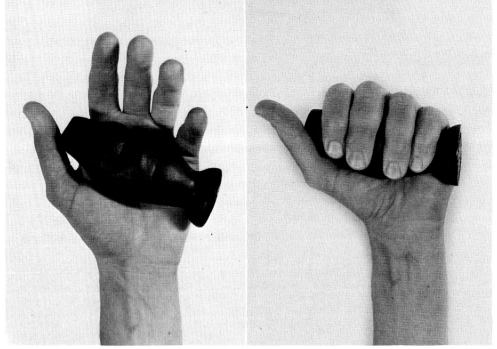

Fig. 20-8. **A,** Variety of devices used to increase joint motion and muscle strength. **B** and **C,** Ideally shaped exercise device to maintain the proper anatomic position of the digits and the arches of the hand. Progressive sizes of this device are used to obtain improved range of motion. Exercises should be continued for at least 3 months after surgery. (**A** to **C** from Swanson, A.B., Swanson, G. de Groot, and Leonard, J.: In Hunter, J.M., et al.: Rehabilitation of the hand, St. Louis, 1978, The C.V. Mosby Co.)

support the bone proximal to the reconstructed joint. With these goals in mind, we devised a "finger gripper" available in three different sizes (Fig. 20-8). Isotonic movements are important for the gliding mechanism of the joint. Isometric exercises, as in grasping around a solid object or therapy putty, are especially good for muscle strengthening. The use of progressively smaller grasping devices, such as wood dowels, can efficiently improve the range of motion. Strengthening of the first dorsal interosseous muscle is important and can be achieved by active abduction exercises of the index finger with or without passive resistance. Abduction and adduction exercises of the digits are also indicated to reinforce the intrinsic muscles.

The patient should use his hand protectively during the early postoperative phase. The postoperative rehabilitation program must be continued for at least 3 months after surgery because of the tendency of the joints to tighten up. It is best to gradually, rather than abruptly, discontinue the exercises and wise to follow a weekly self-evaluation of range of motion. After doing so, the patient can safely use his hand for activities of daily living and vocational skills. However, the patient should continue to exercise and splint as necessary for up to 1 year after surgery. Rough usage of the hand is not recommended.

A very cooperative patient following a good rehabilitation program can obtain an excellent range of motion after implant resection arthroplasty.

Stretching of contractures

Most contractures around joints can be progressively stretched by application of splints or plaster casts; these slowly elongate the tissues without the secondary reactions occurring after overzealous movements that tear the collagen. If bone adhesions are not involved in the contracture, diligent stretching by repeated applications of splints can be of benefit.

Manipulation

Manipulation of joints to correct contracture deformities is usually not indicated. Gentle progressive stretching is preferred. Occasionally, if the contracture has not been long established, gentle manipulation of the joint with or without anesthesia may achieve better positioning of the joint. We have used this technique very infrequently in our practice. If a manipulation is done, temporary fixation in the corrected position is usually indicated.

Rehabilitation techniques are highly individualized for each surgeon. A physical or occupational therapist or other trained personnel, when available, can be of assistance in carrying out postoperative therapy programs. However, close supervision by the surgeon is required to properly adhere to the prescribed program. An understanding of the basic concepts of flexible implant resection arthroplasty and the development of a good rapport with the patient can allow the operating surgeon to obtain ideal results from this method.

REFERENCES

1. Madden, J.W., DeVore, G., and Arem, A.J.: A rational postoperative management program for metacarpophalangeal implant arthroplasty, J. Hand Surg. **2**(5):358, Sept. 1977.
2. Madden, J.W., and Peacock, E.E., Jr.: Studies on the biology of collagen during wound healing: dynamic metabolism of scar collagen and remodeling of dermal wounds, Ann. Surg. **174**:511-520, 1971.
3. Swanson, A.B.: A flexible implant for replacement of arthritic or destroyed joints in the hand, N.Y. Univ. Inter-Clin. Inform. Bull. **6**:16-19, 1966.
4. Swanson, A.B.: Flexible implant resection arthroplasty in the hand and extremities, St. Louis, 1973, The C.V. Mosby Co.
5. Swanson, A.B.: Flexible implant arthroplasty in the hand, Clin. Plast. Surg. **3**:141-157, 1976.
6. Swanson, A.B., de Groot Swanson, G., and Leonard, J.: Postoperative rehabilitation program in flexible implant arthroplasty of the digits. In Hunter, J.M., Schneider, L.H., Mackin, E.J., and Bell, J.A., editors: Rehabilitation of the hand, St. Louis, 1978, The C.V. Mosby Co.

21. Total wrist arthroplasty

Ronald L. Linscheid, M.D.
Robert D. Beckenbaugh, M.D.
James H. Dobyns, M.D.

The total wrist arthroplasty as a substitute for arthrodesis has special attraction for patients with bilateral wrist disease and multiple other involved joints in the upper extremity as in rheumatoid arthritis. Preservation of wrist motion is often attractive to patients because of the easier adaptability of the hand for functional requirements.

CLINICAL SERIES

Between April 1974 and April 1979, 121 wrist arthroplasties using the Meuli device[6-8] (Fig. 21-1), 12 of which were bilateral, were performed. Thirteen wrist arthroplasties using the Volz prosthesis[3] and one Weber prosthesis[9] were performed. During the same period 13 Silastic wrist arthroplasties were done. The indications for total wrist arthroplasty included destruction and deterioration of both intercarpal and radiocarpal joints, malposition of the joint, greatly limited motion, moderate to severe pain, and a need to preserve wrist motion.

The age range was from 16 to 74 years, with an average of 55 years. Eighty percent of the patients were women. The follow-up ranged from 3 to 62 months, with an average of 36 months.

Wrist replacement was performed with standard techniques for total joint replacement through a dorsal incision. The extensor tendons were reflected and sufficient amounts of the carpus and distal radius were resected (Fig. 21-2). The distal ulna was resected if there was substantial destruction, deterioration, or subluxation. The intramedullary cavity of the radius was cleaned of cancellous bone and fatty marrow, and the intramedullary cavity of the second and third or occasionally the third and fourth metacarpals through the remaining portions of the distal carpus were identified and reamed with an air drill or hand reamer. An attempt was made in each instance to line up the third metacarpal and the center of the lunate fossa of the radius for the center of rotation of the wrist. This was usually accomplished by bending of the stems of the device sufficiently to obtain this position. Polymethylmethacrylate cement was injected into the intramedullary cavities, and the proximal and distal components were inserted sequentially; in the case of the Meuli prosthesis the interposed ball was placed on the trunion bearing and the device was reduced after the cement had set. Capsulorrhaphy was followed by replacement of the extensor tendons of the fingers in the fourth compartment and repair of all or a portion of the dorsal carpal ligament to retain the tendons in the compartment.

Certain technical difficulties were appreciated during the course of the series.[1,2,4] This included difficulty in reaming the intramedullary cavity of the second metacarpal, accurate bending of the stems of both the proximal and distal devices, difficulty in reinserting the device in the tested position after cement injection, difficulty in injecting cement to the end of the prepared cavities, and difficulty in maintaining the alignment of the device during insertion and assembly.

Some of these problems were substantially improved with the development of the offset stems for the Meuli device and a single dorsally placed distal stem for both the Meuli and the Volz devices.

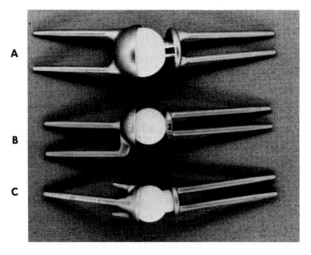

Fig. 21-1. Meuli total wrist prosthesis. **A,** Original model with straight stems. **B,** Revised distal stems with one centered and one offset. **C,** A second revision with a centered single distal stem for the frontal plane and a dorsal offset for the sagittal plane. Bending plates provided with the device may be used to contour the stems to fit the intramedullary cavities of radius and metacarpals.

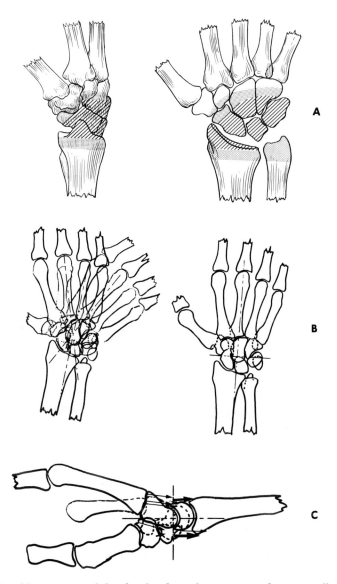

Fig. 21-2. A, Variable amounts of the distal radius, the carpus, and occasionally the distal ulna were removed to provide sufficient space for the prosthesis. **B** and **C,** The moments of force about the wrist are most closely balanced if the center of rotation of the prosthesis lies close to the normal center of rotation of the wrist joint. In both the anteroposterior and the sagittal plane, these appear to be within the capitate bone. (**A** from Beckenbaugh, R.D., and Linscheid, R.L.: Total wrist arthroplasty: a preliminary report, J. Hand Surg. **2**(5):337-344, Sept. 1977; with permission.)

Table 21-1. Total wrist arthroplasty expressed as motion averages (in degrees)

	Preoperative	Postoperative
Dorsiflexion	11	36
Palmar flexion	39	30
Radial deviation	0	11
Ulnar deviation	19	20

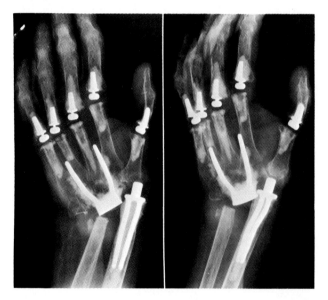

Fig. 21-3. At 1 year after total wrist arthroplasty this patient was noted to have dislocated the implant. She had no pain and was not significantly bothered by the dislocation. She refused further surgery.

RESULTS

The preoperative and postoperative ranges of motion are given in Table 21-1. Pain relief was satisfactory in almost all instances. There was a great variation in grip strength, but it is difficult to assess this parameter because most patients also had substantial involvement of the joints of their hands and often the elbows and shoulders.

COMPLICATIONS

There were three infections, of which two were deep, requiring removal of the prosthesis, and one was superficial responding to local measures. There were nine dislocations, of which three were reduced by closed manipulation and five required open reduction. One was found late but the patient was not bothered by the dislocation and no further treatment was carried out (Fig. 21-3). Most dislocations occurred shortly after surgery within the first 2 weeks.

Loosening of the prosthesis has occurred in five patients (Fig. 21-4). This has been most commonly seen at the distal ends of the stem of the distal component and has been associated in most instances with insufficient cement in the metacarpal intramedullary cavities. Protrusion of a stem through the metacarpal after loosening was seen in one of these patients, but penetration of the stem through the metacarpals at the time of insertion has also occurred in several instances. Usually this is of no particular moment. Fourteen patients developed a malposition of the wrist such that the wrist tended to fall into a fixed position (Fig. 21-5). This occurred in ulnar deviation in 10, as a flexion deformity in two, and an extension deformity in an additional two. Usually the malposition was secondary to difficulty in maintaining adequate centering of the device or rebalancing of the tendons about the wrist. Occasionally it was secondary to bowstringing of the finger extensor tendons or rupture of a wrist extensor.

Four patients developed carpal-tunnel symptoms apparently because of intrusion into the carpal canal by the device. In nine patients there were additional problems from protrusion of a stem, impingement during the extremes of motion, tendon rupture, or adhesions that required additional treatment. One or more of the complications sometimes existed in the same patient.

Reoperations were done in 38 patients, or 36% of the total.[1] Of the first 47 patients, 55% had reoperation, with an average follow-up of 4 years. Of the second 95, reoperation was undertaken for malposition in 12, dislocation in five, infection in three, loosening in five, carpal-tunnel syndrome in four, and miscellaneous reasons in nine. In most instances revision of the arthroplasty was undertaken. Removal of the device alone was done in two. Arthrodesis was done in three. During revision, recentering of the device, recementing, and soft-tissue reconstruction were most often carried out.

The most substantial improvement in technique has been associated with injection of cement under pressure through a syringe to fill the medullary cavities, substitution of the single-stem or offset-stem components, roentgenographic con-

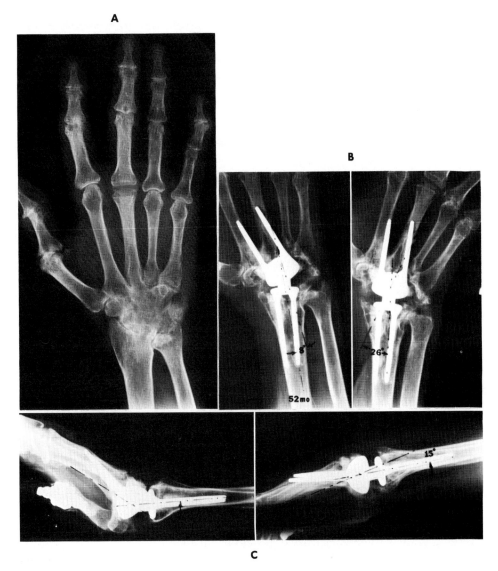

Fig. 21-4. A, This 49-year-old patient originally had synovectomy of the wrist, which deteriorated over the ensuing 4 years. **B,** Total wrist arthroplasty provided her with good function as an operator of business machines for 4 years before loosening of the distal stem in the metacarpal, which necessitated revision. Failure to obtain cement packing past the ends of the stems and into the metacarpals probably contributed significantly to the late loosening. Note satisfactory balance of the wrist obtained by insertion of the original stems at a slight angle; this was accomplished in later instances when the stems of the device were bent. **C,** After revision the range of motion was dorsiflexion 35 degrees, palmar flexion 20 degrees, radial deviation 10 degrees, and ulnar deviation 15 degrees. No pain. Grip strength 12 kg. Moderate heterotopic bone formation a factor in restriction of motion. Well satisfied. Healing of defect in third metacarpal secondary to toggling of stem in **B**.

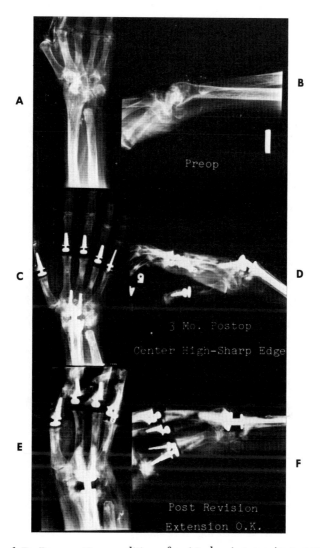

Fig. 21-5. A and **B,** Preoperative condition of wrist showing previous resection of ulnar head, intercarpal collapse, and volar flexed position of wrist. **C** and **D,** Three months after operation, distal component has been inserted in a flexed position resulting in persistent wrist flexion. **E** and **F,** Revision wrist prosthesis. Placement of center of rotation in sagittal plane in a volar position has allowed dorsiflexion and increased range of motion.

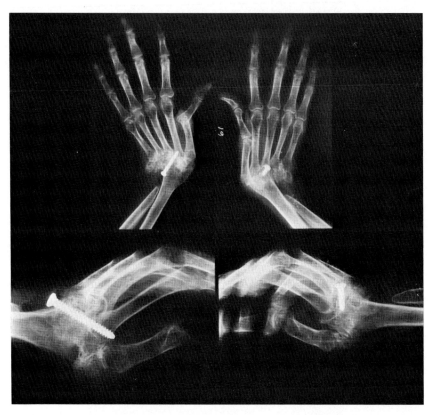

Fig. 21-6. A, Housewife, 53 years old, with progressive multiarticular rheumatoid arthritis. Self-care greatly restricted. Bilateral arthrodeses previously attempted, which proceded to nonunion with noticeable ulnar deviation and dorsiflexion deformities. Resorption of carpals.

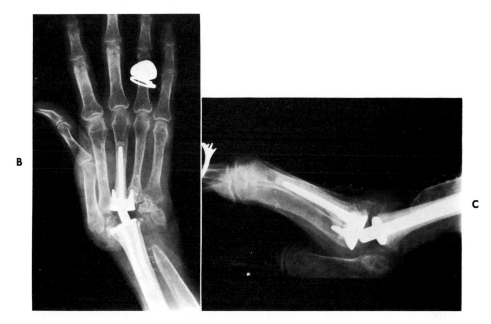

B

C

Fig. 21-6, cont'd. B and **C,** Meuli type of total wrist arthroplasty at 1 year. Improved self-care, feeding, and writing. Moderate but controllable recurrent ulnar deviation. Extensor carpi radialis longus was attenuated at surgery and repaired. Further improvement might have been accomplished by improvement of position and collapse of thumb to increase moments provided by thumb tendons. Slightly increased ulnar placement of prosthesis may have improved balance as well.

trol of position during component insertion, and careful soft-tissue reconstruction and postoperative positioning (Fig. 21-6).

Use of a hinged flexion-extension wrist splint for 4 to 6 weeks after arthroplasty is of some value in allowing soft-tissue stabilization about the wrist.

DISCUSSION

The complication rate and reoperation rate in this series is unacceptably high and reflects technical problems that were encountered during the course of prosthetic development. Despite this, most patients have been reasonably satisfied with the relief of pain and the functional abilities of their wrists. In those patients in whom arthrodesis was done on one side, most prefer the freedom associated with arthroplasty.

Improvement in design and technique has substantially improved the complication and revision rate in the last 2 years.

The biggest remaining factor will be to provide accurate centering of the devices for stability by the tendons crossing the wrist joint. It has been reasonably well established that the normal center of rotation for the wrist lies in the neck and head of the capitate bone in the frontal and sagittal plane respectively.[5,10] The accurate positioning of the device in the frontal plane is somewhat easier with visual alignment than is the placement of the components to place the center of rotation correctly in the sagittal plane because of the exposure offered by the dorsal surgical approach. Offsets built into the stems of both the radial and metacarpal components as well as accurate roentgenographic control during surgery should substantially improve alignment. This, however, does not take into account imbalances in the tendon moments at the wrist produced by the initial disease process. The strengths of the extrinsic tendons crossing the wrist and all soft-tissue contractures must be taken into account during the soft-tissue reconstruction phase.

Most of the presently available wrist prostheses use a ball-and-socket mechanical analog for the wrist. The wrist joint, however, more closely simulates a universal joint with only 2 degrees of freedom.[3] There is therefore a certain amount of rotatory instability inherent in these designs, except for the Weber design.[9] In a few of the patients there has been a tendency for the hand to adapt a mild supine posture on the distal forearm. This can be accentuated by excision of the distal ulna and by laxity of the capsule, particularly on the ulnar side of the joint. For this reason we preserve the distal ulna when possible and attempt a capsulorrhaphy of the joint if there is noticeable laxity. Reconstruction of ulnocarpal stability has been done with a strip of flexor carpi ulnaris sutured into a drill hole in the distal ulna or similar reconstruction of the ulnocollateral ligament complex. Most of the patients who have had wrist replacements are able to induce torque in their hands through forearm rotation. This appears to be attributable to the resistance to supination torque provided by the tendons crossing the wrist. Most of these patients are using their forearms at below normal force, but this is adequate for most self-care tasks. Further study of this aspect of wrist function would be desirable.

Total wrist arthroplasty has had an unacceptably high rate of complications and reoperation in the initial group in this series. Nevertheless, in patients with severe wrist deformity and a need for wrist motion it remains an acceptable procedure with a satisfactory range of motion, excellent pain relief, and substantial working capacity. Improved design and technique should result in greatly improved late results.

REFERENCES

1. Beckenbaugh, R.D., and Linscheid, R.L.: Total wrist arthroplasty: a preliminary report, J. Hand Surg. **2**(5):337-344, Sept. 1977.
2. Beckenbaugh, R.D.: Total joint arthroplasty—the wrist, Mayo Clin. Proc. **54**:513-515, 1979.
3. Lamberta, F.J., Ferlic, D.C., and Clayton, M.: Volz total wrist arthroplasty in rheumatoid arthritis: a preliminary report, J. Hand Surg. **3**(3):245-252, May 1980.
4. Linscheid, R.L.: The mechanical factors affecting deformity at the wrist in rheumatoid arthritis (Abstract), J. Bone Joint Surg. **51A**:790, 1969.
5. Linscheid, R.L., and Beckenbaugh, R.D.: Total arthroplasty of the wrist to relieve pain and increase motion, Geriatrics **31**:48-52, 1976.
6. Meuli, H.C.: Reconstructive surgery of the wrist joint, Hand **4**:88-90, 1972.
7. Meuli, H.C.: Arthroplastie du poignet, Ann. Chir. **27**:527-530, 1973.
8. Meuli, H.C.: Alloarthroplastik des Handgelenks, Z. Orthop. **113**:476-478, 1975.
9. Weber, E.R.: Personal communication, Little Rock, Arkansas, 1979.
10. Youm, Y., McMurthy, R.Y., Flatt, A.E., and Gillespie, T.E.: Kinematics of the wrist. I. An experimental study of radial-ulnar deviation and flexion-extension, J. Bone Joint Surg. **60A**(4):423-431, June 1978.

22. Spherical–Tri-Axial Total Wrist replacement

Chitranjan S. Ranawat, M.D.
Neil A. Green, M.D.
Allan E. Inglis, M.D.
Lee Ramsay Straub, M.D.

Cemented total wrist arthroplasty is a relatively new procedure.[8,10,17] Meuli,[11-13] Volz,[18-20] and Lodi[9] have made significant contributions in this area. All their prostheses, however, lack articular stability, and dislocation of components can occur. The Meuli and Volz wrist replacements do not articulate at the instant center of the wrist in both anteroposterior and lateral planes and thus are incongruent with understood kinesiology.[6] Beckenbaugh and Linscheid[4] of the Mayo clinic reported a revision rate of 35% with the Meuli prosthesis because of dislocation or volar-ulnar settling of the wrist joint.

In an effort to achieve stability and more clearly simulate normal wrist movements, a Spherical–Tri-Axial Wrist replacement has been developed and clinically utilized at The Hospital for Special Surgery.

DESCRIPTION OF PROSTHESIS

The Spherical–Tri-Axial Total Wrist Joint (STW) consists of metacarpal and radial components, a plastic bearing, and axle mechanism. The metacarpal component has a larger stem for the third metacarpal and a small second metacarpal stem. The base plate strengthens the stem and contains the cement. The radial component has an offset stem that placed centrally in the radius automatically positions its articular sphere at the level of the instant center of the wrist, within the capitate bone.[14] There is 12 degrees of palmar tilt to the radial component; thus the axis of rotation is shifted palmarward to augment the wrist extensor lever arm. A plastic bearing of high-density polyethylene fits onto the metacarpal component forming a ball-and-socket joint with the radial sphere. The sides of the bearing limit radioulnar deviation. This articulating mechanism unloads the axle. Together the axle and plastic housing serve to maintain the articulation. A safety device in the form of a restraining ring secures the axle placement.

The prosthesis allows 85 degrees of flexion and extension, 10 degrees of radioulnar deviation, and greater than 10 degrees of axial rotation. Separate right and left replacements are utilized and two sizes, 18 × 18 and 21 × 21 mm, are provided for better fitting of components.

INDICATIONS AND CONTRAINDICATIONS

Total wrist replacement should be offered as an alternative to arthrodesis in severely affected wrists.[1-3,5] It may be utilized after failure of a dorsal stabilization procedure[15] or other wrist arthroplasty. A Spherical–Tri-Axial Wrist implant can be considered in the presence of extensor tendon rupture if the tendon can be repaired or suitable tendon transfers can be performed. This type of wrist extensor tendon repair is often associated with palmar subluxation or dislocation of the wrist.[15]

At the present time we cannot recommend our replacement arthroplasty other than in rheumatoid arthritis. Infection is a contraindication to any total wrist arthroplasty.

OPERATIVE TECHNIQUE

The upper extremity is prepared and draped in the fashion outlined in *Campbell's Operative Orthopaedics*, and a hand table attachment is utilized. We also recommend the use of a pneumatic tourniquet. After the extremity is elevated and exsanguinated and the tourniquet inflated, a straight dorsal incision is made. Careful attention is directed to the isolation and protection of the dorsal ulnar and radial sensory nerves. The dorsal retinaculum is elevated from the radial aspect at the junction of the first and second dorsal compartment. The dorsal retinaculum is raised as a single flap to be utilized later in the closure. Removal of the diseased synovium from the extensor tendons can then be accomplished. The need for tendon repair or transfers is noted and performed at the conclusion of the procedure. The distal 1 to 2 cm of the ulna is isolated and resected (Darrach's procedure) followed by a synovectomy of the distal radioulnar joint. The wrist-joint capsule is opened in a horizontal fashion and raised as two flaps. Synovectomy of the distal radioulnar joint is then completed. A part of the retinaculum and dorsal capsule will be used to stabilize the distal ulna at the end of the procedure, by interposing it between the radius and ulna.

Axial traction is applied to compensate for soft-tissue slack and faciliate proper tendon tension. The block spacer is utilized as a template to mark out the area of bone to be resected from the articular surface of the radius and the carpus so as to provide a trough for the prosthetic mechanism. Once this marking is made, an oscillating saw is used to make the respective cuts.

Metacarpal reamers are used to prepare the canals of the second and third metacarpals to accept the metacarpal component. A trail component determines the proper fit. Similarly, the distal radius is prepared with the radial reamer after a pilot hole is placed in the central portion of its canal. Once reaming is accomplished on both sides, trial components are inserted. There should be full range of motion without pistoning of components. The canals of the metacarpals and distal radius should be carefully irrigated using the Water-Pik and packed with sponges to dry them well. This facilitates better cement filling. The cement is injected into the metacarpals in liquid form (in 1 minute or less) by use of a 10 ml syringe with a plastic intravenous catheter, and it is packed digitally and tamped with the reversed end of a cotton applicator so that a homogeneous column of cement is provided. The metacarpal component is placed with the longer stem into the third metacarpal, and the shorter stem into the second metacarpal. Once this metacarpal component is cemented, the radial component is cemented and all excessive acrylic cement removed. Correct positioning and orientation of the radial component should be rehearsed. If placed correctly, the sphere is offset ulnarward and tilted palmarward. The plastic is placed onto its housing on the metacarpal component, and the articulation is completed with locking of the axle with its plastic cylinder using the metal restraining ring. This accomplished, the total wrist replacement should have a flexion-extension range of motion of approximately 170 degrees, radioulnar deviation of 10 degrees, and a mild degree of supination-pronation to obviate transmission of excessive torque forces to the material interfaces. The tourniquet is released, hemostasis is achieved, and the tourniquet is reinflated. The dorsal capsule is reapproximated tightly with 5-0 Mersilene sutures while the wrist is held in neutral position. The dorsal retinaculum is brought under the extensor tendons and there sutured after a small beltlike portion is saved to provide a covering for the extensor tendons to eliminate bowstringing. This complex provides covering for the prosthesis and reinforcement of the dorsal structures, and it provides a smooth gliding surface for the extensor tendons. Extensor repair and appropriate tendon transfers, if needed, are done at this point. Ruptured wrist extensors are isolated and repaired end to end, or distal ends are sutured for yokelike function. The extensor carpi radialis brevis can be advanced to its insertion using the extensor carpi radialis longus tendon as an intercalary graft.

The small portion of the dorsal retinaculum that was maintained to cover the extensor is now sutured into place. Skin is closed with interrupted sutures, and the patient is placed in a bulky hand dressing in neutral position. The patient remains in the dressing for 3 to 5 days. Thereafter the patient is placed in a splint or cast for 2 to 4 weeks of immobilization to allow good soft-tissue healing. After this, the patient is removed from external support and allowed to go to therapy for rehabilitation. Both active and active-assisted range of motion and use of a night splint are utilized while the patient is gaining strength.

CLINICAL MATERIAL

Our clinical experience includes 12 patients receiving 14 implants. Eleven patients, comprising nine females and two males, had rheumatoid arthritis with an average length of disease of 10 years. Four patients had previous corticosteroid treatment and five had gold salt therapy. The average age at surgery was 61 years.

All patients had a positive latex-fixation test during the course of their disease, as well as an elevated erythrocyte sedimentation rate. One patient had previous meta-carpophalangeal arthroplasties, and one had a previous dorsal stabilization procedure. Two patients had previous total knee replacement. Pain at rest and at work was the chief complaint among the majority of patients. All had limited active range of motion. Three patients had preoperative rupture of the wrist tendons, and one patient had bilateral rupture of the extensor carpi radialis brevis and longus muscles requiring an end-to-end reanastomosis of the extensor carpi radialis brevis tendon. A second had the extensor carpi radialis longus tendon used as a graft for the extensor carpi radialis brevis. The third patient had the flexor digitorum superficialis of the ring finger transferred to the distal stump of the extensor carpi radialis brevis tendon. Three patients had extensor digitorum communis tendon ruptures that were treated by a transferal of the distal tendon to an intact adjacent extensor tendon. One patient, who did not have rheumatoid arthritis, developed traumatic arthritis 10 years after a Colles' fracture. He had severe functional and roentgeno-graphic destruction of the wrist joint. In his case an implant arthroplasty was used rather than an arthrodesis.

Method

All patients were followed and evaluated by one of us. Nine patients were followed for 3 months to 2 years and 4 months. Roentgentograms were obtained preoperatively in the anteroposterior, lateral, flexion, and extension planes (Fig. 22-1, *A* and *B*). Severe wrist deformity with associated pain and limitation of motion correlated well with the amount of volar and ulnar subluxation of the radiocarpal joint and destruction of the distal radioulnar joint. Criteria for assessment of success of total wrist arthroplasty were in the areas of pain relief, active range of motion, and overall functional improvement of the hand with regard to activities of daily living.

Results

Overall results have been good. Of the nine patients followed, eight had no pain to mild pain of the wrist at rest or at work. One patient with severe pain preoperatively complained of moderate pain postoperatively, assessed to be associated with elbow synovitis and ulnar neuropathy at the elbow for which she declined surgical therapy. Seven patients had an average increase in both active flexion and extension of 21.3 and 32.5 degrees respectively (Fig. 22-2). One patient who had an extension deformity preoperatively gained a more functional flexion-extension motion without increasing her total arc. A second lost 30 degrees of active extension. These two patients, however, had improvement in alignment and functional use of their hands for activities of daily living.

Because of polyarthropathy, grip strength improved modestly, usually only a few pounds. There were no infections or component failures. An anteroposterior and lateral roentgenogram in active flexion and extension were obtained during

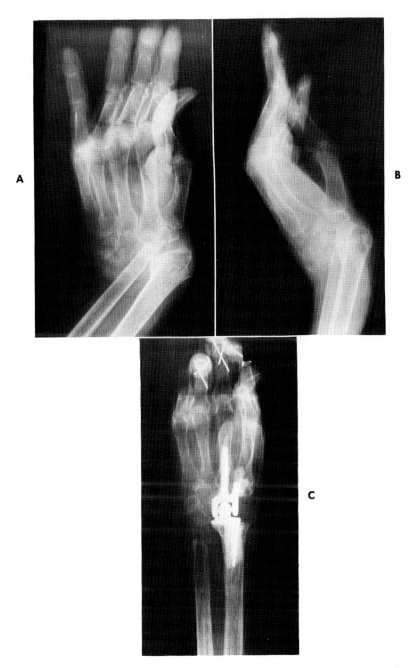

Fig. 22-1. A 75-year-old male patient with a 15-year history of rheumatoid arthritis. **A,** Anteroposterior roentgenogram of the hand and wrist demonstrating carpal destruction and radiocarpal dislocation. **B,** Lateral roentgenogram shows swan-neck deformity in fingers. **C,** Postoperative anteroposterior roentgenogram with implanted arthroplasty. Wrist alignment is restored. *Continued.*

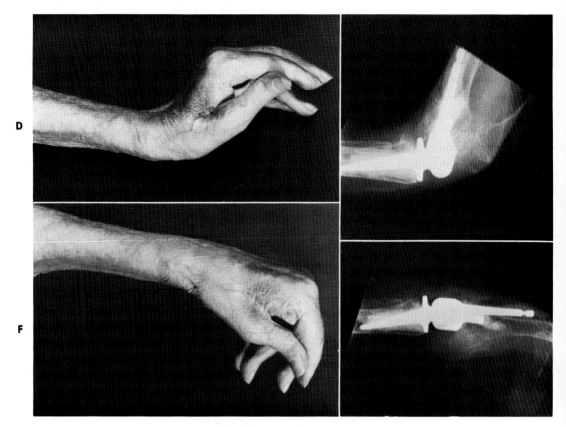

Fig. 22-1, cont'd. D, Active extension. **E,** Lateral roentgenogram showing active extension. **F,** Active flexion. **G,** Lateral roentgenogram during active flexion.

postoperative rehabilitation (Fig. 22-1, C to G). All patients showed good cement filling of the distal radius; however, four of our early patients showed incomplete cement filling of the metacarpals around the tips of the implant.

DISCUSSION

Preservation of painless and stable joint motion, especially in individuals with multiple arthropathy, is of paramount importance.[5] Although arthrodesis usually gives relief of pain, the loss of motion must not be ignored. One should remember that a small arc of painless motion in the wrist will increase finger reach by several centimeters.

Swanson[16] has adroitly summarized the wrist and digital deformities in rheumatoid arthritis. In the design of the Spherical–Tri-Axial Total Wrist we have systematically endeavored to correct these deformities while balancing forces to provide controlled movement. A cemented prosthesis should provide good alignment

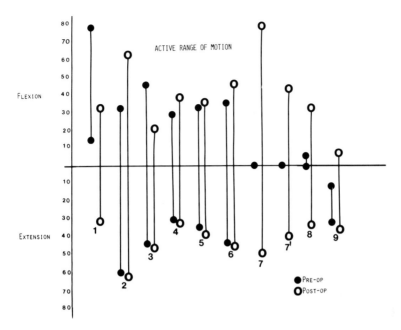

Fig. 22-2. Preoperative and postoperative flexion-extension and arc of motion.

and pain-free range of motion. The advantages of the Spherical–Tri-Axial Total Wrist are many. It prevents dislocation of components and ulnar drift because it is articulated. Torque forces are reduced because the articulation is located at the instant center of the wrist. This lessens stress concentration at material interfaces, reducing the opportunity for loosening. Although the wrist does not function as a weight-bearing joint, the tension and compression forces are considerable. However, using his joint replacement, Volz[18] has demonstrated that the force needed to loosen the components within the cement was only 3 kg less than the force needed to fracture the bone. A 5-year follow-up study will be necessary for accurate assessment of the magnitude of this problem.

Cement technique, especially in the metacarpals must be meticulous. The injection technique for cementing has been used by Lee et al.[7] in total hip replacement and has good application here. They demonstrated that careful removal of debris from the intermedullary canal by a pulsating wash, followed by drying of the cancellous bone and injection of low-viscosity acrylic polymer under pressure gives a multifold increase in the strength of cement fixation of components. The Spherical–Tri-Axial design allows stress to be dissipated primarily into the supportive soft-tissue structures. This is accomplished by careful capsular closure and subsequent reinforcement by the transposed extensor retinaculum. Cast immobilization avoids stretching of the repair during wound healing.

The articulated prosthesis restores the alignment of the extensor mechanism and contributes to a functional increased extensor lever arm (by the palmar tilt of the radial component). Wrist and digital function, particularly in fine movements, becomes once again possible.

Although the Spherical–Tri-Axial Total Wrist implant does not provide a normal wrist mechanism, we believe that it is an important reconstructive alternative to arthrodesis in severe rheumatoid arthropathy.

REFERENCES

1. Beckenbaugh, R.D.: Die GSB-Endoprothese des Handgelenks, Z. Orthop. **113**:473, 1975.
2. Beckenbaugh, R.D.: New concepts in arthroplasty of the hand and wrist, Arch. Surg. **112**:1094-1098, 1977.
3. Beckenbaugh, R.D.: Total joint arthroplasty, Mayo Clin. Proc. **54**:512-515, 1979.
4. Beckenbaugh, R.D., and Linscheid, R.L.: Total wrist arthroplasty: a preliminary report, J. Hand Surg. **2**:337-344, 1974.
5. Cooney, W.P., III: Total joint arthroplasty, Mayo Clin. Proc. **54**:495-499, 1979.
6. Hamas, R.S.: A quantitative approach to total wrist arthroplasty: development of a "precentered" total wrist prosthesis, Orthopedics **2**:245-255, 1979.
7. Lee, A.J.C., Ling, R.S.M., and Vangala, S.S.: Some clinically relevant variables affecting the mechanical behavior of bone cement, Arch. Orthop. Traumatic Surg. **9**:1-18, 1978.
8. Linscheid, R.L., and Beckenbaugh, R.D.: Total arthroplasty of the wrist to relieve pain and increase motion, Geriatrics **31**:48-52, 1976.
9. Lodi, G.: Personal communication, 1978, Buenos Aires, Argentina.
10. Mantero, R., Bertolotti, G.L., and Ferrari, G.L.: Meuli's total prosthesis in severe rheumatoid osteoarthrosis of wrist, Ital. J. Orthop. Traumatol. **3**:47-51, 1977.
11. Meuli, H.C.: Arthroplastie du poignet, Ann. Chir. **27**:527-530, 1973.
12. Meuli, H.C.: Alloarthroplastik des Handgelenks, Z. Orthop. **113**:476-478, 1975.
13. Meuli, H.C.: Der totale Gelenkersatz für das Handgelenk, Ther. Umsch. **35**:366-371, 1978.
14. Ranawat, C.S.: Anatomical considerations and design features of total wrist joint, Orthop. Nurs. J. **6**:61-65, 1969.
15. Straub, L.R., and Ranawat, C.S.: The wrist in rheumatoid arthritis, J. Bone Joint Surg. **51A**:1-20, 1969.
16. Swanson, A.B.: Flexible implant arthroplasty for arthritis disability of the radiocarpal joint, Orthop. Clin. North Am. **4**:383-394, 1973.
17. Taylor, J.A.: Total wrist arthroplasty (Meuli) for the treatment of advanced rheumatoid arthritis, J. Am. Osteopath Assoc. **78**:267-272, 1978.
18. Volz, R.G.: The development of a total wrist arthroplasty, Clin. Orthop. **116**:209-214, 1976.
19. Volz, R.G.: Total wrist arthroplasty, Clin. Orthop. **108**:180-189, 1977.
20. Volz, R.G.: Clinical experiences with a new total wrist prosthesis, Arch. Orthop. Unfallchir. **85**:205-209, 1976.

23. Total wrist arthroplasty: a clinical and biomechanical analysis

Robert G. Volz, M.D.

In 1973 work was begun at the Arizona Health Sciences Center on the development of a cementable total wrist prosthesis.[19] Based upon the concepts successfully employed by Charnley at the hip, the implant represented a cobalt-chrome metallic prosthesis that articulated against an ultrahigh molecular weight polyethylene interface. The necessity for a total wrist prosthesis was based upon the observation that for some patients, because of occupational or vocational needs, the preservation of a pain-free stable arc of wrist motion was essential for the implementation of fine motor control of the hand and fingers.[1,16] Additionally it was observed that a loss of wrist motion compromised not only digital dexterity but also strength of grasp.[17]

ANATOMY AND KINESIOLOGY

Before the development of a prosthetic design, the anatomy and kinesiology of the normal carpus was carefully studied. From the anatomic studies undertaken, it was observed that the wrist represents a joint complex of rather remarkable flexibility and stability, considering that it is composed of seven small articulating bones and one sesamoid, which when examined separately possess no significant mechanical stability one to the other.

An analysis of the carpal motion revealed that movement occurs predominantly between linked segments represented by the proximal and distal carpal rows. Movement between these linked segments always occurred in an integrated fashion. Thus, as the hand is placed in a position of radial deviation, the proximal carpal row moves ulnarward while the distal row is displaced radialward. These diametric shifts in proximal and distal rows are reversed with ulnar deviation (Fig. 23-1). It was also noted that with radioulnar deviation, the proximal and distal carpal rows move essentially in a single plane with one exception, that being the displacement of the distal pole of the scaphoid. With radial deviation, the distal pole of the scaphoid is flexed toward the palm because of a compromise in space about the radial side of the carpus. With ulnar deviation, the distal pole of the scaphoid is drawn into an approximate position of neu-

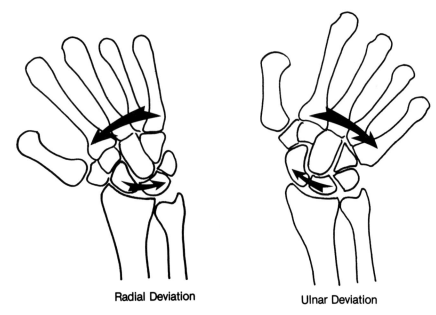

Radial Deviation   **Ulnar Deviation**

Fig. 23-1. Diametric motion occurs between the proximal and distal carpal row with radial ulnar deviation of the hand. With radial deviation the proximal carpal row moves in an ulnarward direction while the distal carpal row moves in a radialward fashion. With ulnar deviation shifts in the proximal and distal carpal row occur in opposite directions.

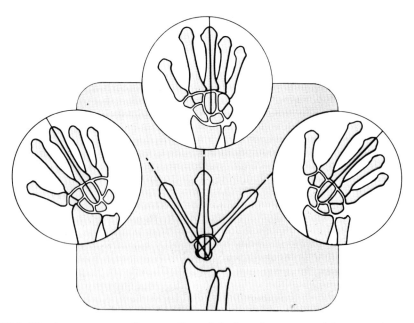

Fig. 23-2. The instant center of motion for radial ulnar deviation and flexion and extension of the carpus is located in a multicentered focus within the proximal pole of the capitate bone.

trality with reference to planes of flexion and extension and in such a position a truer appraisal of its anteroposterior configuration is possible by roentgenographic examination. The total arc of radioulnar deviation is approximately 50 degrees, with 15 degrees being in a radial direction and 35 degrees ulnarward. The instant center or axis of motion for radioulnar deviation is located within the proximal pole of the capitate bone (Fig. 23-2).

Inspection of the proximal pole of the capitate bone suggests that the capitate-scaphoid-lunate articulation resembles a ball-and-socket joint capable of rotational motion.[3] Although small amounts of rotation are possible and perhaps do exist in some individual wrists, from a practical point of view rotational motion does not occur through the carpal complex. Rotation of the hand instead results from motion arising at the proximal and distal radioulnar joints and is dependent on a maintenance of their normal alignment. The wrist is therefore a joint of biplane motion that encompasses radioulnar deviation, palmar flexion and extension, and a combination of these planes of motion, circumduction.[6]

Many authors have analyzed the contribution of the two carpal rows to the total arc of flexion and extension, and considerable discrepancy in such motion has been noted, a fact that probably only underscores the normal variation in the range of motion seen in the populace at large. Sarrafin reported the average total arc of carpal flexion and extension to be 120 degrees, with ranges varying from 69 to 181 degrees.[15] Because of the slight volar tilt of the distal radial plate, the arc of flexion exceeds the range of extension by an average of 10 degrees. In a study of 55 normal wrists, the greatest contribution to extension was made by the proximal carpal radial articulation (66.5%), whereas the greatest component to flexion arose from the distal carpal row (60%) (Fig. 23-3). As with radioulnar deviation, the axis of motion for flexion and extension of the carpus is located eccentrically within the proximal and palmar area of the capitate.[18,20]

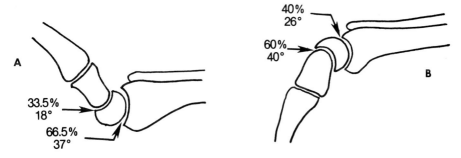

Fig. 23-3. The contribution of the radial carpal and midcarpal articulation to the planes of carpal flexion and extension are shown. The majority of carpal extension, **A**, occurs at the radial carpal articulation, whereas the greater component of carpal flexion, **B**, occurs at the midcarpal interface.

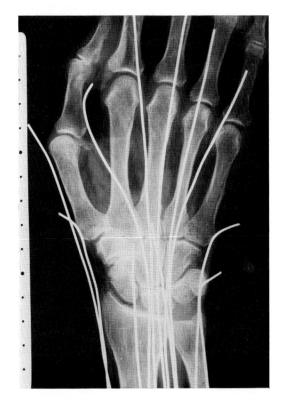

Fig. 23-4. Wires were placed within the tendon sheaths of the respective tendons crossing the carpus. The roentgenogram identifies the lever-arm length of these respective tendons as the arm acts upon the instant center of motion located within the proximal pole of the capitate.

Stability of the carpal complex is derived in part from the precisely opposed multifaceted articular surfaces and from several important intracapsular and inter-osseous ligaments.[11] The three flexors and three extensors of the wrist also serve as important dynamic stabilizers for the carpus.[3-5,7-10,14] In their absence, motor imbalance frequently results often with an eventual compromise of stability, which may lead to subluxation and dislocation. The planes of motion arising between the second to fifth metacarpals and their respective carpal bones were also analyzed. For all practical purposes no motion was observed either between the second metacarpal and the trapezoid or the third metacarpal and its respective carpal bone, the capitate.[13,19] Significant motion, however, does exist between the fourth and fifth metacarpals and the hamate. The preservation of this motion is therefore essential in permitting cupping motions of the palm and adduction of the fourth and fifth fingers.

Motor control of the carpus is predominantly relegated to a subconscious level though obviously volitional control over the respective wrist motors is, of course,

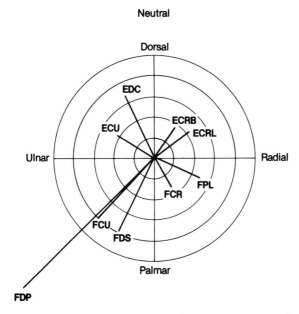

Fig. 23-5. A vector-force analysis of the musculotendinous units crossing the carpus discloses that the summation of forces tends to place the wrist in a position of flexion and ulnar deviation. The magnitude of force for each respective musculotendinous unit (abbreviated) was computed by measurement of the potential force generated by each muscle times its lever arm of action upon the instant center of motion. *E*, extensor; *F*, flexor; *C*, carpi or else communis; *D*, digitorum; *R*, radialis; *B*, brevis; *L*, longus; *S*, superficialis; *P*, pollicis; *U*, ulnaris.

possible. But in most hand activities concentrated efforts are devoted to the control of finger motors. In the normal wrist, closing motions of the hand evokes considerable activity among wrist extensors with the extensor carpi radialis brevis predominating. As finger-flexor activity increases, the extensor carpi ulnaris is recruited followed by the extensor carpi radialis longus. With the decrease in activity of long finger flexors, the extensor carpi radialis longus is the first to become quiescent. With opening motions of the hand, one wrist extensor, the extensor carpi ulnaris, and one wrist flexor, the flexor carpi ulnaris, participate actively.[9,12]

An analysis of the muscle vector forces acting upon the instant center of motion of the wrist was also studied. For determination of the potential deforming force of each muscle as it acted upon the instant center of motion of the wrist, the motor potential of each muscle was multiplied by the lever arm distance from its point of crossing the carpus to the instant center of motion located within the capitate (Fig. 23-4). The mean vector force and its magnitude was then calculated for each muscle and plotted in relationship to the planes of radioulnar deviation and palmar flexion and extension (Fig. 23-5). From this study it was noted that the flexor carpi ulnaris is the most powerful of all wrist motors tending to place the wrist in a position of flexion and ulnar deviation. Further the summation of all muscle forces crossing the carpus is one that tends to facilitate placement of the wrist in a position of flexion and ulnar deviation.

PROSTHETIC DESIGN

As a result of these studies, a semiconstrained two-component prosthesis designed in 1973 provided essentially for the two planes of motion observed at the wrist—palmar flexion and extension—and radioulnar deviation (Fig. 23-6). The prosthetic design further permitted skeletal fixation by intramedullary stem technique. The original metacarpal component possessed two prongs intended for insertion within the second and third carpometacarpal heads, whereas the radial

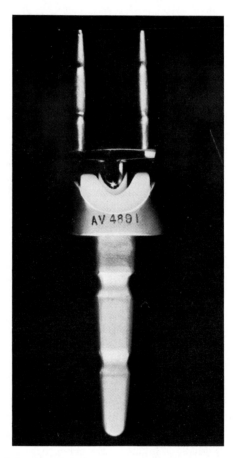

Fig. 23-6. The original design of the Arizona Medical Center Total Wrist prosthesis is shown. The interface represents a toroid sector, which is a sphere with two different radii. The interface permits 90 degrees of flexion and extension and 50 degrees of radio ulnar deviation. Considerable stability is achieved by the design of the interface. Two metallic prongs of the metacarpal component are intended for insertion in the second and third carpometacarpal medullary canals.

component was designed to be inserted within the distal radial medullary canal (Fig. 23-7). Because the normal carpus represents a complex of three skeletal segments composed of the distal radius and the proximal and distal carpal rows, the substitution of a single interface prosthesis for a double interface type of joint coupling would logically result in a lessened arc of motion if any degree of stability were to be achieved. The interface design of the Arizona Medical Center prosthesis with its two different radii allows for 50 degrees of radioulnar deviation and 90 degrees of palmar flexion and extension. Later as it became apparent with clinical usage that the prosthetic design had placed the instant center of motion too far radialward thus enhancing ulnar deviation, a metacarpal component with a single prong was designed to permit a more precise restoration of the instant center of motion for the carpus (Fig. 23-8). Additionally the intramedullary stems of all components were offset toward the dorsal direction by 1.5 mm. This effectively placed the instant center of motion farther toward the palm; thus the lever arm of the inherently weaker wrist extensors over the wrist flexors was enhanced.

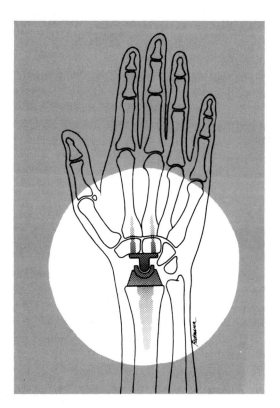

Fig. 23-7. Diagram showing the proper location of the double-pronged wrist prosthesis after resection of the scaphoid, lunate, and the proximal one half of the capitate.

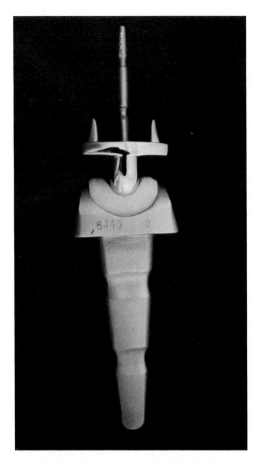

Fig. 23-8. Later modification of the Arizona Medical Center Total Wrist prosthesis. The metacarpal component now has a single prong, which more precisely locates the instant center of motion in its anatomic location. The prong should be inserted within the medullary canal of the capitate third metacarpal.

SURGICAL TECHNIQUE

A straight vertically placed incision over the dorsal aspect of the carpus made parallel to the third metacarpal is used for exposure. The extensor tendons are retracted to the radial and ulnar aspect of the wound after the dorsal carpal ligament has been carefully freed from its radial border and is reflected ulnarward. The dorsal capsule is then elevated and reflected radialward. The scaphoid, lunate, and head of the capitate are then excised (Fig. 23-9). If limitation of motion persists, it may be necessary to resect a portion of the triquetrum. With disruption or appreciable arthritic involvement of the distal radioulnar joint, excision of the distal end of the ulna should be performed. The indications for usage of the single-pronged metacarpal component are (1) translocation of the carpus ulnarly, (2) sub-

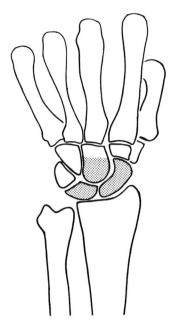

Fig. 23-9. *Stippled area,* Minimal amount of bone that must be resected to provide suffi-cient space for implantation of the prosthesis. On occasion a portion of the hamate and the triquetrum should also be resected.

luxation or dislocation of the carpus, and (3) the presence of imbalance or disrup-tion of the wrist motors. If the single-pronged metacarpal component is to be em-ployed, a single drill hole is placed across the resected bed of the capitate into the third metacarpal medullary canal. A reciprocating rasp is then used to enlarge this hole until a sufficiently enlarged bed exists permitting insertion of the prosthesis. The distal end of the radius is then reamed until a sufficient canal has been created to permit insertion of the appropriately sized radial component. A trial fit of both prostheses is then undertaken, and if the range of motion appears to be limited, particularly toward the arc of extension, incision or excision of the volar capsule is performed. After proper irrigation of the respective bone beds, the component parts are cemented into place after injection of cement by syringe technique. Care-ful closure of the capsule is essential to ensure stability of the prosthesis with acute flexion. Soft dressings incorporating a volar splint are worn for a period of 7 to 10 days. Active motion is begun when sufficient healing has occurred.

CLINICAL MATERIAL

An analysis of 100 patients undergoing total wrist replacement with the Arizona Medical Center design during the years 1974 to 1979 was recently completed. Fifteen surgeons collaborated in the study, all agreeing beforehand to the completion of a standardized analysis form that documented preoperative, operative, and postoperative data in addition to periodic roentgenographic evaluation.

The criteria for appropriate patient selection were identified at the outset of the study. Patients who were being considered as candidates for total wrist replacement were required to show far-advanced destructive changes to the carpus to an extent that arthrodesis would be viewed as an appropriate mode of therapy. Candidates, however, were also expected to exhibit a need for the preservation of some arc of pain-free wrist motion because of occupational or recreational needs or because of the presence of associated hand and finger disability. Specific contraindications were identified as (1) prior or suspected infection, (2) loss of wrist extensor activity, (3) significant unrestorable hand or finger dysfunction, (4) paralysis or, (5) a lifestyle that would predictably subject the implant to hazardous stresses.

One hundred patients underwent implantation of 111 prostheses. I operated on 45 patients who were designated as "group 1" and the remaining 55 patients were managed by the other 14 collaborating surgeons and were identified as "group 2." The breakdown of these two patient groups was helpful in providing a comparison of the postoperative results achievable.

The age distribution of the 100 patients range from 19 to 82 years, with a mean of 53.8 years. Forty-eight percent of the patient population were males, and 52% where females. Eighty-three patients presented with rheumatoid arthritis, 15 with degenerative osteoarthritis, and two with psoriatic arthritis. The postoperative follow-up period ranged from 12 to 52 months, with a mean of 30.8 months (Table 23-1). The most predictable postoperative result observed was relief of pain, with the degree of pain relief being nearly identical between the two groups (Table 23-2). The next most predictable postoperative result was a useful stable arc of motion. Because the design of the implant interface allows for no more than 90 degrees of palmar flexion and extension, it was obvious that some patients who presented postoperatively with an arc of flexion and extension greater than 90 degrees would predictably show a decrease in the arc of motion postoperatively. Therefore the percent change in arc of motion postoperatively was analyzed after the patient population was divided into three sets, that is, those presenting with 0 to 30 degrees, 30 to 90 degrees, and greater than 90 degrees of arc of flexion and extension

Table 23-1. Length of follow-up study

	Cases	Percent
Greater than 60 months	2	2
48-60 months	21	19
36-47 months	27	24
24-35 months	38	34
12-23 months	23	21
	111	
Mean 30.8 months		

preoperatively. The percent change noted postoperatively is shown in Table 23-3. The patient set exhibiting the greatest improvement in arc of motion was not surprisingly those with the least amount of motion preoperatively (0 to 30 degrees). Table 23-4 lists the change in the arc of motion seen with respect to radioulnar deviation and pronation and supination. Patients with destructive changes to the distal radioulnar joint generally underwent resection of the distal ulna at the time

Table 23-2. Relief of pain*

	Group 1	Group 2
Preoperative 3.9	4	3.8
Postoperative 1.3	1.4	1.2

*Ratings: (1) none, (2) occasional or mild, (3) moderate, (4) serious, and (5) incapacitating

Table 23-3. Range of motion

Type of motion	Cases	Preoperative	Postoperative	Percent change
Flexion-extension				
Arc 0° to 30°				
Group 1	14	17°	42°	+147
Group 2	7	18°	47°	+161
Arc 30° to 90°				
Group 1	17	51°	54°	+3
Group 2	30	47°	60°	+27
Arc 90° +				
Group 1	1	110°	98°	−10
Group 2	3	98°	70°	−18

Table 23-4. Range of motion

Type of motion	Cases	Preoperative	Postoperative	Percent change
Radioulnar				
Group 1	26	24°	28°	+16
Group 2	34	25°	32°	+28
Pronation-supination				
Arc 0° to 90°				
Group 1	7	53°	108°	+103
Group 2	8	45°	124°	+175
Arc 90° +				
Group 1	25	112°	160°	+42
Group 2	7	130°	147°	+13

Table 23-5. Results

	Patients	Average percentage
Excellent	48/100	48
Good	38/100	38
Poor	8/100	8
Failure	6/100	6

of total wrist arthroplasty. This procedure was belived to be responsible for the improved arc of pronation and supination observed postoperatively.

The overall postoperative result was tabulated by each surgeon according to the degree of pain relief, change in range of motion, stability and balance to the wrist, and overall functional improvement in wrist and hand activities. Grasp-strength measurements were not specifically obtained preoperatively and postoperatively because many patients presented with far-advanced extensive metacarpophalangeal and proximal interphalangeal joint disease. A tabulation of the results observed among the 100 patients with a postoperative follow-up study of 12 months or longer reveals that 48% were excellent, 38% good, 8% poor, and 6% failures (Table 23-5).

COMPLICATIONS

A listing of the complications encountered among the patient study is shown in Table 23-6. Motor imbalance was the most frequently observed postoperative problem, with 18% exhibiting this condition. By definition, motor imbalance was the inability of the patient to volitionally bring the wrist to a neutral position. Thirteen patients displayed a tendency for the hand to drift into ulnar deviation, and five lacked any arc of extension postoperatively (Table 23-7). It should be emphasized that motor imbalance was only observed in patients with rheumatoid arthritis who preoperatively presented with the following findings: (1) roentgenographic evidence of an ulnarly translocated, subluxated, or dislocated carpus, (2) a resting posture of flexion with or without a fixed flexion contracture of the hand, (3) a grasp pattern of finger flexor and wrist flexor activity rather than finger flexor and wrist extensor activity, and (4) a loss of volitional wrist extensor activity.

The second most frequently encountered postoperative problem was that of an inadequate range of motion (Table 23-8). Among the six patients presenting with this problem, all had essentially no wrist motion preoperatively. This failure to gain an adequate range of motion in some patients points to the fact that both the wrist flexors and the wrist extensors function with a very short lever arm upon the axis of motion. Additionally it was believed that many patients presented with considerably weakened wrist extensors secondary to far-advanced arthritic change and disuse. Six patients exhibited some difficulties with wound healing, the majority occurring in patients with rheumatoid arthritis who were taking an excess of 10 mg of prednisone daily and who displayed pronounced atrophy of skin and soft

Table 23-6. Complications

	Number of cases	Percentage of all cases
Motor balance	20/111	18
Inadequate range of motion	6/111	5
Wound healing	6/111	5
Postoperative dislocation	4/111	4
Wound infection	2/111	2
Implant loosening	1/111?	1

Table 23-7. Motor imbalance* (in 20 patients, or 18%)

Plane	Cases	Revised
Ulnar deviation	13	3
Lack of extension	5	3
Lack of flexion	1	
Radial deviation	1	1

*Definition: lack of motion in any plane or extreme imbalance in any plane.

Table 23-8. Inadequate range of motion

Six patients	6%	
Average preoperative arc	5°	(0° to 10°)
Average postoperative arc	7°	(0° to 10°)

tissues. The abandonment of a curvilinear dorsal incision for a straight dorsal midline incision, which destroyed fewer of the small venous structures, did much to lessen the problem of wound healing. The avoidance of a postoperative wound hematoma and restraint in allowing early wrist motion were also believed to be important considerations if wound healing were not to be jeopardized.

Four patients had a single episode of prosthetic dislocation, three of which occurred in the immediate postoperative period while the patient was awakening from the anesthetic. Only one dislocation occurred later at the 6-week postoperative interval. No patients have experienced a second or recurrent episode of dislocation. The identifiable cause for the immediate postoperative dislocation was believed to be a contracted volar capsule, which tended to function as a tether as the wrist was being splinted in dorsiflexion at the time the operative dressing was being applied. Excision or incision of the volar capsule at the time of surgery has tended to eliminate this problem in our experience. Two patients developed a postoperative infection. Both required removal of the prosthetic component. One patient, a 19-year-old male, who had suffered a large open laceration and loss of the distal part of the ulna from a motorboat propeller accident, presumably was infected at the time of implantation. Studies later documented that cultures of *Pseudomonas* had been recovered at the time of skin grafting but such information was not made available to the surgeon performing the arthroplasty. One patient with rheumatoid arthritis has shown painful impingement of the greater multangular bone against the radial component because of proximal migration of the base of the thumb. Roentgenograms, however, show an excessive amount of resection to the trapezoid, which was believed to account for the loss of stability to the trapezium.

The issue of the development of a radiolucent line with or without clinical evidence of loosening was also carefully evaluated. Few patients have exhibited any evidence of radiolucency, though when present this has tended to occur most commonly on the metacarpal side. Only one patient has shown evidence of clinical loosening, and this was about the metallic intramedullary prong, which was incorrectly inserted into the fourth metacarpal canal. Intramedullary stem fixation within the fourth and fifth metacarpal canals has always been cautioned against because of the considerable degree of motion that normally occurs between these metacarpals and the hamate with certain hand motion.

An analysis of the factors leading to the identification of a postoperative failure disclosed that three were attributable to motor imbalance, two an infection, and one a failue of wound healing. Among these six patients with a failed result, five required prosthetic removal (83%), two had motor imbalance, two an infection, and one a failure of wound healing. Three of these five patients were managed with an interpositional bone graft arthrodesis that went on to a solid bony union whereas two patients were left with a fibrous ankylosis. One patient who was taking large doses of steroids because of rheumatoid arthritis and subsequently failed to adequately heal the surgical incision and who required removal of the prosthesis was quite satisfied with the results, which was a fibrous ankylosis. The patient later requested that the opposite wrist be operated upon, but this the treating physician declined to do so.

DISCUSSION

Perhaps of greatest pertinence to any discussion of total wrist arthroplasty is the question of the need for preservation of a pain-free stable wrist. Experience certainly shows that arthrodesis of the wrist is a satisfactory salvage procedure to resolve the problem of pain associated with usage of a damaged and unstable carpus. But for certain patients, the permanent loss of wrist motion served as a distinct handicap because accommodative motion cannot be gained from joints more proximal or distal to the carpus.[19] Thus certain occupations and vocations place a demand upon the preservation of a pain-free stable arc of wrist motion. Additionally patients who exhibit diffuse joint dysfunction of the upper extremity secondary to inflammatory arthritis, especially at the metacarpophalangeal and interphalangeal joints, are aided in hand function by the preservation of even a small arc of wrist motion. This observation has been identified by Clayton[2] and others in a review of patient preferences where an arthrodesis and arthroplasty of the carpus was present bilaterally.

From our experiences to date, the most difficult problem associated with total wrist replacement is the attainment of a well-balanced volitionally controlled wrist joint. Many patients with far-advanced arthritic changes were observed to have lost volitional control of the wrist extensors. Grasping activities of the fingers and hands were thus perfromed with a synergistic interplay between the finger flexors and wrist flexors rather than between finger flexors and wrist extensors as observed in the normal setting. When examined by an electromyograph, some patients displayed no electrical activity in the wrist extensors with closing motions of the hand. This loss of volitional wrist extensor activity presumably arose secondary to disuse and the inhibitory effects of carpal pain. Additionally, the original metacarpal component placed the instant center of motion too far radialward. This merely enhanced the mechanical advantage of the already dominant flexor carpi ulnaris in allowing for ulnar deviation postoperatively. As a result, some patients displayed a tendency for the hand to drift into flexion and ulnar deviation postoperatively. The employment of a single pronged metacarpal component placed within the third metacarpal canal has during the past 2 years greatly resolved the problem of motor imbalance.

Thus total wrist replacement has in our experience and in the experience of others to date proved to be a predictable, acceptable, and safe means of treatment for the patient requiring a pain-free, stable, and mobile wrist joint. Problems of infection, loosening, and dislocation appear not to be significant ones at least at this time. The low incidence of loosening may in part be attributable to the observation that the wrist is generally loaded in a static fashion whereas other joints of the body are loaded in a dynamic fashion. Additionally, many of the patients with rheumatoid arthritis undergoing this type of reconstruction exhibit sufficient metacarpophalangeal and interphalangeal joint disease that significant grip strengths are not attainable. The preservation of a pain-free, stable arc of motion in these patients, however, does augment finger and hand function.

REFERENCES

1. Boyes, J.H.: Bunnell's surgery of the hand, ed. 4, Philadelphia, 1964, J.B. Lippincott Co.
2. Clayton, M.L.: Personal communication, 1978, Denver, Col.
3. Cyriax, E.: The rotatory movements of the wrist, J. Anat. **60**:199, 1925.
4. Destat, E.: Injuries of the wrist, a radiological study, New York, 1926, Paul E. Hoeber, Inc., Medical Book Dept. of Harper & Bros.
5. Flatt, A.E.: The care of the rheumatoid hand, ed. 3, St. Louis, 1974, The C.V. Mosby Co.
6. Howitz, T.: An anatomic and roentgenologic study of the wrist joint, Surgery **7**:773, 1940.
7. Landsmeer, J.M.F.: Studies in the anatomy of articulation, 1 and 2, Acta Morphol. Scand. **3**:287, 1961.
8. Lewis, O.J., Hamshere, R.J., and Bucknill, T.M.: The anatomy of the wrist joint, J. Anat. **106**:539-552, 1970A.
9. Long, C.: Electromyographic kinesiology of the wrist: normal and abnormal motor control in the upper extremity, Social Rehabilitation Services, Grant no. RD-2377-M, p. 26-31, 1970.
10. MacConaill, M.A.: The mechanical anatomy of the carpus and its bearings on some surgical problems, J. Anat. **75**:166, 1941.
11. Mayfield, J.D., Johnson, R.P., Kilcoyne, R.F.: The ligaments of the human wrist and their functional significance, Anat. Rec. **185**:417-428, 1976.

12. McFarland, G.B., Krusen, U.L., and Weathersby, H.T.: Kinesiology of selected muscles acting in the wrist: electromyographic study, Arch. Phys. Med. Rehabil. **43:**165-171, 1962.
13. McMurtry, R.Y., and Youm, Y.: Wrist motion, a new approach, J. Bone Joint Surg. **57A:**727, 1975.
14. Radonjic, D., and Long, C.: Kinesiology of the wrist, Am. J. Phys. Med. **50:**57-71, 1971.
15. Sarrafian, S., Melamed, J., and Goshgarian, G.M.: Study of wrist motion in flexion and extension, Clin. Orthop. Rel. Res. **126:**153-159, 1977.
16. Steindler, A.: Kinesiology of the human body, ed. 3, Springfield, Ill., 1970, Charles C Thomas, Publisher.
17. Straub, L.R., and Ranawat, C.S.: The wrist in rheumatoid arthritis, J. Bone Joint Surg. **51A:**1, 1969.
18. Volz, R.G.: Clinical experiences with a new total wrist prosthesis, Arch. Orthop. Unfallchir. **85:**205-209, 1976.
19. Volz, R.G.: The development of a total wrist arthroplasty, Clin. Orthop. **116:**209-214, 1976.
20. Youm, Y., McMurtry, R.Y., Flatt, A., and Gillespie, T.E.: Kinematics of the wrist, J. Bone Joint Surg. **60A:**423-431, 1978.

24. Metacarpotrapezial arthroplasty

Ronald L. Linscheid, M.D.
William P. Cooney III, M.D.
James H. Dobyns, M.D.

TOTAL JOINT DESIGN

A total joint design for the metacarpotrapezial joint was devised in an attempt to improve our results at this joint from those previously obtained by various types of replacement or excisional arthroplasty[6,10-13,21,24] and in those patients in whom arthrodesis[17] seemed a poor choice of treatment.[16] It seemed to us that retention of the trapezium was desirable when possible to retain stability of the radial aspect of the wrist and thumb. Resection of a small segment of the base of the first metacarpal appeared to reduce long-term thumb axis instability and provide for improved thumb strength in pinch and grasp.

In the design of a device for total joint replacement an attempt was made to ensure that positioning of the forces about the metacarpotrapezial joint bore a close relationship to their normal balance around the contact point[7,8,15,19,20,23] (Figs. 24-1 and 24-2). We believed that access at the base of the metacarpal would be limited and might result in the distal component being positioned under the dorsoradial cortex of the metacarpal if suitable provision for displacement of the joint contact were not provided in the design. If the metacarpal component axis were allowed to remain aligned with the dorsoradial cortex of the metacarpal,[5] the moment arm of the abductor pollicis longus would be considerably shortened and the flexor moments of the tendons and muscles crossing the joint would be enhanced resulting in a flexion deformity. To obviate this, we decided to design an asymmetric metacarpal component that would hold a captive ball of the trapezial component (Fig. 24-3). Previous work of Pieron[20] has shown that the contact area of the metacarpotrapezial joint outlined an area closely over the center of the trapezial saddle. This area is readily identified at the time of surgery and allows for drilling a hole in the cortex without disrupting the remainder of the cortex or the ligamentous support of the trapezium. The offset of the metacarpal component would then place the center of rotation near its normal position. The protrusion of the trapezial ball above the trapezial articular surface, however, does induce torque on the trapezial fixation during metacarpal angulation (Fig. 24-4). It also diminishes the similar torque on the metacarpal fixation, which is inherent in designs with an elongated metacarpal stem.

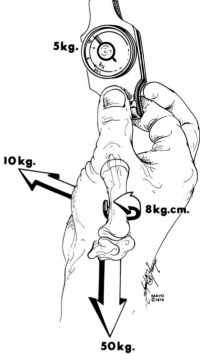

Fig. 24-1. The forces on the metacarpotrapezial joint during apposition pinch tend to be significant multiples of the pinch force. They average a joint compressive force 10 times greater, a subluxation force twice as great, and equally strong torque forces. The ability to resist forces of this magnitude places a significant requirement on a total joint system.

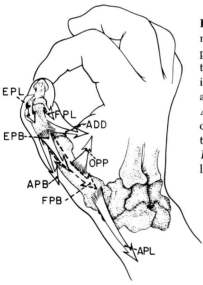

Fig. 24-2. The forces acting on the joint are transmitted through the tendons that cross the metacarpotrapezial level. In order for these tendinous forces to remain balanced so that the thumb can maintain its usual position, the contact area must be placed accurately within the joint. *ADD*, Adductor pollicis; *APB*, abductor pollicis brevis; *APL*, abductor pollicis longus; *EPB*, extensor pollicis brevis; *EPL*, extensor pollicis longus; *FPB*, flexor pollicis brevis; *FPL*, flexor pollicis longus; and *OPP*, opponens pollicis.

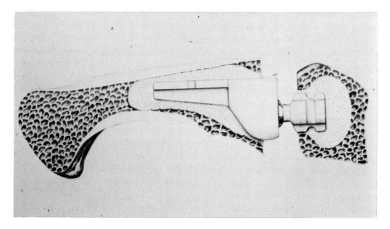

Fig. 24-3. The present device was designed with an asymmetric metacarpal plastic component to ensure correct positioning of the contact point in the metacarpal bone and with a metallic trapezial component designed for precise centering within the articular surface of the trapezium.

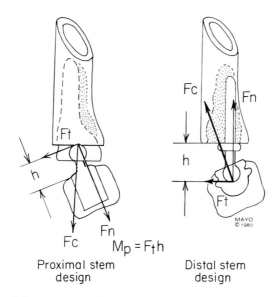

Proximal stem
design

Distal stem
design

Fig. 24-4. A stemmed design must, of necessity, result in torque on the stemmed component equal to the length of the stem protruding from the cement-bone interface and the component of force perpendicular to the joint contact force. The resistance of cement-bone interface is less in the proximal stem design because of the diminished height of the trapezium, whereas in the distal stem design the longer intramedullary cavity of the metacarpal provides the possibility for developing greater resistive moment. Correct positioning of the distal stem may be more of a problem in the latter design. Fc, Joint compressive force; Fn, component of force normal to prosthesis; Ft, component of force perpendicular to prosthesis; h, stem height; Mp, moment acting on extended stem of prosthesis, which must be resisted by cement-bone interface.

CLINICAL MATERIAL

Review of the metacarpotrapezial arthroplasty of the Mayo design showed 77 patients who had a 1 year follow-up study and 45 patients with a follow-up of 2 years or greater. Of the patients with at least a 2-year follow-up, there were 39 women and six men ranging in age from 46 to 80 years, with an average of 59 years. Thirty devices were implanted in the right and 15 in the left hand. The duration of symptoms of the patients ranged from 4 to 75 months, with an average

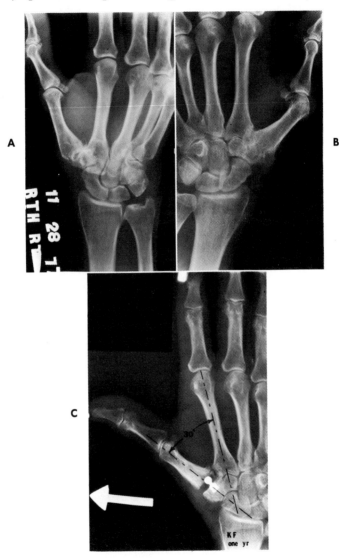

Fig. 24-5. Active 69-year-old woman with arthrodesis of left metacarpotrapezial joint, which had provided adequate strength. She wished to preserve thumb motion in her right dominant hand. **A,** Metacarpotrapezial degenerative changes, narrowed joint space, partial radial subluxation of first metacarpal, mild hyperextension deformity at metacarpophalangeal joint. **B,** Arthrodesis of left metacarpotrapezial joint. **C,** Abduction parallel to palm.

duration of 32 months. Thirty-seven thumbs showed degenerative changes of the metacarpotrapezial joint; there were two with traumatic arthritis and six with rheumatoid arthritis. Ten patients had previous surgery on the joint. In four this was a failed implant and in one a failed arthrodesis. Four patients had previous carpal tunnel release and one a de Quervain's release.

On examination there was a significant dorsoradial protuberance of the base of the first metacarpal in almost all patients. Six patients had an extension contracture at the metacarpophalangeal joint with a duckbill type of collapse deformity secondary to the dorsoradial dislocation at the metacarpotrapezial joint. Extension at the metacarpotrapezial joint was usually limited. Preoperative pinch strength in apposition averaged 2 kg (Fig. 24-5).

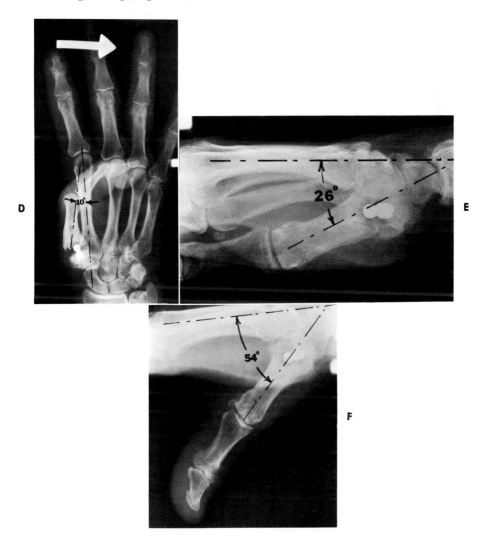

Fig. 24-5, cont'd. **D,** Adduction. **E,** Adduction perpendicular to palm. **F,** Abduction perpendicular to palm. Patient had 4 kg pinch strength, good pain relief, and good functional result, which persisted to 3 years postoperatively.

Most patients had a period of conservative care including splinting, cortisone injections, and restricted usage without significant benefit.

OPERATIVE TECHNIQUE

The metacarpotrapezial joint of the thumb was exposed through an incision on the subcutaneous surface of the first metacarpal, which angled sharply at the wrist crease and proceeded approximately 1 cm toward the thenar crease before extending again proximally. The dorsoradial digital nerve was identified and retracted dorsally. The capsule of the metacarpotrapezial joint was opened radial to the abductor pollicis longus insertion on the base of the metacarpal. Less than 1 ml of joint fluid and a mild chronic synovitis were usually noted. There were occasionally loose osteocartilaginous bodies and frequently large osteophytes extending radially from both the trapezium and metacarpal. Subperiosteal dissection of the base of the first metacarpal around approximately one half the circumference was performed, and 4 to 5 mm of the base of the metacarpal was removed with a sagittal cut saw. The center of the trapezium was identified and a drill hole made with an air burr. Care was taken to preserve subchondral bone plate of the trapezium. The diameter of the hole in the cortex was made a fraction larger than the diameter of the proximal component. Cancellous bone in the trapezium was removed with curved curettes. Curettage was continued until trial fitting of the proximal component allowed the shoulder of the proximal component to rest level with the trapezial surface. The intramedullary cavity of the metacarpal was then reamed with an air drill, and the metacarpal component trial was fitted. The asymmetric base of this metacarpal component is turned to parallel the palm. The components were then assembled to judge the adequacy of resection and motion. In general, the larger of the two sizes was used for men and medium sized to large for women, whereas the small components were reserved for small women.

The trapezial component was cemented into place by injection of methyl methacrylate into the trapezium under pressure and insertion of the proximal component perpendicular to the trapezial surface. After this has set, cement was then injected into the metacarpal and the distal component inserted and held. The components were assembled by snap fitting the trapezial ball into the metacarpal socket. Inherent stability is then obtained. Passive motion was tested, and if necessary, loose cement or trapezial surface was removed with an osteotome until motion appeared full and unimpeded. The capsule was closed with reconstruction of soft tissue including repair of the radial ligament and advancement of the abductor pollicis longus. Dressings were then applied.

Postoperatively motion was begun between the fourth and seventh day. A protective Orthoplast splint was worn except during the exercise periods for 3 weeks, at which time the splint was discarded and full active motion begun.

RESULTS

Postoperative motion[1,2] was for the most part quite satisfactory, with palmar abduction averaging 48 degrees, radial abduction 39 degrees, and opposition of the thumb tip to the fifth metacarpal head obtainable in most patients[3] (Fig. 24-5). Strength in pinch and grasp improved with postoperative pinch strength in apposition averaging 3.9 kg, ranging from 1 to 12 kg, and complications were seen in several patients (Fig. 24-6). Heterotopic new bone formation usually at the ulnar base of the metacarpal was seen in nine instances and appeared mildly symptomatic in three. Seen in three instances was loosening of the cement, or the device

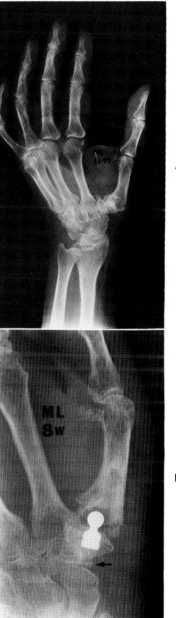

Fig. 24-6. A, Degenerative joint disease of metacarpotrapezial joint. **B,** Eight weeks postoperatively there was continued pain, redness, and limited motion. *Arrow,* Apparent extrusion of cement into scaphotrapezial joint. This cement was removed. Small area of chondromalacia on scaphoid noted. Subsequent sharp improvement in range of motion, little discomfort, good motion, and satisfactory function.

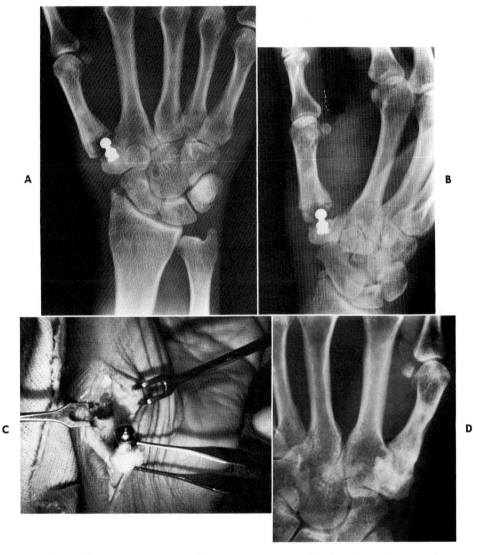

Fig. 24-7. A and **B**, Persistent pain after metacarpotrapezial arthroplasty. **C**, Reexploration showed the trapezial component had loosened. Subsequently arthrodesis of the metacarpo-trapezial joint using intercalated bone graft was performed with satisfactory result. **D**, One year after interpositional arthrodesis with iliac donor site.

Table 24-1. Metacarpotrapezial arthroplasty (results: patient's evaluation/surgeon's evaluation)

	Excellent	Good	Fair	Poor
Rheumatoid arthritis	1/0	2/3	1/1	2/2
Degenerative joint disease	24/19	9/11	2/3	2/4
Traumatic arthritis		1/0	1/1	
TOTAL	25/19	12/14	4/5	4/6

with the cement, that required reoperation and revision (Fig. 24-7). A lucent line was seen in 12 instances, but it was asymptomatic. A neuropathy of the radial dorsal digital nerve to the thumb occurred in several patients. This generally subsided spontaneously over a few weeks to months. There was one dislocation that was reduced. Four patients had late complaints of discomfort that appeared to arise at the scaphotrapeziotrapezoidal joint, but they have not required further treatment. Two patients had discomfort that they located deep in the thenar eminence and that was aggravated by action of the flexor pollicis longus. The exact nature of this pain has not been determined and has not required further treatment. Erosion of the trapezial component through the cortex occurred in two of the patients with rheumatoid disease.

An evaluation of results was given by both the patient and the doctor on the basis of pain, range of motion, and strength, as noted in Table 24-1.

DISCUSSION

The large number of operative procedures[1-3,6,10-14,17,18,21,22,24] recommended for treatment of metacarpotrapezial arthrosis attest to a continued dissatisfaction with the present treatment modalities. Neither satisfactory schema of pathogenesis or a universally satisfactory prophylaxis for prevention of metacarpotrapezial arthritis is available.[9] Most treatment modalities are therefore directed at improved function and pain relief for the joint with established arthritic changes. There is an increasing realization that the arthritic changes in the contiguous joints and particularly the scaphotrapeziotrapezoidal joint play a part in the range of symptoms and may be implicated in the pathogenesis. Later in this series a few patients were examined for stability of their trapezium at surgery. In several of these cases there appeared to be a distinct laxity of the trapezial stability from the second metacarpal and trapezoid. Whether this was a result of the underlying arthrosis or it was a precipitating cause was not determined. The trapezium is cantilevered radially from the trapezoid and second metacarpal. If its ligamentous constraints loosen under the compressive stress[4] from the first metacarpal under usage, it may rotate to encourage translation of the first metacarpal base as well as change the dynamics at the scaphotrapezoid articulation. Such changes, if true, should introduce factors to be considered in the pathogenesis of degenerative changes of the metacarpotrapezial joint as well as in the treatment methods.

Metacarpotrapezial arthrodesis[17] generally offers strength at the expense of motion of the thumb, and for many patients the instability to retract the thumb is a distinct handicap. If there is significant scaphotrapezial change, symptoms may continue.

Resection of the trapezium[6,11,12] results in loss of strength because of shortening of the thumb axis and the tendency for the thumb to go into a duckbill deformity, which is hard to control. Besides this instability, the metacarposcaphoid joint can become painful with the passage of time. Silastic replacement[10,14,21,22] of the trapezium has produced satisfactory results, but stability at the scaphoid surface has been difficult to achieve without resorting to a variety of ligamentous reconstructions and capsulorrhaphies. Interpositional arthroplasties using fibrous material[6,12] or silicone rubber[1,13,14] have enjoyed popularity by their advocates but not widespread acceptance.

There have been a number of designs for total joint arthroplasty at the metacarpotrapezial joint, almost all of which have used a ball-and-socket design.[5] In most, the ball has been placed on the metacarpal component and the socket within the trapezium. The metacarpotrapezial joint is a complex saddle (universal) joint with 2 degrees of freedom that is not easily reducible to a mechanical equivalent. However, the substitution of a ball-and-socket joint offers a reasonable analog since rotation is maintained by thenar muscles. By the nature of the various designs, the contact area will sit either above the surface of the trapezium as in the present design or beneath the surface of the trapezium as in other designs (Fig. 24-4). The constraint to prevent subluxation of the metacarpal on the trapezium is transferred to the cortical surface of the trapezium through the cemented-in device. The reliance on joint constraint through the bone-cement interface rather than a partial reliance on ligamentous restraints may be a weakness in the system.

Loosening of the bone-cement interface, as in most total joint systems, would appear to be the essential weakness of this approach to metacarpotrapezial arthroplasty. We believe that retention of a strong cortex and subchondral bone of the trapezium, except at the site of proximal component insertion, would help to lock the cement and prosthetic device into place and resist stress more reliably. The technique for centering the device by placement of the drill hole in the central part of the trapezial articular surface and the use of an offset metacarpal component has appeared to reliably balance the tendinous forces around the base of the thumb so that secondary collapse position has not been a problem.

Pain relief and range of motion in general have been satisfactory. Pinch strength has been somewhat less than anticipated, ranging about 50% better than preoperatively but just over 50% of normal.

Certain technical difficulties are inherent with the procedure. These are (1) the surgical problem in drilling the trapezial hole perpendicular to the line of surgical access to the joint, (2) adequate cement packing of the trapezium, (3) critical alignment of the trapezial component, (4) prevention of impingement at the extremes of motion between the metacarpal component and trapezial component, (5) retained cement in the joint, and (6) the possibility of loosening of the device with time.

Salvage after failure of such an arthroplasty can be achieved either with fibrous arthroplasty or arthrodesis (Fig. 24-7, *D*).

Usage of total joint replacement arthroplasty at the metacarpotrapezial joint is probably best limited to patients with bilateral disease, minimal scaphotrapezial joint involvement, and a requirement for a satisfactory range of motion with moderate strength in the older population group. Patients with pronounced osteopenia from osteoporosis or rheumatoid disease are not good candidates for prosthetic replacement because of the danger of erosion and in the latter the presence of pantrapezial disease.

REFERENCES

1. Ashworth, C.R., Blatt, G., Chuinard, R.G., and Stark, H.H.: Silicone rubber interposition arthroplasty of the carpometacarpal joint of the thumb, J. Hand Surg. 2:345, 1977.
2. Aune, S.: Osteoarthritis of the first carpometacarpal joint: an investigation of 22 cases, Acta Chir. Scand. 109:449-456, 1955.
3. Burton, R.I.: Basal joint arthrosis of the thumb, Orthop. Clin. North Am. 4:331-348, 1973.
4. Cooney, W.P., and Chao, E.Y.S.: Biomechanical analysis of static forces in the thumb during hand function, J. Bone Joint Surg. 59A:27-36, 1977.
5. de la Caffinière, J.Y.: L'articulation trapézo-métacarpienne: approche biomécanique et appareil ligamentaire, Arch. Anat. Pathol. (Paris) 18:277-284, 1970.
6. Dell, P.C., Brushart, T.M., and Smith, R.J.: Treatment of trapeziometacarpal arthritis: results of resectional arthroplasty, J. Hand Surg. 3:243-249, 1978.
7. Duparc, J., et al.: A biomechanical study of the first metacarpal bone movements, Rev. Chir. Orthop. 57:1-12, 1971.
8. Eaton, R.G., and Littler, J.W.: A study of the basal joint of the thumb, J. Bone Joint Surg. 51A:661-668, 1969.
9. Eaton, R.G., and Littler, J.W.: Ligament reconstruction for the painful thumb carpometacarpal joint, J. Bone Joint Surg. 55A:1655-1666, 1973.
10. Ferlic, D.C., Busbee, G.A., and Clayton, M.L.: Degenerative arthritis of the carpometacarpal joint of the thumb: a clinical follow-up of eleven Niebauer prostheses, J. Hand Surg. 2:212-215, 1977.
11. Froimson, A.: Tendon arthroplasty of the trapeziometacarpal joint, Clin. Orthop. 70:191, 1970.
12. Gervis, W.H.: Excision of the trapezium for osteoarthritis of the trapeziometacarpal joint, J. Bone Joint Surg. 31B:537-539, 1949.
13. Kessler, I.: Silicone arthroplasty of the trapeziometacarpal joint, J. Bone Joint Surg. 55B:285-291, 1973.
14. Kessler, I., and Axer, A.: Arthroplasty of the first carpometacarpal joint with a silicone implant, Plast. Reconstr. Surg. 47:252-257, 1971.
15. Kuczynski, K.: Carpometacarpal joint of the human thumb, J. Anat. 118:119-126, 1974.
16. Linscheid, R.L., and Dobyns, J.H.: Total joint arthroplasty—the hand, Mayo Clin. Proc. 54:516-526, 1979.
17. Muller, G.M.: Arthrodesis of the trapeziometacarpal joint for osteoarthritis, J. Bone Joint Surg. 31B:540-542, 1949.
18. Murley, A.H.G.: Excision of the trapezium in osteoarthritis of the first carpometacarpal joint, J. Bone Joint Surg. 42B:502-507, 1960.
19. Napier, J.R.: The form and function of the carpometacarpal joint of the thumb, J. Anat. 89:362-369, 1955.
20. Pieron, A.: Biomechanics of the hand, Int. Surg. 60:9-11, 1975.

21. Poppen, N.K., and Niebauer, J.J.: "Tie-in" trapezium prostheses: long-term results, J. Hand Surg. 3:445-449, 1978.
22. Swanson, A.B.: Disabling arthritis at the base of the thumb: treatment by resection of the trapezium and flexible (silicone) implant arthroplasty, J. Bone Joint Surg. 54A:456-471, 1972.
23. Van Wetter, P.: The range of action of the thumb and its limitations, Ann. Chir. 28:851-853, 1974.
24. Weinman, D.T., and Lipscomb, P.R.: Degenerative arthritis of the trapeziometacarpal joint: arthrodesis or excision? Mayo Clin. Proc. 42:276, 1967.

25. Flexible implant arthroplasty of the radiocarpal joint: surgical technique and long-term results

Alfred B. Swanson, M.D.
Genevieve de Groot Swanson, M.D.

Rheumatoid arthritis is a frequent cause of severe wrist impairment. It may affect the soft tissues and the joints of the wrist, including the radiocarpal, inter-carpal, and radioulnar, singly or in combination.[6,21,23,24,27,29] The destructive rheumatoid synovitis causes loosening of ligaments and erosive changes of bones, disturbing the multiple-link system of the wrist joint.[11,16,26,28,41] In some cases spontaneous fusion of the wrist may occur before subluxation. In severe cases complete dislocation of the wrist may result. Loosening of the ligaments on the radial aspect of the joint is common and allows ulnar displacement of the proximal carpal row; radial deviation of the hand on the forearm may follow. The associated subluxation of the distal radioulnar joint causes a loss of stability on the ulnar aspect of the wrist. Loosening of the palmar radiocarpal ligament allows collapse of the long axis and buckling of the radiocarpal link system. However, palmar subluxation of the proximal row on the radius is more common.

Many different procedures have been proposed for treatment of the rheumatoid wrist.[1-3,5,7,19,20,22] Arthrodesis of the wrist has been the commonly accepted procedure for treatment of the severely involved rheumatoid arthritic wrist,[4,10,13,18,25] the concept being that a stable wrist is needed for transmission of forces to the digits and for useful strong function to occur in the hand. A mobile wrist is necessary for performance of activities of daily living, particularly in the placement of the hand to the body surfaces. The obvious ideal method is one that would provide both stability and mobility, durability and salvageability. We have attempted to develop a reliable yet simple arthroplasty method for the radiocarpal joint.

Functional adaptations of the hand are greatly facilitated by wrist motion, especially flexion, even if very limited. A few degrees of wrist movement will increase the reach of the fingers in space by 5 to 6 cm to greatly improve their functional potential. The need for some degree of wrist motion, especially flexion, is particularly important if disabilities of the finger or of other proximal joints of the upper extremity are present such as those often seen in the rheumatoid arthritic patient. Personal hygiene can be a problem for patients with fused wrists, especially if they are stiff in the extended position. The majority of hand adaptations are associated with forearm supination and wrist flexion.

CONCEPT AND METHOD

Stability of the wrist is important for normal function of the extrinsic muscles of the fingers. A reconstructive procedure must provide, in a disabled wrist, reasonable stability and strength with enough mobility to assist in hand adaptations. In light of our experience gained with the development of the finger joint implant, the concept of a flexible intramedullary stemmed hinged implant was applied to the wrist joint.[30,33,34,37-39] A double-stemmed flexible hinge of silicone rubber for the radiocarpal joint was developed in 1967 to be used as an adjunct to resection arthroplasty of the wrist. Four different implant models were designed and tested in order to determine the best possible configuration of the midsection. The best model has a barrel-shaped midsection slightly flattened on the dorsal and volar surfaces. The core of the implant contains a Dacron polyester reinforcement to provide axial stability and resistance to rotatory torque. Since 1974, this implant model has been made of high-performance silicone elastomer and has been mechanically tested to more than 200 million flexion repetitions to 90 degrees without evidence of material fatigue or fracture. The implant has barium in it to improve its visibility on roentgenograms and is available in five anatomic sizes (Fig. 25-1).

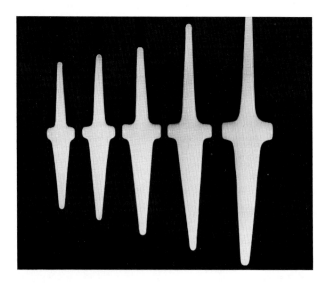

Fig. 25-1. Intramedullary, stemmed, flexible hinge implant of silicone rubber used as an adjunct to resection arthroplasty of the radiocarpal joint. The core of the implant contains a Dacron polyester reinforcement to provide greater axial stability and resistance to rotary torque. This implant is available in five sizes and is made of high-performance silicone elastomer.

The implant acts as a flexible hinge to help maintain an adequate joint space and alignment while supporting the development of a new capsuloligamentous system; it allows vertical and lateral movements through its flexible midsection and stems. This implant is used with a proximal row resection, which includes a resection of the base of the capitate bone.[8,14] The distal implant stem is directed through the capitate into the third metacarpal and the proximal into the intramedullary canal of the radius. This positions the implant very well in respect to the normal appropriate area for bending. It has been demonstrated that the axis of motion of the wrist is at the level of the head of the capitate bone.[12,15,17] However, most of these wrists are severely diseased and the normal radiocarpal and intercarpal articular movements have been altered. The flexible hinge has an advantage over rigid implants because its flexibility allows it to adjust to the required axis of rotation with little resistance; the fact that the stems are not fixed further allows this adjustment as demonstrated on cinefluoroscopy studies. Furthermore, this procedure is essentially retrievable. In the event of a fracture the implant is easily replaced, and if fusion becomes indicated, this can easily be done with a bone graft. Observation of our own cases over a period of more than 10 years has shown that there has been excellent tolerance by the host tissues to the implant, which is an excellent indication of its biomechanical acceptability.[40] The reinforced capsule and the balanced musculotendinous system are very important for the stability and the durability of the arthroplasty. The degree of stability and mobility, durability and biologic tolerance obtained with this technique to date has been most encouraging.[36]

SURGICAL TECHNIQUE
Indications

The wrist implant arthroplasty is indicated in cases of instability of the wrist because of subluxation or dislocation of the radiocarpal joint, severe deviation of the wrist causing musculotendinous imbalance of the digits, stiffness or fusion of the wrist in a nonfunctional position, and stiffness of a wrist when movement is a requirement for hand function.[9,34,36]

We believe that the wrist reconstruction should be usually performed before surgery of the finger joints when indicated. This procedure is contraindicated in young patients with open epiphyses, in those with inadequate skin, bone, or neurovascular system, and in those with irreparable tendon damage. We do not recommend this method for patients who are heavy manual workers.

Technique

A straight longitudinal incision is made over the dorsal wrist, with care being taken to preserve the superficial sensory nerves. The extensor retinaculum is incised as to prepare a radially based flap between the first and second dorsal compartments. Another retinacular ligament flap can be prepared to relocate the extensor carpi ulnaris tendon in associated implant reconstructions of the ulnar head[32,35] (Fig. 25-2, *A*). Synovectomy of the extensor compartments is performed

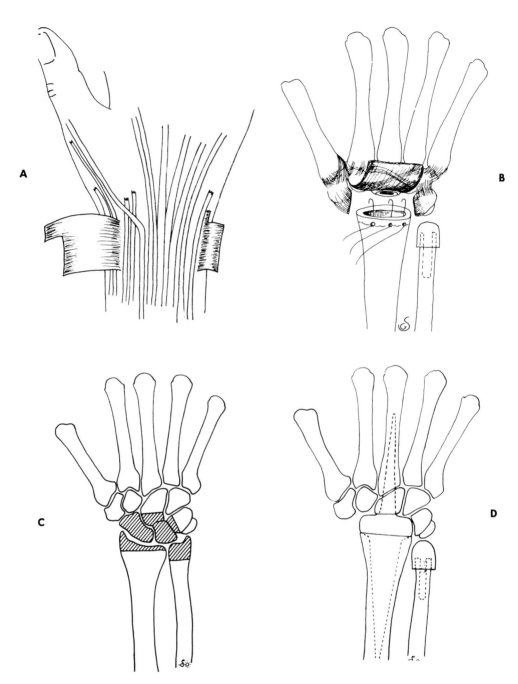

Fig. 25-2. **A,** Preparation of the extensor retinaculum flap based between the first and second dorsal compartments. A small distal flap is used as a pulley for relocation of the extensor carpi ulnaris tendon in associated reconstruction of the distal radioulnar joint. **B,** Preparation of a distally based radiocarpal flap by elevation of the dorsal capsuloligamentous structures from the underlying radius and carpal bones. **C,** Usual area of resection of the distal radius, ulna, and carpal bones in preparation for the wrist implant arthroplasty. **D,** The proximal stem of the wrist implant fits into the intramedullary canal of the radius, and the distal stem is inserted through the capitate bone into the intramedullary canal of the third metacarpal. The silicone rubber ulnar head implant is also shown in place.

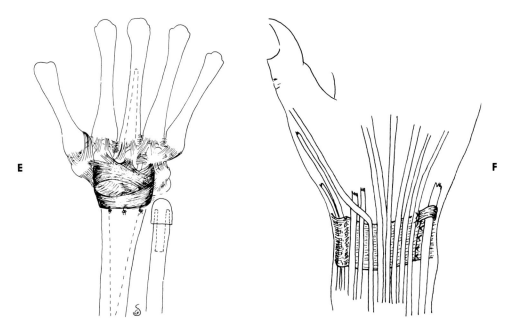

Fig. 25-2, cont'd. **E**, The radiocarpal capsuloligamentous flap is firmly sutured over the wrist implant. Sutures (3-0 Dacron) are passed through small drill holes in the dorsal cortex of the radius by use of an inverted knot technique. **F**, The extensor retinacular flap is placed over the wrist joint under the extensor tendons. The small distal retinacular flap is used to relocate the extensor carpi ulnaris tendon over the distal ulna as illustrated.

with care being taken to remove the synovium only. The dorsal capsuloligamentous structures are carefully preserved for later resuture, and they are reflected from the radius so that a distally based flap is left (Fig. 25-2, *B*).

A part of the proximal carpal row is usually absorbed, and the remnants are displaced palmarward on the radius. Resection of the remaining lunate is carefully done with a rongeur. Part of the distal scaphoid, capitate, and triquetrum can be retained in some cases (Fig. 25-2, *C*). Injury to the underlying tendons and neurovascular structures should be avoided. The end of the radius is squared off to fit against the distal carpal row. The distal row of carpal bones should be left intact because of their importance in maintaining the stability of the metacarpal bases. The radiocarpal subluxation should be completely reduced.

The intramedullary canal of the radius is prepared with a broach, curette, or air drill to receive the proximal stem of the implant. If there has been a pronounced radiocarpal dislocation with subsequent soft-tissue contracture, it is preferable to shorten the distal radius rather than remove more of the carpal bones. The distal stem of the implant fits through the capitate bone into the intramedullary canal of the third metacarpal (Fig. 25-2,· *D*). The intramedullary canal of the third metacarpal is prepared by carefully passing a wire or very thin broach through the capitate bone and the base of the metacarpal and into its canal. A Kirschner wire can be passed into the metacarpal and out through its head to verify the intramedullary orientation. An air drill may be used for the final reaming procedure.

The distal ulna is trimmed back to about 1 cm from the distal end of the radius and capped with a silicone rubber ulnar head implant. The hand is then centralized over the radius. The proximal stem of the wrist joint implant is inserted first into the intramedullary canal of the radius, and the distal stem is then introduced through the capitate and into the intramedullary canal of the third metacarpal. Enough bone should have been removed so that extension of the wrist is possible on passive manipulation. Usually 1 to 1.5 cm of separation between the bone ends is adequate. The capsuloligamentous structures are firmly sutured over the implant. Sutures are passed through small drill holes in the dorsal cortex of the radius to assure a good capsular fixation (Fig. 25-2, *E*). The repair should be tested so that approximately 45 degrees of extension and flexion and 10 degrees of ulnar and radial deviation are possible on passive manipulation.

The previously prepared extensor retinaculum flap is brought down over the wrist joint under the extensor tendons and sutured in place to provide further capsular support (Fig. 25-2, *F*). The pull of the extensor tendons of the wrist joint are then evaluated, and they are shortened or transferred as required to obtain wrist extension without lateral deviation. The extensor carpi radialis longus tendon may be transferred under the extensor carpi radialis brevis tendon to attach to the third metacarpal by a suture through the bone or interwoven into the brevis tendon distal attachment. The extensor tendons of the digits are repaired if necessary. We frequently may use one of the flexor superficialis muscles as a tendon transfer to reconstruct ruptured extensor digitorum communis tendons. If isolated extensor tendons are ruptured, side-to-side suture can be performed. Ruptures of the extensor pollicis longus tendon can be repaired by transferal of the extensor indicis proprius tendon. The reconstruction of the distal radioulnar joint is completed by use of a retinacular flap from the sixth dorsal compartment to relocate dorsally the extensor carpi ulnaris tendon.

The wound is closed in layers, and a drain or suction drainage is inserted subcutaneously. The usual voluminous conforming hand dressing is applied, including a plaster splint with the wrist in neutral position. The extremity is maintained in an elevated position for 3 to 5 days with an arm sling, with the patient being at bed rest. A short arm cast, with the wrist in neutral position, is then applied and fitted with outriggers to hold rubber band slings to keep the fingers in extension if the tendons have been repaired. This is worn for approximately 2 to 4 weeks. We desire a good ratio of stability and mobility. A joint that is too loose may be unstable. We attempt to obtain 50% to 60% of normal flexion-extension movements as the goal.

Postoperative care

The patient should be started on an exercise program after cast removal to obtain active flexion and extension. If there is a tendency for tightness, some active

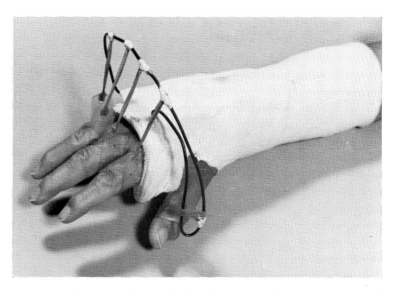

Fig. 25-3. Outrigger devices can be attached to the cast (or a dynamic brace) to help support finger extension if the extensor tendons have been repaired.

and passive stretching exercises are prescribed. If the extensor tendons have been repaired, finger extension can be supported by the outrigger devices attached to the cast or a dynamic brace (Fig. 25-3).

RESULTS

A detailed survey of 76 wrists operated on in our clinic was carried out in 1977. The results of a 1978 field-clinic computer study involving 301 wrists are briefly discussed.

Grand Rapids 1977 Study

Materials and methods. A flexible-hinge radiocarpal implant arthroplasty was carried out in 76 wrists in our clinic. This series included 59 patients (17 bilateral reconstructions). There were 45 females and 14 males, ranging from 20 to 74 years of age for an average age of 53. The pathologic process resulted from rheumatoid arthritis in 63 wrists, from psoriatic arthritis in 3 wrists, from scleroderma in 2 wrists, from osteoarthritis in 6 wrists, and there were sequelae of poliomyelitis in one wrist and of arthrogryposis in one other wrist. The duration of the pathologic process ranged from 4 to 52 years for an average duration of 19 years. A follow-up study of 6 months to 1 year was available in 20 wrists; 21 wrists were followed up to 2 years, 17 wrists up to 3 years, and 18 wrists from 3 years to 91 months. The group of 56 wrists followed from 12 to 91 months, averaged 34 months of follow-up.

The patients were thoroughly assessed before and after surgery on specially designed forms. The anatomic evaluation included measurements of grasp strength

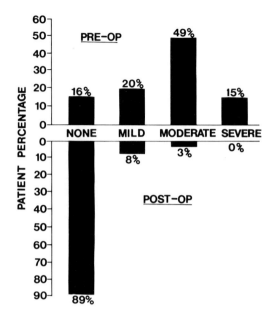

Fig. 25-4. Preoperative and postoperative joint evaluation (Grand Rapids series) for flexible implant wrist arthroplasty.

and range of motion. The functional evaluation included rating and questioning the patients on their performance of activities of daily living, as well as pain and cosmetic improvement. Roentgenograms taken before surgery and serially after surgery were also available for analysis. Cinefluoroscopy studies were also obtained.

A total of 30 wrists were operated on with implants made of silicone elastomer no. 372, and 46 wrists with implants made of high-performance silicone elastomer. For various reasons, the use of an ulnar head implant reconstruction was not indicated in 23 of the 76 operated wrists.

Pain. The pain was classified according to the degree that it interferes with the individual's performance of his activities as follows: (1) Minimal: Is it annoying? (2) Mild: Does it interfere with activity? (3) Moderate: Does it prevent activity? (4) Severe: Does it prevent activity and also cause distress?

Preoperatively, there was no pain in 16% of the wrists, mild pain in 20%, moderate pain in 49%, and severe pain in 15% of the wrists. After surgery an improvement was noted: 89% of the operated wrists were pain free, only 8% had a mild pain, and 3% had moderate pain on prolonged activity, but none had severe pain (Fig. 25-4).

Cosmetic result. The cosmetic improvement was evaluated from both the patient's and examiner's point of view on rest and activity and was rated on a point system. A minimum improvement was given 1 point, moderate improvement 2 points, and great improvement 3 points; the maximum possible points is 12 and would correspond to a great improvement (3 points) on both rest and activity from the patient's

Table 25-1. Preoperative and postoperative range of motion of flexible-implant wrist arthroplasty (Grand Rapids series)

	Flexion	Extension	Ulnar deviation	Radial deviation	Pronation	Supination
Preoperative	38°	6°	18°	4°	65°	58°
Postoperative	41°	21°	18°	9°	72°	57°

and examiner's observations. In the 76 operated wrists, the postoperative cosmetic improvement ranged from 6 to 12 points for an average of 9.8 points.

Range of motion. The preoperative and postoperative ranges of motion are shown for the 76 reconstructed wrists in Table 25-1. The average postoperative flexion was 41 degrees and extension 21 degrees. It is to be noted that the greatest improvement was obtained in the direction of extension, with a gain of 15 degrees. The average degrees of pronation, radial deviation, and flexion were also improved postoperatively (Figs. 25-5 and 25-6). An average supination of 57 degrees and an ulnar deviation of 18 degrees show little or no change as compared to the preoperative values and are very functional values.

Strength of grasp. The grasp strength was measured before and after surgery with a Jamar hydraulic dynamometer. This value averaged 7 pounds preoperatively and 12 pounds postoperatively. It is to be noted this group of patients had associated rheumatoid finger and tendon involvement, which can significantly affect the power of grasp. The moderate increase of strength noted is related to the improved position, stability, and freedom of pain of the wrist.

Complications and revision procedures. There were no postoperative infections. A delay in wound healing requiring no secondary procedure was noted in 3 wrists; there were 2 with rheumatoid arthritis involvement and one with psoriatic arthritis.

Postoperative problems requiring a revision procedure were present for 8 wrists in 7 patients, one being reoperated on bilaterally. There were 3 fractured implants made of the original elastomer, one case of tendon imbalance with recurrent ulnar deviation, and 4 cases of tendon imbalance and recurrent synovitis.

Associated tendon surgery. Associated tendon reconstruction was required in 24 of the 76 wrists and comprised the following:

Repair of the extensor carpi radialis brevis and longus tendons in two cases
Transfer of the brachioradialis tendon to the wrist extensors in one case
Transfer of the extensor carpi radialis longus to the base of the third metacarpal in one case
Transfer of the extensor carpi radialis longus to the extensor carpi radialis brevis by interweaving of the tendons in three cases
Repair of a ruptured extensor pollicis longus by transfer of the indicis proprius tendon in three wrists
Transfer of the extensor carpi ulnaris to the extensor digitorum in three wrists
Transfer of the flexor superficialis tendon of the ring finger to the extensor digitorum in four cases

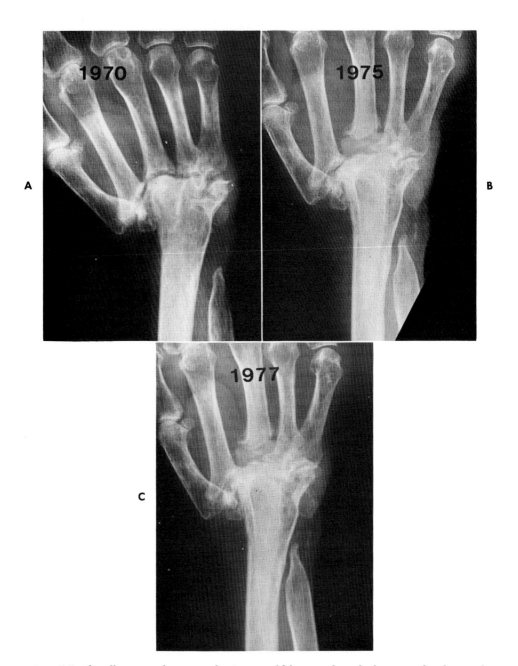

Fig. 25-5. This illustrates the cases of a 51-year-old housewife with rheumatoid arthritis who had a previous wrist synovectomy and ulnar head resection. She presented for wrist joint pain and instability. **A,** Preoperative roentgenogram showing a severe absorption of the carpal bones and radial deviation of the wrist. She underwent a wrist reconstruction with the flexible implant in 1970. **B** and **C,** Roentgenograms at 5 and 7 years after surgery showing the implant in position. There is evidence of bone formation around the stems of the implant and maintainance of a joint space with no evidence of unusual bone changes around the midsection. She has a pain-free, stable wrist with 20 degrees of extension, 35 degrees of flexion, 5 degrees of ulnar deviation, and 15 degrees of radial deviation.

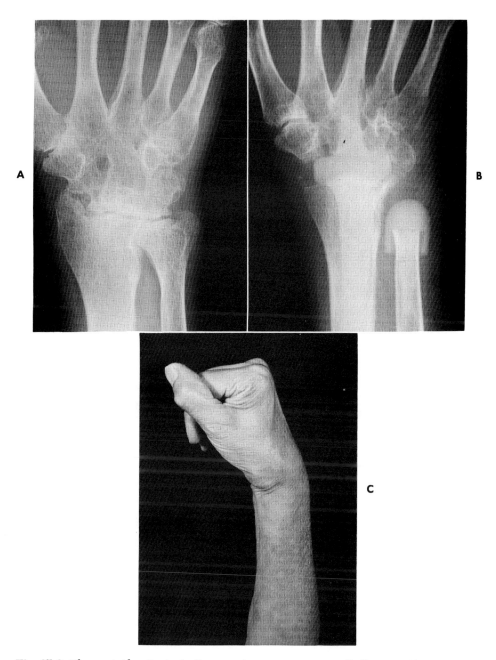

Fig. 25-6. Rheumatoid patient. **A,** Preoperative roentgenogram. **B,** Postoperative roentgenogram. **C,** Range of flexion. *Continued.*

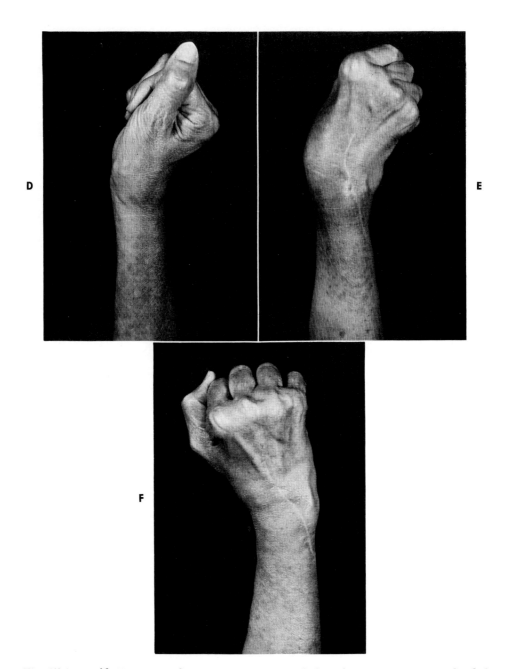

Fig. 25-6, cont'd. D, Range of extension. **E,** Range of ulnar deviation. **F,** Range of radial deviation.

Side-to-side transfer of the tendons of the extensor digitorum in three cases
Rerouting of the extensor carpi ulnaris as a routine in all cases
Repair of the ruptured extensor carpi ulnaris in two cases
Lengthening of a contracted flexor carpi ulnaris in two wrists

Roentgenologic survey. Postoperative roentgenograms of the wrist were routinely reviewed and compared at 3-month, 6-month, and yearly intervals. The films were evaluated for evidence of recurrent deformity, loss of the joint space, and bone resorption around the stems or at the junction of the of the implant midsection. Bone production around the stems or at the midsection level was evaluated.

The development of a thin bone plate around the intramedullary stems of the implant and a smooth remodeling of bone next to the midsection were routinely seen. There was one case with bone growth across the implant midsection to form a fusion of the wrist in a patient with scleroderma. An adequate joint space was maintained in all the other wrists. There were no cases of increasing bone absorption around the stems or midsection of the implant. In two cases the distal stem of the implant was not properly fitted in the third metacarpal and protruded through its side wall. There were no significant clinical or roentgenologic consequences from this technical error.

Field-clinic computer study

The results obtained by 41 participating field-clinic surgeons in 301 flexible-implant wrist arthroplasties were retrieved in 1978. This study included 101 silicone elastomer no. 372 implants and 200 high-performance silicone elastomer implants. The parameters of evaluation included pain relief and wrist stability and mobility (Tables 25-2 to 25-4). The complications and revision procedures were also reported (Tables 25-5 and 25-6). The slight discrepancies in the total number of cases reported in Table 25-2 to 25-6 are attributable to incomplete information received in certain cases. The results shown in these tables are self-explanatory.

Table 25-2. Pain relief (field-clinic survey of 1978)

	Original implant	High-performance implant	Combined results
Good	92	180	272
Fair	4	15	19
Poor	1	1	2
Unsatisfactory	3	4	7
TOTAL	100	200	300

Table 25-3. Wrist stability (field-clinic survey of 1978)

	Original implant	High-performance implant	Combined results
Good	87	191	278
Fair	5	6	11
Poor	4	2	6
Unsatisfactory	5	1	6
TOTAL	101	200	301

Table 25-4. Range of motion (field-clinic survey of 1978)

	Original implant	High-performance implant	Combined results
Good	55	125	180
Fair	33	60	93
Poor	7	14	21
Unsatisfactory	4	1	5
TOTAL	99	200	299

Table 25-5. Complications (field-clinic survey of 1978)

	Original implant	High-performance implant	Combined results
Dislocation	1	0	1
Fracture	7	1	8
Infection	1	0	1
Recurrent deformity	8	4	12
Other	2	1	3
TOTAL	101	200	301

Table 25-6. Revision procedures (field-clinic survey of 1978)

	Original implant	High-performance implant	Combined
Fracture	6	0	6
Fusion for ambulatory aid	1	0	1
Recurrent deformity or synovitis	3	2	5
TOTAL	101	205	306

DISCUSSION

The flexible intramedullary stemmed wrist joint implant can be a worthwhile adjunct to resection arthroplasty procedures in cases of severely involved and unstable rheumatoid arthritic wrists. Clinically it maintains the relationship of the carpus and radius and allows motion of the wrist joint in all planes. The formation of a surrounding capsuloligamentous system provides adequate stability of the wrist in rheumatoid cases. The functional adaptation of the hand of these patients has been facilitated by the movement and good stability of the wrist provided by this reconstructive method. Ideally, a range of motion of 45 degrees of dorsiflexion and 45 degrees of palmar flexion, with 10 degrees of radioulnar deviation should be achieved. This implant arthroplasty method has not been used for the heavy worker in our clinic though some of our patients have returned to manual occupations in factory and office jobs not requiring heavy lifting. One patient with bilateral wrist arthroplasties for degenerative arthritis has returned to his job as a welder.

An important and unique factor that is typical of silicone implant arthroplasty is that this method does not require cement or significant bone resection so that in case of infection or implant failure, the implant can be simply removed or replaced as necessary or the procedure can be converted to an arthrodesis by bone grafting if desired.

Experience with the use of this method of arthroplasty for the radiocarpal joint indicates that satisfactory wrist mobility, stability, and pain relief can be obtained. The procedure is retrievable and acceptable for both the patient's function and the surgeon's requirements. It is our opinion that the wrist flexible-implant resection arthroplasty method has a place in the reconstruction and rehabilitation program of the upper extremity and has decided advantages over wrist arthrodesis, pseudarthrodesis, or other arthroplasty procedures.

REFERENCES

1. Adamson, J.E., Horton, C.E., and Crawford, H.H.: The surgical reconstruction of the rheumatoid hand, Southern Med. J. **57:**928-933, 1964.
2. Albright, J.A., and Chase, R.A.: Palmar-shelf arthroplasty of the wrist in rheumatoid arthritis: report of nine cases, J. Bone Joint Surg. **52A:**896-906, 1970.
3. Boyes, J.H.: Bunnell's surgery of the hand, ed. 5, Philadelphia, 1970, J.B. Lippincott Co.
4. Campbell, C.J., and Keokarn, T.: Total and subtotal arthrodesis of the wrist, J. Bone Joint Surg. **46A:**1520-1533, 1964.
5. Campbell, R.D., and Straub, L.R.: Surgical considerations for rheumatoid disease in the forearm and wrist, Am. J. Surg. **109:**361-367, 1965.
6. Chaplin, D., Pulkki, T., Saarimaa, A., and Vainio, K.: Wrist and finger deformities in juvenile rheumatoid arthritis, Acta Rheum. Scand. **15:**206-223, 1969.
7. Clayton, M.L.: Surgical treatment at the wrist in rheumatoid arthritis: a review of thirty-seven patients, J. Bone Joint Surg. **47A:**741-750, 1965.
8. Crabbe, W.A.: Excision of the proximal row of the carpus, J. Bone Joint Surg. **46B:**708-711, 1964.
9. Cregan, J.C.F.: Indications for surgical intervention in rheumatoid arthritis of the wrist and hand, Ann. Rheum. Dis. **18:**29-33, 1959.
10. Dupont, M., and Vainio, K.: Arthrodesis of the wrist in rheumatoid arthritis, Ann. Chir. Gynaecol. Fenn. **57:**513-519, 1968.
11. Ehrlich, G.E., Peterson, L.T., Sokoloff, L., and Bunim, J.J.: Pathogenesis of rupture of extensor tendons at the wrist in rheumatoid arthritis, Arthritis Rheumat. **2:**332-346, 1959.

12. Flatt, A.E.: Personal communication, 1975, Iowa City, Iowa.

13. Haddad, R.J., and Riordan, D.C.: Arthrodesis of the wrist, J. Bone Joint Surg. **49A:**950-954, 1967.

14. Jorgenson, E.C.: Proximal row carpectomy: an end result study of 22 cases, J. Bone Joint Surg. **51A:**1104-1111, 1969.

15. Kaplan, E.B.: Functional and surgical anatomy of the hand, ed. 2, Philadelphia, 1965, J.B. Lippincott Co.

16. Kessler, I., and Vainio, K.: Posterior (dorsal) synovectomy for rheumatoid involvement of the hand and wrist, J. Bone Joint Surg. **48A:**1085-1094, 1966.

17. Lewis, O.J., Hamshere, R.J., and Bucknill, T.M.: The anatomy of the wrist joint, J. Anat. **106:**539-552, 1970.

18. Liebolt, F.L.: Surgical fusion of the wrist joint, Surg. Gynecol. Obstet. **66:**1008-1023, 1938.

19. Lipscomb, P.R., and Henderson, E.D.: Surgical treatment of the rheumatoid hand, J.A.M.A. **175:**431-436, 1961.

20. Marmor, L.: Surgery of rheumatoid arthritis, Philadelphia, 1967, Lea & Febiger.

21. Martel, W., Hayes, J.T., and Duff, I.F.: The pattern of bone erosion in the hand and wrist in rheumatoid arthritis, Radiology **84:**204-214, 1965.

22. Milford, L.W.: The hand. In Crenshaw, A.H., editor: Campbell's operative orthopaedics, ed. 5, St. Louis, 1971, The C.V. Mosby Co.

23. Moberg, E., Wassen, E., Kjellberg, S.R., Zettergren, L., Scheller, S., and Aschan, W.: The early pathological changes in rheumatoid arthritis, Acta Chir. Scand. Suppl. **357:**142-147, 1966.

24. Ranawat, C.S., Freiberger, R.H., Jordan, L.R., and Straub, L.R.: Arthrography in the rheumatoid wrist joint, J. Bone Joint Surg. **51A:**1269-1281, 1969.

25. Robinson, R.F., and Kayfetz, D.O.: Arthrodesis of the wrist, J. Bone Joint Surg. **34A:**64-70, 1952.

26. Savill, D.L.: Synovectomy of the wrist joint. In Early synovectomy in rheumatoid arthritis, Amsterdam, 1967, Excerpta Medica Foundation.

27. Steindler, A.: Arthritic deformities of the wrist and fingers, J. Bone Joint Surg. **33A:**849-862, 1951.

28. Straub, L.R., and Wilson, E.H., Jr.: Spontaneous rupture of extensor tendons in the hand associated with rheumatoid arthritis, J. Bone Joint Surg. **38A:**1208-1217, 1956.

29. Straub, L.R., and Ranawat, C.S.: The wrist in rheumatoid arthritis, J. Bone Joint Surg. **51A:**1-20, 1969.

30. Swanson, A.B.: Silicone rubber implants for replacement of arthritic or destroyed joints in the hand, Surg. Clin. North Am. **48:**1113-1127, 1968.

31. Swanson, A.B.: Finger joint replacement by silicone rubber implants and the concept of implant fixation by encapsulation, International Workshop on Artificial Finger Joints, Ann. Rheum. Dis. **28**(suppl.): 47-55, 1969.

32. Swanson, A.B.: The ulnar head syndrome and its treatment by implant resection arthroplasty, J. Bone Joint Surg. **54A:**906, 1972.

33. Swanson, A.B.: Flexible implant arthroplasty for arthritic finger joints—rationale, technique and results of treatment, J. Bone Joint Surg. **54A:**435-455, 1972.

34. Swanson, A.B.: Flexible implant arthroplasty in the hand and extremities, St. Louis, 1973, The C.V. Mosby Co.

35. Swanson, A.B.: Implant arthroplasty for disabilities of the distal radioulnar joint, Orthop. Clin. North Am. **4:**373-382, 1973.

36. Swanson, A.B.: Flexible implant arthroplasty for arthritic disabilities of the radiocarpal joint, Orthop. Clin. North Am. **4:**383-394, 1973.

37. Swanson, A.B.: Flexible implant arthroplasty in the hand, Clin. Plast. Surg. **3:**141-157, 1976.

38. Swanson, A.B.: Reconstructive surgery in the arthritic hand and foot, Ciba Clin. Symp. **31**(6), 1979.

39. Swanson, A.B., and de Groot Swanson, G.: Flexible implant resection arthroplasty: a method for reconstruction of small joints in the extremities, AAOS Instructional Course Lectures, **27:**27-60, St. Louis, 1978, The C.V. Mosby Co.

40. Swanson, A.B., Meester, W.D., de Groot Swanson, G., Rangaswamy, L., and Schut, G.E.D.: Durability of silicone implants—an in vivo study, Orthop. Clin. North Am. **4:**1097-1112, 1973.

41. Vainio, K.: Synovectomies of the hand and wrist in rheumatoid arthritis. In Tubiana, R., editor: The rheumatoid hand, Groupe d'Etude de la Main, Monograph No. 3, pp. 111-114, Paris, 1969, L'Expansion.

Index